HEALTH
INFORMATICS

HEALTH INFORMATICS
A Systems Perspective

Gordon D. Brown • Timothy B. Patrick • Kalyan S. Pasupathy

AUPHA

Health Administration Press,
Chicago, Illinois

Association of University Programs in Health Administration,
Arlington, Virginia

17   16   15   14   13   5   4   3   2

Library of Congress Cataloging-in-Publication Data

Health informatics : a systems perspective / edited by Gordon D. Brown, Timothy B. Patrick, and Kalyan S. Pasupathy.
   p. cm.
 Includes bibliographical references and index.
 ISBN 978-1-56793-435-9 (alk. paper)
 1. Medical informatics. 2. Information storage and retrieval systems--Medicine. 3. Medical informatics--Case studies. 4. Information storage and retrieval systems--Medicine--Case studies. I. Brown, Gordon D. II. Patrick, Timothy B. III. Pasupathy, Kalyan S.
 R858.H3478 2012
 362.1068'4--dc23
                     2012022497

The paper used in this publication meets the minimum requirements of American National Standard for Information Sciences—Permanence of Paper for Printed Library Materials, ANSI Z39.48-1984. ♾™

Acquisitions editor: Carrie McDonald; Project manager: Jane Calayag; Typesetting: Virginia Byrne; Cover: Marisa Jackson

Found an error or a typo? We want to know! Please e-mail it to hap1@ache.org, and put "Book Error" in the subject line.

For photocopying and copyright information, please contact Copyright Clearance Center at www.copyright.com or at (978) 750–8400.

Health Administration Press
A division of the Foundation of the American
   College of Healthcare Executives
One North Franklin Street, Suite 1700
Chicago, IL 60606–3529
(312) 424–2800

Association of University Programs
   in Health Administration
2000 North 14th Street
Suite 780
Arlington, VA 22201
(703) 894–0940

To students who have the vision and courage to lead profound change in the health system.

To Parker, Jackson, Henry, Samuel, Eleanor, Gwyneth, and Declan
and to their generation. May they inherit a health system characterized by many of the
qualities envisioned in this book.

BRIEF CONTENTS

DETAILED CONTENTS

PREFACE

Health Informatics: A Systems Perspective is written to introduce students in health services management and the health professions to the transforming power of health informatics. It is unique in that it can reach a broad range of healthcare professionals and students in various academic programs, including medicine, nursing, health policy, and information technology. Unlike traditional informatics books that in their application to specific professions tend to differentiate and separate them, this book focuses on health informatics as the basis for interprofessionalism and collaboration.

For readers who are pursuing a degree in a clinical area, the book can be used alongside informatics articles that apply specifically to their area of study. The book is ideal for courses that explore the foundational concepts of health informatics and the common framework for building more effective informatics capabilities.

Health Informatics: A Systems Perspective challenges the traditional perspective of applying information technology (IT) to better inform existing patterns of practice. Here, we argue that IT can fundamentally transform the structure of clinical processes and the organizations that support them. We explore health IT from a systems perspective and view it as a disruptive technology and thus one that is inherently transformational. The concepts discussed in this book are based on sound theory and evidence from a range of disciplines, drawing on the accumulated knowledge and experience from inside and outside the healthcare field.

This book presents a new conceptual model of informatics, including bioinformatics (cellular level), medical and nursing informatics (clinical level), and public health informatics (population level). In addition, it introduces health systems informatics (dynamic systems), which adds to and alters previous conceptions. Specifically, the book discusses the following:

- Operational issues, including building clinical vocabularies and databases (Chapter 2), implementing electronic medical records (Chapter 3), creating a corporate culture for knowledge workers (Chapter 10), using consumer and e-health applications (Chapter 11), protecting security and privacy (Chapter 13), and understanding IT valuation and financing (Chapter 14)

- The complexity and potential of evidence-based clinical decision support systems in medicine (Chapter 5) and nursing (Chapter 6) and the increasing importance of genomic medicine for health professionals and patients (Chapter 12)
- Systems theory, including the science of clinical decision making (Chapter 4), the dynamics of clinical work processes (Chapter 7), knowledge-based decision making and knowledge management (Chapter 8), and the application of advanced analytics such as predictive modeling and data mining (Chapter 9)

We encourage readers to deepen their understanding of the topics discussed by further searching the literature and by demonstrating their ability to develop and defend evidence-based solutions to complex problems. Concepts in each chapter are supported by current or classic literature, and a robust list of references is included at the end of the book. In addition, the book offers the following:

- Learning objectives, a listing of the take-away lessons and points in each chapter
- Key concepts, a listing of the major topics or terms discussed in each chapter
- Sidebars, extra information or practical discussions related to a specific concept in the chapter
- Chapter discussion questions, a framework for reviewing, conceptualizing, or articulating the concepts and issues presented in the chapter
- Case studies, real-world applications of the theories and challenges discussed in the chapter; each case study is accompanied by discussion questions to test the reader's understanding
- Glossary, a collection of the definitions of the book's main concepts and terminologies

To assist instructors in developing material for teaching this book and in guiding the text discussions, we have created Instructor Resources. To access the Instructor Resources, text adopters may e-mail hap1@ache.org. The Instructor Resources include the following:

- The authors' responses to the chapter discussion questions in each chapter
- Guidance on how the case studies may be used
- The authors' responses to the case study discussion questions in each chapter
- PowerPoint slides of the exhibits in the text, which may be used as supplements to the classroom discussion and lecture

In preparing this book, we approached both academics/professors and leading healthcare practitioners to contribute their expertise and thus provide a balanced theoretical and practical perspective. All of our contributing authors have taught graduate courses, and some have led the design and management of academic programs. They represent a wide range of disciplines and bring many years of varied experience to this undertaking. We knew that writing a multidimensional but highly integrated book was going to be a challenge, but we all agreed that the result would be beneficial and the experience enjoyable. We hope that the reader finds the culmination of our work—*Health Informatics: A Systems Perspective*—to be equally beneficial and valuable.

Gordon Brown
Timothy Patrick
Kalyan Pasupathy

June 2012

INTRODUCTION TO HEALTH SYSTEMS INFORMATICS

Gordon D. Brown, Kalyan S. Pasupathy, and Timothy B. Patrick

Learning Objectives

After reading this chapter, students should be able to

- Conceptualize health informatics and differentiate it from bioinformatics and medical informatics as an analytical framework
- Explain the interdependencies between management information systems and informatics
- Develop a conceptual understanding of the transforming power of information technology
- Differentiate the application and functions of electronic medical records, electronic health records, and electronic personal health records
- Understand the use and potential of clinical information technology and decision support tools in process and performance improvement

---

KEY CONCEPTS

- Health informatics, medical and nursing informatics, and bioinformatics
- Transformational change
- Electronic medical records, electronic health records, and electronic personal health records
- Clinical decision support systems
- Clinical data standards

Introduction

The term *informatics* was first applied four decades ago with a specific focus on the structure and properties of scientific information. The need for standards and vocabularies for information in the biological sciences was recognized in order to develop and apply complex, computer-based computational analyses and models. The application of informatics in the biological sciences is generally referred to as *bioinformatics*. The analysis of sequences of the three billion chemical base pairs that make up human DNA would not be possible without complex algorithms and powerful computers.

In clinical sciences, informatics has been used for more than three decades and reflects the growing application of computers to clinical trials and the analysis of pathological tissues and radiological films. Clinical applications of computational tools are generally labeled "medical informatics," but with major and minor specialized foci such as nursing informatics, pathology informatics, or rehabilitation informatics. The field of medical informatics has primarily focused on digitizing medical records in hospitals and large medical clinics, and it currently serves as a national health policy priority in the United States and many other countries.

The concept of health informatics has come to suggest a broad perspective, but it lacks a definition and conceptualization that is generally accepted in the field, except when used as one of a number of synonyms for medical informatics. The term is used interchangeably with health information technology (IT) and e-health and thus inappropriately describes the term as any application of advanced IT to any healthcare delivery process.

In this book, **health informatics** refers to the application of multidisciplinary sciences to transform (not just automate) the structure and behavior of health-related systems, organizations, and individuals (including patients, professionals, and support personnel) who interact to provide personalized care. This systems concept draws on biological, clinical, engineering, social, and behavioral sciences. A fundamental assumption of health informatics in this sense is that, whether or not the implementation of IT can be said to *cause* changes in the health system, it enables a profound shift in how health services are organized and delivered at the organization, system, and individual levels. The health system has lagged behind most sectors in adopting advanced IT, and its primary focus has been on automating existing technical processes, such as digitizing medical records and clinical decision support. Health systems change will be realized through the vision and innovation of health leaders who recognize and embrace the transforming power of IT.

This book focuses on the basic concepts of health informatics relevant to health professionals. Mastery of the knowledge and skills necessary to lead an IT transformation will require advanced preparation in a relevant university program. Health systems leaders should have a basic understanding of information and computer technologies and a mastery of the social, behavioral, and systems sciences related to the transformational science of IT. The relevant social, behavioral, and systems sciences are based on sound theory and evidence but must be considered within the context of advanced IT. Theories and concepts based on old paradigms represent fossilized thinking.

All health professionals, workers, managers, and IT specialists should learn the basics of health informatics and how it affects their work. Individuals who are focused on applying IT only to the technical aspects of their jobs will be unable to provide leadership or even to adapt easily to the rapidly changing clinical work environment.

Evolution of Information Technology in Healthcare

Electronic information systems have been applied to the business side of the health enterprise for half a century. Like organizations in the commercial sector, healthcare organizations applied IT first to payroll, billing, and accounting and then later to personnel administration and supply chain management. These areas (unlike medical services) were suited for electronic data processing because they possessed standardized vocabularies, well-defined data structures, and repetitive processes. These functions could be automated using standards broadly accepted in the business world.

For example, the importance of generally accepted standards for accounting and finance was recognized in the late 1930s and led to the establishment of the Committee on Accounting Procedures and subsequently the creation of the generally accepted accounting principles (GAAP)—standardized measures and reporting of financial information. GAAP were established to facilitate financial analysis and communication within the business sector. These standards were not initiated with the computer in mind, but standardization greatly facilitated later application of computer technology. The business side of the health enterprise thus evolved with a corporate orientation, while the clinical side maintained an individual, professional perspective. This clash of cultures is still prominent in the health system and directly affects the architecture, use, and effectiveness of IT.

On the clinical side, the emergence of the health insurance industry required some standardization of medical services. Clinicians initially resisted the idea of health insurance as a third party because it interfered with the doctor–patient relationship, but insurance became a financial necessity. In order for insurance companies to reimburse hospitals and clinicians for the units of care they provided, the companies needed a process for translating medical diagnoses and procedures into codes that represented a uniform classification of diseases. To meet this need, the American Medical Association (2011) developed **current procedural terminology** (CPT). The purpose of the CPT coding was financial and not clinical, and as such it did not violate the clinical decision process. CPT gave rise to the profession of medical coders and professional associations such as the **American Health Information Management Association**. The role of professional coders is expanding as the health sector moves to develop standardized clinical guidelines and protocols used as the basis for assessing clinical quality.

The initial application of computers to the accounting and finance functions in hospitals made IT a function structured under the finance department. That early business orientation became the root of subsequent problems (e.g., integrating business IT with clinical IT, conceptualizing IT as clinical decision support rather than management technology) when IT expanded to clinical applications. In the beginning, IT was identified as a data-processing function and thus was staffed with technically trained personnel.

Management Information Systems Versus Informatics

With the development of competencies necessary for applying IT to business functions, the discipline of management information systems (MIS) emerged. MIS evolved as part of the standard business curriculum. It was structured initially as an area of concentration but not as a separate degree program (as was medical informatics); later, it developed into a degree program in many universities. No record exists that the term *informatics* was used in the MIS program to label the concentration in business, most likely because MIS was considered as an integrated management function and not focused on the structure and properties of information. The separation of informatics from MIS was consistent with the separation of the business function from the clinical function in healthcare organizations. Health informatics, however, requires the full integration of the clinical and business functions because clinical systems cannot be transformed without also transforming the financing, human resources, and IT functions as well as the basic structure of the organization (see Chapters 4 and 7 for further discussions).

Scientific Basis of Health Informatics

A.I. Mikhailov of the Scientific Information Department of the Moscow State University coined "informatics" in his 1968 book *Oznovy Informatiki* (Foundations of Informatics) (Collen 1995). Adopted from the Russian words *informatik* and *informatikii*, the term is defined as a study of the "structure and general properties of scientific information and the laws of all processes of scientific communication" (Collen 1995, 39). This definition establishes **informatics** as the study of linguistics applied broadly to scientific language. Informatics applies the study of morphology (the formation and composition of words) and syntax (the rules that determine how words combine into meaning) to analyze biological and clinical databases. As such, informatics combines basic and clinical sciences with computational science, particularly computer science.

Informatics was historically viewed as a form of computational linguistics, the statistical or rule-based modeling of scientific information. The *Oxford English Dictionary* defined informatics as the "discipline of science which investigates the structure and properties of scientific information, as well as the regularities of scientific information activity" (Collen 1995, 39). Informatics has evolved as a separate science within the domains of basic and clinical sciences. Other areas of science have adopted the root word *informatics*, such as geoinformatics, which deals with the science and structure of spatial information.

Bioinformatics and Clinical Bioinformatics

In the health field, the *Oxford English Dictionary's* definition applies primarily to bioinformatics. **Bioinformatics** is a discipline that combines the biological sciences (microbiology, biochemistry, physiology, and genetics) with computational fields (such as statistics and computer science). The focus of bioinformatics is on the management, analysis, and interpretation of data from biological experiments and observational studies (Moore 2007). There is debate whether bioinformatics constitutes a set of computational tools for biological scientists (computational biology) or is a separate discipline (bioinformatics) (Stein 2003; Lakhno 2010; Martin-Sanchez and Hermosilla-Gimeno 2010). This debate will continue as the bioinformatics field evolves into specialized areas of scientific inquiry. Clinical bioinformatics and biomedical informatics are rapidly emerging fields in translational science and are focused on the use of genomics and proteomics data integrated with clinical data to provide molecular diagnostics, pharmacogenomics, and evidence-based clinical outcomes. Bioinformatics continues to evolve by incorporating diverse technologies and methodologies from disparate fields to apply advanced computational and informational tools to biomedical research (Fenstermacher 2005; Sarkar et al. 2011).

Bioinformatics is the most advanced area of informatics mainly because biological data are standardized and available in extremely large quantities, and the analytical process is primarily computational. One might regard bioinformatics with its focus on computational biology as peripheral or unrelated to the topic of health informatics, yet IT enables bioinformatics (and medical informatics as well) to transcend the laboratory and go directly to clinical decision making and to individual patients and consumers. There is considerable potential for bioinformatics to be a transformational science, and that is explored in Chapter 12.

Medical Informatics

Medical informatics was founded on logic consistent with the *Oxford English Dictionary* definition. It deals with the "structure and properties of scientific information"—in this instance, clinical information generated from clinical trials and medical records. The primary sources of data are the clinical trials that involve large population samples, and these sources are quite different from translational informatics in that they are much less structured and more dispersed and make access to large databases more difficult. In addition, medical informatics includes clinical decision support, which inherently involves the structure of the clinical decision process. Medical informatics generally includes imaging informatics and clinical informatics. Imaging informatics focuses on pathology and radiology, converting film documents and anatomical slides into digital format to facilitate the transmission, storage, and computer enhancement of images for the purpose of in-depth analysis. Unlike bioinformatics (which focuses on molecular and cellular processes), imaging informatics focuses on tissues and organs. Imaging informatics and clinical informatics integrate computational sciences and clinical decision making to analyze the relationship between clinical interventions and outcomes.

The application of computers to clinical medicine and nursing requires that diagnostic information and chart notes contained within medical records be digitized. Developing the **electronic medical record** (EMR) has proven to be a monumental task, as the structure of clinical information lacked a basic vocabulary and data standards essential for a unified language explored in Chapter 2. These tasks have served as the primary focus of the field of medical informatics over the past few decades. Chapter 3 explores the complexity and utility of converting from paper to EMR and presents alternative approaches to this difficult task. The orientation of clinical informatics is on automating the traditional structure of medical information and applying it to diagnosis and treatment. In hospitals and clinics, this means digitizing the traditional medical record.

Models for informatics research and education are varied among universities and are adapted to the core competencies of faculty and the unique structures of each university. Informatics programs are generally interdisciplinary but are limited to the computational, biological, and clinical sciences. The appropriate foundational disciplines depend on the special focus of faculty and academic programs, which to this point have been structured around the integrated concept of bioinformatics.

Biomedical Informatics

Bioinformatics and medical informatics applied to the basic and clinical sciences have fostered the concept of a single science and profession: biomedical informatics (Friedman et al. 2004). The biomedical field has identified a distinct set of competencies and dedicated degree-granting programs. Professional societies have developed that bestow fellowship status to senior scholars and practitioners who have made significant contributions to the science. Membership associations, such as the American Medical Informatics Association (www.amia.org), have formed to support practitioners and students of computational science in the clinical setting.

Biomedical informatics has evolved as a separate and distinct science from MIS, which generally does not use the term *informatics*. MIS is the application of advanced information technology to functional areas of both product and service organizations, including accounting and finance, marketing, strategy, purchasing, supply, and operations management. In the health field, the application of MIS to operations management has been restricted to the business function of the organization and thus is separate from the clinical function. This is the classical view in healthcare, where the responsibilities of clinical professionals are distinct from those of the rest of the organization (Brown, Stone, and Patrick 2005, 31–50).

The Biomedical Information Science and Technology Initiative (BISTI), formed by the National Institutes of Health, issued a report on the field of informatics applied to health and labeled it as biomedical informatics (Friedman et al. 2004). The report recognized four primary concentrations in the field: bioinformatics, imaging informatics, clinical informatics, and public health informatics (see Exhibit 1.1). The respective foci of these areas were molecular and cellular, tissues and organs, individual patients, and population and society. The report also delineates the core body of knowledge in biomedical informatics. Biomedical methods, techniques, and theories that serve as core competencies include algorithms, data structures,

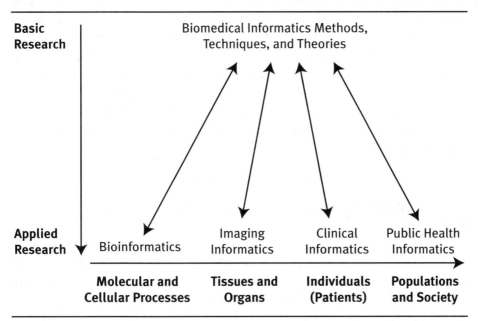

EXHIBIT 1.1
Biomedical
Informatics

Source: Friedman et al. (2004). Reprinted with permission from Hanley & Belfus, Inc.

database design, ontology/vocabulary, knowledge representation, programming languages, software engineering, modeling, and simulation (Friedman et al. 2004, 171). Inclusion of the competency area of cognitive and human factors and interfaces broadens the concept, recognizing not only the structure and properties of scientific information but the use of scientific information by practitioners to inform decision making and change decision-making behaviors.

As mentioned, medical informatics is consistent with the *Oxford English Dictionary* definition of informatics ("structure and properties of scientific information") in that medical informatics combines clinical and computational sciences. The computer became a tool used (frequently with great reluctance) by doctors, nurses, and other health professionals to structure, store, retrieve, process, and distribute clinical data. Digitizing information brought about changes in "cognitive and human factor interfaces," but the changes were limited to clinical decision making by health professionals within their fairly traditional roles. Such changes may be characterized as evolutionary and transactional in nature, rather than transformational or innovative from a systems perspective (Christensen, Bohmer, and Kenagy 2000; Herzlinger 2006; Strange, Ferrer, and Miller 2009; Havighurst 2008). Considerable focus is given to human–computer interface, studying how clinical information is stored, retrieved, and processed for maximum utility. This competency was intended to alter the decision-making behavior and not the decision responsibility of health professionals or the structure of the clinical decision process. However, the availability of electronic information did enable more and better information to be processed in a readable form, allowing health professionals to improve the service and care given to patients. Biomedical informatics was not considered a technology for restructuring but informing the clinical decision processes. Chapters 5 and 6 give perspective on the applications of informatics to the clinical areas of medicine and nursing. Applications of IT designed to change the structure of the clinical process inherently introduce the broader behavioral, social, and systems sciences and provide the basis for exploring health informatics as a transformational science.

Health Systems Informatics as a Transformational Science

Medical informatics shares properties with but is substantially different from bioinformatics in that the application of medical informatics may involve noncomputational decision-making models (and, some would argue, primarily noncomputational models). Clinical science, in addition to using computation, includes the art of clinical practice applied by a wide range of specialties to a wide range of patients and treatment processes across many professions and organizations. In the past, informatics was relegated to automating and administering existing clinical processes (Stead 2005). The power of digitized clinical information, however, lies not only in automating existing processes but also in transforming the fundamental structures of those processes. Greater value can be derived from transforming or restructuring, not just automating, clinical processes.

The BISTI report's inclusion of cognitive/human factors and interfaces as a core competency was intended to understand how physicians change their behavior by using computer technology in their practice. However, the application of advanced information technology inherently broadens that focus—from the structure and properties of clinical information to the structure and properties of health systems. The broadened focus extends to disciplines and sciences traditionally considered outside of informatics, such as industrial engineering, social and behavioral sciences, complex adaptive systems, systems engineering, organization design, and human behavior. These disciplines allow informatics to be applied to complex social systems. In addition, they are linked to information science, which allows the automation *and* transformation of existing decision and work processes.

We extended the biomedical informatics model developed by Friedman and colleagues (2004) based on the BISTI report (Exhibit 1.1) to include complex adaptive systems (see Exhibit 1.2). Our extension does not imply that the original model is not complex and creative, but it exists within the paradigms of medical and biological sciences. The Friedman model correctly depicts the linear relationship of the core body of science and the application of science to the four domains—bioinformatics, imaging informatics, clinical informatics, and public health informatics. For example, in the area

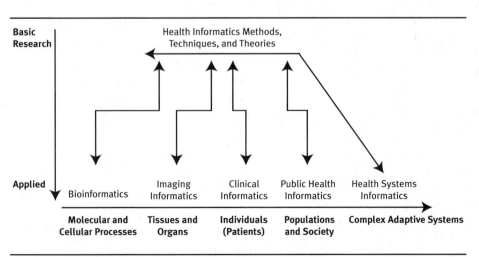

EXHIBIT 1.2
Health Informatics: The Transforming Power of HIT

Source: Adapted from Friedman et al. (2004).

ILLUSTRATION OF TRANSFORMATIONAL CHANGE

Understanding the extended biomedical informatics model (Exhibit 1.2) requires an understanding of the difference between change that automates processes and change that transforms those processes. Transformation enabled by information technology is the key concept in health informatics. An example can be taken from the banking industry. Before the development of the automated teller machine (ATM), banking transactions entailed going to the bank and dealing with a teller who stood behind a counter. Withdrawing cash from a checking account, for example, involved visiting a branch between the hours of 9:00 AM and 4:00 PM, filling out a withdrawal slip, and joining a queue to wait for the next available teller. The withdrawal slip gives the pertinent information to the teller, who then counts out (often twice to avoid an error) the appropriate amount of cash to dispense.

The ATM was conceived to automate this process. Initially, the ATM was placed behind the counter to support the teller. The teller would take the customer's credit card, swipe it through the machine, receive the money, and count out the money to the customer. In addition, the ATM provided a daily accounting of all transactions. One reason banks closed at 3:00 PM was to enable tellers to count the cash and complete the accounting for the day. The advent of the machine meant the tellers did not have to perform this count. In this way, the ATM was transactional: It automated the work process but did not transform it. Note that one (or micro) change, even a radical one, does not constitute a transformation. A true transformation entails a macro (or systems) change.

Some bright, visionary clerk questioned why the ATM was not placed in front of the counter to allow the customers to swipe their card and receive their cash and receipt directly. Management and executives argued that customers would not trust a machine to accurately count their money, although engineers emphasized that machines were actually more accurate than people in performing this task.

(continued)

of clinical informatics, the EMR requires doctors to use the computer for charting and to inform their decisions, among others; this use changes clinical behaviors but in itself does not change the structure of the clinical process. If those doctors apply the methods, techniques, and theories of complex adaptive systems, the doctors' decisions and work processes are altered. The extended model, expressed in a nonlinear manner, adds a conceptual dimension. It does not merely add an application, but it also affects all other relationships, which reflects its disruptive, transforming nature and the profound change it could bring to health system structure and function. Simply, the inclusion of complex adaptive systems extends the concept of biomedical informatics to form health informatics as a transformational science.

Health informatics is viewed as an automating and a transformational science, with a focus on the structure of the clinical process and support from a range of relevant disciplines and professions. Traditional informatics scholars and practitioners have resisted the use of health informatics as a label for the broader focus of the field, although professional associations such as the American Medical Informatics Association have adopted the label in recent years to describe the scope of their journal and national meetings. The resistance is understandable because the generalized label widens the competencies and core faculty composition of educational programs, making the health informatics field an interdisciplinary area of study rather than a distinct profession within the biological and clinical sciences.

However, the broader focus emphasizes the importance of informatics competency among health services managers, policymakers, and other health professionals. It acknowledges the natural and inherent integration of the clinical function with the design and management of complex organizations and systems, a link that clinicians have resisted and to which managers have acquiesced, perpetuating the cultural divide in many healthcare organizations. Furthermore, health informatics enables a reconceptualization of the role of the patient and family in clinical decision making and the clinical process.

The transforming power of IT enables change that will be highly disruptive to the system and will require visionary, innovative, and highly skilled leaders. Such a change will be deemed appropriate if it adds value in terms of improving health system performance, such as achieving higher patient satisfaction. Would today's healthcare leaders have the commitment and competencies to bring about this profound change? That is the question for those to whom this book is directed.

In addition, money transactions were thought to be a personal experience and thus customers would not be comfortable interacting with a machine. The fear was that the ATM would destroy the banker–customer relationship. The clerk was persistent, however, and the change-resistant president reluctantly agreed to test restructuring the process by placing an ATM in front of the counter. Customers flocked to it because of its convenience.

Once the machine was moved to the front of the counter, the movement spread. It could be found outside neighborhood branches and street corners and was available 24 hours a day. The transformation of the banking industry was on. Now, one can access her bank even at shopping malls and in a foreign country, where the local currency at the current exchange rate is dispensed and the US bank account is debited within minutes.

The ATM is an information technology that transformed financial functions, jobs, institutions, and customers. Health leaders and practitioners have envisioned electronic systems as a means to automate transactions rather than transform work processes. Although extremely disruptive to the old (but beloved) ways of doing things, the application of electronic information systems has great value in organization transformation. This is the work of both organization leaders and health professionals in the future.

Advances in Health Informatics

The first major development in informatics thinking was in public health and occurred long before the computer was envisioned. In the early 1800s, public health workers in many countries saw the need to develop a common vocabulary for classifying diseases and causes of death so that nations throughout the world could establish surveillance programs. The first initiative to standardize clinical information (or provide a common vocabulary) was the **International Classification of Diseases** (ICD), developed by the International Statistical Congress in 1853 and maintained by the World Health Organization (2012). The ICD could be considered the first medical informatics initiative, and it proved to be difficult to develop because of the different perspectives and judgments by clinicians and nations on disease classifications and terms. Despite the initial difficulty, the ICD did not alter the structure of the clinical decision process and was easier to establish than measures for clinical processes and outcomes. The technical complexity and political resistance to the ICD was a precursor to the standardization of clinical processes and outcomes.

The public health focus on surveillance as an outcome measure is still prevalent in the United States and most countries, as evidenced by the presence of many registries. Registries are operated by federal, state, and local governments; universities; nonprofits; private groups; and hospitals. Each registry focuses on a disease (e.g., hemophilia), a group of similar diseases (e.g., cancer), or an exposure (e.g., a toxin like PCB found in hazardous-waste sites). There is data standardization within each registry, and data sources are disaggregated to provide a summary of incidence and prevalence. Outcomes data, however, are difficult to link to individual clinical decisions. The aggregation of data and increased use of outcomes information will be facilitated by advanced information technology. In the future, registries can be generated from individual medical charts, and the clinical areas can learn much from the public health registries on data standards and quality.

Evolution of Medical Informatics

Medical informatics evolved in the clinical area (initially in laboratories) in part as a result of the existence of standardized data, repetitive processes, and standard outcomes—all of which are important qualities to computational analysis and reporting. Physicians demand standardized tests and outcomes so that they can interpret results, regardless of where the tests are completed. Radiology also met these conditions but lagged because imaging informatics needed massive computer storage and processing capacity. While physicians in pathology and radiology were passionate about standardization and measurement, those in direct patient care recognized variability and inflexibility—not good qualities for computer applications. It is not surprising then that the early work on medical informatics involved physicians such as Donald A. B. Lindberg, a pathologist at the University of Missouri. This first generation of physicians in medical informatics developed and tested the application of artificial intelligence and other technologies in direct patient care and achieved promising results (Kingsland 1985). Broad application of these methods required digitizing medical information and using it to transform clinical decision making, both areas of considerable complexity as they are partly technical and partly behavioral.

Electronic Medical Record

The idea of the EMR has been around for half a century, conceived in the 1960s by visionaries such as Dr. Lawrence Weed (Jacobs 2009). Automating the medical record was hampered not only by the lack of computing power but also by considerable resistance from those in direct patient care to accept and use a unified terminology and clinical practice guidelines. EMR plays a role in clinical decision support, and several concepts served as pathways for the development of electronic clinical decision support systems in the United States and in other countries.

Integrating Records

In the past few decades, EMRs have been installed primarily in large institutions—mainly hospitals—and limited to these institutions because of their high cost and because of these organizations' commitment to maintaining comprehensive and accurate medical records for inpatients. Medical records provided documentation for financial reimbursement and for patient treatment and progress. Quality recordkeeping became an accreditation requirement, although it was not unusual for a patient to have more than one medical record—one for each nursing unit to which the patient was admitted. In this way, records were viewed from the perspective of individual encounters.

When records were converted to the electronic system the individual copies spread throughout the organization became integrated, which was a significant step in the development of decision support. The integration of records revealed recordkeeping irregularities, such as records maintained under the name of the insured instead of the patient. For example, a hospital record shows the name and other information of the father (who is the insurance holder) but not the mother (who delivered the baby and received inpatient care). This made sense from a reimbursement perspective but not from a clinical perspective. Needless to say, the integration of medical information within a hospital was not a trivial task. An organization's EMR should consist of a patient's comprehensive health information, which is entered, integrated, managed, and accessed by authorized clinicians, nurses, coders, and other health professionals.

Changing Focus

The focus of EMRs is on the institution; that is, the EMR (like the paper record) was created for one organization and not shared or integrated with other information systems. Moreover, leaders were reluctant to apply the electronic system to how clinical decisions were made because they saw information technology as an automating rather than a transforming device. In other words, the EMR was acquired, financed, implemented, and maintained to automate clinical data and support clinical decision making, not to transform clinical processes. Managers assumed the responsibility for selecting a vendor to create the information system, securing necessary financial resources, developing an effective implementation strategy, staffing project initiatives, and training users. Training frequently focused on learning technical skills, although the greater EMR challenge revolved around changing the values and behaviors of highly independent health professionals, such as physicians. For managers the EMR became synonymous with e-health. Managers, thus, believed that once the EMR was installed and operating the organization had entered the "information age." The development of health information exchanges (discussed later), which were designed to integrate EMRs across various institutions, enabled the transfer of information from one organization to the next but did not change the perception that EMR is a decision support technology.

Converting paper records into digital format was in itself a monumental task, given that common clinical terminology and data standards did not exist. This complex, new information system, in turn, produced a need for hospitals and clinics to train their health professionals on using the technology to document clinical findings. All of these have proven to be difficult changes for everyone, especially highly trained health professionals. Compounding these challenges are issues of privacy and security, which are heightened in healthcare because of the danger of unauthorized access to highly personal health information. Many health information technology specialists approached the security and privacy issues as if these concepts were unique to the healthcare industry, although other sectors have gained considerable experience and knowledge about security and privacy (see Chapter 13).

Valuing the EMR

The economic assumption is that the EMR's value accrues primarily to the hospital or clinic, and thus the institution should bear the cost burden. This is a limited perspective on information technology. Digital patient record or EMR is increasingly recognized as providing great value not only to the institution or practice that owns and operates the system but also to other parties, including the individual or patient who traverses several facilities and providers, the insurance companies and other payers that have a financial stake in holding institutions accountable for quality and cost, and the public health surveillance programs. (The valuation of EMR in a society is complex and is discussed in Chapter 14.)

Electronic Health Record

Electronic health record (EHR) is sometimes used interchangeably with EMR, but the two differ conceptually, although both have a singular institutional focus. EHR is based on the medical record but includes documentation of the clinical workflow and provides alerts, reminders, therapy plans, and medication orders. As such, EHR is a more comprehensive picture of the clinical process, but individual clinicians retain the responsibility for it.

One example of EHR is the **computerized physician-order entry** (CPOE). CPOE provides a protocol to be followed when making clinical decisions, such as prescribing drugs. The most invasive feature here is the inclusion of decision rules and guidelines, culled from the best available evidence from population studies, to inform clinical decision making (see the National Guideline Clearinghouse at www.guideline.gov). These rules and guidelines can serve as a basis for the clinician or the organization in evaluating clinical outcomes and outcome–process relationships. Clinical decision support is a major disruptive change in that it invades the domain of the individual clinician, who is an autonomous decision unit. (The complexity of how information technology intrudes on the autonomy of clinicians and its implications on health organizations and systems are discussed in Chapter 4.)

As mentioned, EHR is embedded with evidence-based decision rules and prompts that inform clinical decision making. (The level of evidence to support a clinical decision is a complex and controversial issue and is explored in Chapters 5 and 6.) Clinical decision support focuses primarily on the clinical encounter (a micro process)—when a patient with a given symptom consults a doctor or a nurse. The clinical guideline presented to diagnose and treat the patient on the basis of this initial encounter typically includes information derived from the patient's medical record, such as previous or existing medical conditions, drug and other complications, allergic reactions, interventions, and so on. In addition, the record might include knowledge from clinical trials or some evidence gained from other medical centers. The level of evidence, the medical specialty of the party that generated the evidence, and the judgment of the attending clinician are all attributes of clinical decision support.

Each institution determines the degree to which clinical guidelines are applied and institutionalized (enforced), but in general the attending physician has the prerogative to override the guideline in the best interest of the patient. Even so, the use of EHR to provide guidelines for decision making is a significant invasion of the individual clinician's decision-making authority and requires changing the processes and behaviors within healthcare institutions (as discussed in Chapter 4). In addition, as healthcare organizations become more directly accountable for clinical outcomes, they also become accountable for macro (or overall) clinical processes, including following protocols and using measures of macro clinical processes as benchmarks of quality. This situation presents considerable potential for institutional conflict and stress and requires the creation of new structures and culture based on values and common commitment instead of hierarchical structures, power relationships, and standardized rules (as discussed in Chapters 7 and 8).

Changing macro clinical decision processes is transformational and thus has profound implications for clinical education and practice, health system financing, and the design and management of healthcare organizations. It replaces the culture that has existed for decades and each facet of the institution.

Electronic Personal Health Record

An **electronic personal health record** (e-PHR) is an individual's digital medical record that conforms to nationally recognized interoperability standards and is managed, shared, and controlled by the individual (patient). The patient-driven orientation of e-PHR introduces a profound change to how health services are structured and coordinated and how data are collected and applied. Most healthcare institutions cite patient-centered care as an organization value, but this is typically limited to patient involvement in the clinical encounter and does not extend to the entire macro clinical process, which might include care from outside the institution. Such a focus is admirable, but it is not totally patient centered. A true patient-centered approach covers the entire care process, particularly for chronic illness, and e-PHR contains information on such areas as nutrition, exercise, health risks, and immunizations—elements that are not currently in the EMR or EHR. Patient-centered care requires the clinical process to be restructured around the patient, not the health information system.

Under EHR, evidence-based protocols and guidelines are used to inform and support clinical decisions, but EHR does not fundamentally alter the structure of the decision process. For example, the handoff between the consulting and referring physicians and the involvement of health professionals in the decision process are not substantially altered. To move to an e-PHR, the institution must modify its structure and manage how professionals work within that new structure (as discussed in Chapter 7). Under e-PHR, the structure of the clinical process and clinical information is designed around the patient, to address areas of integration and continuity as a dimension of quality. Here, clinical protocols or pathways inform and bring evidence to the decision process of not just one health practitioner but all the health professionals involved in the patient's care. Such integration results in an e-PHR that documents a wide range of health services, including the use of sensors, care offered in homes, evidence-based processes, and nontraditional treatments or interventions (see Chapter 11).

Simply, e-PHR represents a paradigm shift in the delivery of health services and is not just technological innovation. It exemplifies what is technologically possible with an electronic information system when an organization restructures its clinical processes with the patient in mind. This restructuring requires a systems change, not just a unit-by-unit or clinician-by-clinician adjustment (see Chapter 7).

Health Information Exchange

Health information exchange (HIE) is a framework that enables the movement of patient health data and information across organizations that are geographically dispersed by using nationally recognized standards. HIE both connects disparate information systems and potentially offers a design for information systems that support connected communities of practice.

Today's national investment in health IT is focused on patient information exchange. HIE has consisted of numerous initiatives with many different labels, but they have all had a general pattern of development. When one speaks of HIE as a program, it generally refers to the current federal initiative. Considerable public and private investment in HIE has been made, such as a $300 million allocation from the American Recovery and Reinvestment Act of 2009 (Blumenthal 2009).

The earliest HIE model was the *community health information network* (CHIN), which was organized for the purpose of developing interorganizational patient information arrangements. CHIN had a low survival rate, in part because it was a bit ahead of its time, when the technological and organizational structures were not yet viable. According to Chin (2004, 1), "most CHINs never moved beyond planning because they carried price tags of tens of millions of dollars, participants had different agendas, projects were driven by vendors or health systems, and the technology was inadequate." Even then, however, CHIN understood that the value of health information increases as it is exchanged and used, and electronic information systems make this inevitable and recognize the technical, political, structural, financial, and cultural constraints that must be overcome. One must use caution when criticizing CHINs, given their technical and financial challenges as well as the political power of individual hospitals and clinics, but the leaders' lack of vision was a point of concern.

Another HIE model was the *regional health information organization* (RHIO). RHIO retained much of the structure of CHIN but called for more involvement from regional hospitals and clinics. Efforts to stimulate and adopt health IT met with limited success, in part because of lack of financing, which pushed the main financial burden onto regional providers (Adler-Milstein, Landefeld, and Jha 2010). Chapter 14 addresses the issue of valuation and financing.

CHIN and RHIO were important in conceptualizing an information system that served more than one institution. However, the resulting systems were initially designed as "closed systems," which retained much of the structural characteristics of institution-based IT—except on a larger scale. They could be conceptualized as interorganizational information systems rather than true regional systems. Their contributions included the recognition and development of common terminology and data standards to facilitate interoperability and information exchange among disparate and numerous IT systems. Given the lack of national commitment and investment in a national health infrastructure, the pattern of developing and implementing IT strategies incrementally can be defended.

With funding from the American Recovery and Reinvestment Act of 2009, HIE evolved from a concept to a program (US Congress 2010). The new HIEs are built on the basis of a national information infrastructure with increased federal financing (discussed in Chapter 8). These HIEs could improve clinical care because they allowed clinicians to access comprehensive documentation on previous diagnoses, treatments, prescriptions, and tests. Again, the purpose here is to better serve patients, but this model should not be considered patient centered if it consists only of the integration of institution-centric information systems like the EMR and the EHR. With HIE, the scientific and practitioner communities could access national medical databases for clinical research and the best clinical evidence based on large sample populations. The public health service could use integrated information systems for public health surveillance purposes by gathering and linking data from medical records, illness registries, and the National Health Interview Survey conducted by the US Census Bureau.

Federal legislation has been proposed to ensure that RHIOs can be interconnected, which would provide the foundation for a national health network (see the Health Information Technology Promotion Act of 2006). This national network recognizes that the value of information decreases if its movement is restricted by organizational, geographic, temporal, and professional boundaries. The evolution of the information infrastructure is based on three assumptions:

1. All patient information is retained at the institutional level but accessible through a regional information exchange.
2. Data vaults developed by RHIOs could be accessed across regions.
3. Internet-based or cloud computing information systems would provide protected access to patient information. (This topic is further explored in Chapter 15.)

These patient data and information exchange systems raise the important issues of privacy and security (discussed in Chapter 13).

HIE is a framework not only for building an information exchange and presenting clinical guidelines but also for providing the structure for a team of health professionals or a community of practice. **Accountable care organizations** (ACOs) might be conceptualized to support such structures. Mandated by the 2010 health reform legislation, an ACO is a designation that offers financial incentives to institutions that provide quality, safe, and effective care to Medicare and Medicaid beneficiaries while keeping down operational costs. ACOs could serve as the basis for reporting clinical information and as the organizing structure for delivering clinical services. If information can be moved across geographic, temporal, and institutional boundaries, healthcare delivery teams can form communities of practice that transcend professional boundaries. A **community of practice** that uses advanced IT could be easily formed and changed. An individual practitioner might function within many ACOs tailored to individual patients and their health conditions. The health data exchanged in an ACO would be elevated—from information on the patient to information that supports the clinical decision process. Patients then would be part of the community of practice and would be coproducers of health services, making such a system truly patient centered.

This is a transformational model in that information systems can become patient oriented without diminishing the institutional and clinician orientation. Clinical decision making and the structure of the clinical process would be designed around the individual patient and would be enabled by information exchange. Information exchange would serve as the basis for forming clinical teams and structuring and supporting clinical decision making. Such systems are transformational in nature and truly bring the health system into the information age (see Chapters 7, 8, and 9).

Conclusion

This chapter traces the development of the application of computers in the healthcare field. The historic antecedents have been on two fronts. First was the movement to standardize terms related to disease and causes of death to enable statistical analysis of trends and comparative analysis. This movement resulted in the International Classification of Diseases. Second was the increasing power of computers that enabled basic scientists to explore the structure of scientific information, giving rise to the term *informatics* and the field of bioinformatics. The advances in computer processing have enabled the subsequent application to support clinical decision making in both medicine and nursing. Such application has been a great technical challenge but has led to the development of common clinical terms and replacing paper charts with the EMR.

This book views informatics from a systems perspective. It considers IT as a transforming, not just an automating, science. Historically, the informatics perspective in the health field has been one of adapting IT to existing structures of clinical decision processes, organizations, and the system as a whole. Certainly this has not been a trivial task, and we acknowledge the changes that have been made in decision support at the bedside and the sharing of information among practitioners and organizations. This change perspective has been incremental to a large degree and adaptive (i.e., how IT can be adapted to the structure of the current system, its organizations, professionals, financing, and licensing and regulatory procedures).

The primary focus of this book is on transformation. Specifically, we ask how we might design a health system using advanced IT and how we might adapt the existing structures to that new design. This approach is not purely hypothetical. Our goal here is to present to leaders a vision of what the future healthcare system might look like, which would guide change and investment in the process. Thus, we extend the core competencies in health informatics beyond clinical vocabularies, data structures, computational science, knowledge representation, and so on in an effort to increase emphasis on open systems theory; simulation and modeling; change theory; the design and behavior of complex organizations; communications; and organizational values, ethics, and culture.

Chapter Discussion Questions

1. How has the concept of MIS been applied traditionally in the health system?
2. What are the conceptual differences between EMR, EHR, and e-PHR?
3. How do bioinformatics, clinical informatics, and public health informatics differ from health informatics?
4. What are the limitations of the RHIO given what we know about the value of information? Discuss the logic of why RHIOs were developed.
5. Why did medical informatics evolve separately from MIS?
6. Develop and present arguments for why information systems are a disruptive technology in healthcare organizations.

CASE STUDY   Dog Days and Information Technology

Gordon D. Brown

Joe is a young computer engineer who developed a microchip that consisted of an integrated circuit designed to be implanted in pets. The chip is small but can contain a considerable amount of information, such as the animal's name; the owner's name, address, and phone number; and the veterinarian's name, address, and phone number. The chip uses a passive radio frequency identification technology and can be read with a basic scanning device. Such devices can be purchased by humane societies and veterinarians. One of Joe's marketing pitches is to tell humane societies that a local ordinance encourages or requires all outplaced animals to be implanted with a microchip.

Joe is ecstatic about his technological breakthrough, and given that the United States has nearly 200 million pet dogs and cats he estimates that he would soon launch into the economic stratosphere, like what happened to Steve Jobs and Bill Gates. The plus side is that his innovation presents no controversial or animal-cruelty issues. Production costs are modest, although Joe does invest heavily in marketing the product on the web, in print media, and at animal shows. In his marketing material, he cites that the implant is a method for verifying owners. He also promotes the chip to customs officials, who need to check the animal's vaccination and health records.

The implantable microchip becomes an instant success with animal owners and veterinarians, but its sales growth overwhelms Joe's ability to produce and distribute the product on his own. He expands his investment in production and sales and establishes multiple distribution channels. He is on track to reach his economic goals.

Meanwhile, Jennifer is a young engineer who owns a pet. She created a microchip that can be loaded or programmed with information and worn by the pet externally (not implanted), making the information easy to update. Access to the chip is protected by a password set by the owner. A veterinarian or anyone given access can read the information contained in the chip. Most significantly, the chip can be read by GPS, which enables tracking the location of the animal. This feature is especially important when the pet goes missing, as local pet clubs and their members could get involved in the search or recovery efforts because the chip sends alerts of where the animal is currently located or is moving.

(continued)

Jennifer markets to pet-insurance companies, which find the tracking system handy in reducing the risk of registered animals being lost or abducted. The insurance companies also use the health information embedded in the chip to set policy rates and coverage limits. In addition, she has explored whether the pet identifying number constitutes legal proof of ownership. If not, the number and related information might be sold to pet food and health product marketers, which could translate to a financial bonanza. She regularly checks the law concerning the right to privacy for animals.

Today, Joe works for a large technology company. He is trying to repay the considerable debts he incurred from his failed venture, an enterprise bested by Jennifer's more sophisticated product.

Case Study Discussion Questions

1. Apply the concepts of automating as opposed to transforming a process in this case.
2. What is the transforming power of information technology in this case, and why is it sometimes difficult to envision?
3. How do aspects of electronic information raise legal and ethical issues?

BIOMEDICAL VOCABULARY AND STANDARDS: INFORMATION BUILDING BLOCKS

2

Timothy B. Patrick

Learning Objectives

After reading this chapter, students should be able to

- Understand the importance of concept-based controlled biomedical vocabularies
- Explain the basic aspects of the vocabulary problem and its relation to interoperability of information
- Understand the basic components of controlled vocabularies
- Explain the basic uses of controlled vocabulary
- Relate controlled vocabulary to metadata
- Explain the basic principles of vocabulary mapping

KEY CONCEPTS

- Concept-based controlled biomedical vocabulary
- The vocabulary problem
- Primary and secondary uses of coded data
- Metadata
- Interoperability
- Vocabulary mapping

Introduction

"For often good and sufficient reasons, centres representing the various subject fields would continue to use a variety of subject indication languages, corresponding to a variety of needs. Accordingly, communication through the use of a possible standard indexing language, which all participating centres would use for subject description of documents, was ruled out."
—Coates, Lloyd, and Simandl (1979)

"Two conflicting interests drive the development and use of controlled vocabularies. On the one hand, communities develop controlled vocabularies specific to their concepts, terminology, and needs as a means both of accessing data that is important to them and of codifying the content specific to their domain. On the other hand, searchers and those who support them want to use a single search to find resources in databases serving different domains and accessed by different controlled vocabularies, across which there may be no consensus regarding concepts, terminology, and knowledge organization."—National Information Standards Organization (2005)

"An official of the Centers for Disease Control (CDC) stated that he understood the term 'bad blood' was a synonym for syphilis in the black community. [Charles] Pollard replied, 'That could be true. But I never heard no such thing. All I knew was that they just kept saying I had the bad blood—they never mentioned syphilis to me, not even once.'" —Jones (1982)

This chapter explores the key aspects of using a concept-based controlled biomedical vocabulary (or for short, **controlled vocabulary**) to express biomedical and health information or to serve, as the chapter title suggests, as building blocks of information. Controlled vocabulary is a set of multiword terms and relationships purposely selected to express thematically related concepts and the associations among them. The discussion thus focuses on one of the most far-reaching and pressing problems for the management of biomedical and health information: the vocabulary problem.

In brief, the **vocabulary problem** is a clash of opposing forces of control and decentralization. General standards for controlled schemes for naming and describing things are useful, but so is the decentralization of the production and management of information. The quotations at the beginning of the chapter indicate potential effects of this clash of opposing forces. The simultaneous drives to control and to decentralize can limit integration and interoperability of data across systems, persons, and organizations as well as limit communication among healthcare professionals and laypersons. Unlike many business areas, such as accounting and finance, standardized biomedical vocabularies are relatively new and still in development. One must understand the complexity and utility of how biomedical databases are constructed to become an informed user or manager.

This chapter provides a brief introduction to the components of a concept-based controlled biomedical vocabulary. Next, two basic ways a controlled vocabulary may be used in the management of biomedical and health information are described. The discussion then relates controlled vocabulary to metadata. The chapter concludes with an explanation of interoperability and vocabulary mapping (or schemes for moving) in semantically and practically appropriate ways, from one controlled vocabulary to another.

Components of a Concept-Based Controlled Biomedical Vocabulary

The basic features of a controlled vocabulary serve as the architecture of biomedical information and include the following:

- Thematically restricted set of precoordinated concepts
- Set of terms (multiword noun phrases) selected purposely from natural language and serves as names of the precoordinated concepts
- Preferred name for each precoordinated concept
- Set of semantic relationships defined for the set of precoordinated concepts
- Set of names for the relationships
- Set of alphanumeric identifying codes for the precoordinated concepts
- Set of alphanumeric identifying codes for the terms
- Set of alphanumeric identifying codes for the relationships
- Set of rules for building postcoordinated concept expressions using the precoordinated concepts and relationships (optional feature)
- Set of entry terms (optional feature)
- Rules for the application of the vocabulary (optional feature)

Precoordinated Concepts

The basic unit of meaning in a controlled vocabulary is the concept. Concepts are unique and, although they may be replaced by other concepts, never change in meaning (Cimino 1998). A controlled vocabulary is typically focused on some more or less specific subject domain or domain of practice. For example, a controlled vocabulary might be focused on health services and contain concepts concerning healthcare services, providers, or programs, such as health professional, physician, primary care physician, hospital, outpatient clinic, or support group. These concepts are said to be precoordinated because they form the basis of the vocabulary and are the building blocks of more complicated expressions of meaning. In a way, **precoordinated concepts** are like the atoms of the controlled vocabulary.

Terms

Terms are names for the precoordinated concepts. Typically, several terms are associated with a concept, with one selected as the preferred name for the concept and the remaining terms treated as synonyms for the preferred name.

For example, for the concept *primary care physician*, the preferred name might be "primary care physician" and a synonym for the preferred name might be "PCP."

Semantic Relationships

Semantic relationships link concepts and may be hierarchical or nonhierarchical. Examples of a hierarchical relationship are "is-a" and "is a subtype of." Examples of a nonhierarchical relationship are "is clinically associated with" and "sponsors." Consider the hypothetical example of a controlled vocabulary for healthcare services. In such a vocabulary, the concept *physician* might stand in the relationship "is-a" to the concept *health professional*. Similarly, the concept *hospital* might stand in the relationship "sponsors" to the concept *support group*. Exhibit 2.1 depicts these types of relationships.

Alphanumeric Codes

Typically precoordinated concepts, terms, and semantic (hierarchical or nonhierarchical) relationships are associated with alphanumeric codes of some sort. For example, the concept *healthcare provider* might be associated with the alphanumeric code "C0001," while the term "healthcare provider" might be associated with the alphanumeric code "T4567." A key consideration in the design of the codes is whether they are pure identifiers of their associated concepts and terms or whether they carry other data, such as information about hierarchical relationships among concepts. For example, if the concept *physician* stands in the relationship "is-a" to the concept *healthcare provider*, we might assign hierarchical codes to those concepts—C0001 to *healthcare provider* and C0001.1 to *physician*. There are advantages for computer processing of codes in such a scheme, but there are also considerable disadvantages, particularly regarding whether a concept may participate in multiple hierarchies (Cimino 1998).

EXHIBIT 2.1
Example of
Semantic
Relationships

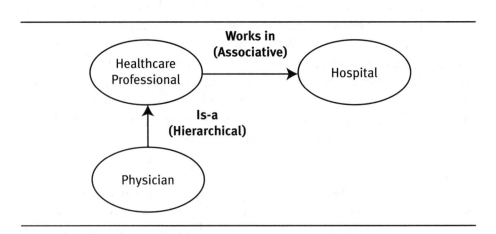

Postcoordinated Concepts

As mentioned, the precoordinated concepts form the basis of the controlled vocabulary, serving as the building blocks of more complicated expressions of meaning. Precoordinated concepts are combined with semantic relationships to form **postcoordinated concepts**. For example, the concept *obesity* might be combined with the concept *heart disease* using the semantic relationship "clinically associated with" to form this postcoordinated meaning:

Obesity clinically associated with heart disease.

Some controlled vocabularies include, in addition to the rules for combining concepts and relations, specific grammar rules or syntax for creating those expressions. The controlled vocabulary SNOMED CT (developed and maintained by the International Health Terminology Standards Development Organisation; see www.ihtsdo.org) is an example of a vocabulary that has both semantic rules for combining concepts and relations to form postcoordinated meanings and grammar rules for creating expressions of them. For example, clinical finding concepts may be combined with the attribute "due to" and an event concept to express a postcoordinated meaning. Thus, the clinical finding concept *bruise of head* could be combined with "due to" and the event concept *accident while engaged in sports activity*. Specific grammar rules could then be used to form an expression of the postcoordinated meaning:

262528003|bruise of head|:42752001|Due To|=57701003| accident while engaged in sports activity|

Entry Terms

Entry terms are multiword terms that are not part of the controlled vocabulary proper (i.e., not used to express or represent information) but provide an entry point to the vocabulary. For example, a controlled vocabulary of diseases might include an entry term "sugar diabetes" to support use of the vocabulary by laypersons. "Sugar diabetes" is not a term in the controlled vocabulary proper, but it provides an entry point to it. If, for example, the vocabulary were used to index medical literature about diseases, users familiar only with the term "sugar diabetes" could do a search, based on this term, for information indexed or coded with the controlled vocabulary term "diabetes mellitus."

Rules for the Application of the Vocabulary

The last component of a controlled vocabulary consists of rules for applying and using the concepts and terms. Pragmatics, a subfield of linguistics, considers those aspects of language that take into account the context and goals of the language users. We may think of the consideration of the rules for applying a vocabulary as a kind of pragmatics component of controlled vocabulary. Medical Subject Headings (MeSH) is the controlled vocabulary used by the National Library of Medicine to index biomedical literature in the PubMed system (National Library of Medicine 2010a; 2011). One example of a rule for applying a vocabulary is the following "Annotation" from MeSH for the concept *meta-analysis* (National Library of Medicine 2010b):

> This heading is used as a Publication Type; for original report of the conduct or results of a specific meta-analysis study; a different heading META-ANALYSIS AS TOPIC is used for general design, methodology, economics, etc. of meta-analyses.

International Classification of Diseases, 10th revision, Clinical Modification (ICD-10-CM) is the clinical modification of ICD-10 used to classify morbidity (NCHS 2011; World Health Organization 2007). Following is another example of a rule for applying a vocabulary, taken from the rules for using the ICD-10-CM code:

> I21 ST elevation (STEMI) and non-ST elevation (NSTEMI) myocardial infarction.

The rules specify this:

Use additional code, if applicable, to identify

- Exposure to environmental tobacco smoke (Z77.22)
- History of tobacco use (Z87.891)
- Occupational exposure to environmental tobacco smoke (Z57.31)
- Status post administration of tPA (rtPA) in a different facility within the last 24 hours prior to admission to current facility (Z92.82)
- Tobacco dependence (F17.-)
- Tobacco use (Z72.0)

Two Basic Uses of Controlled Vocabulary

Controlled vocabulary has two basic uses in representing and managing information. The first use is to express, in a highly structured and controlled way, new information. The second use is to classify or otherwise represent existing information.

For example, codes from the controlled vocabulary SNOMED CT may be used to express facts about a particular patient in a clinical information system. A physician might enter into the electronic medical record (EMR) a diagnosis for a patient using the SNOMED CT preferred concept description *myocardial infarction* using the SNOMED CT concept code

22298006. Another controlled vocabulary could be used to classify or otherwise represent (in a highly structured way) that existing information. For example, the diagnostic information entered into the EMR by the physician using the SNOMED CT concept *myocardial infarction* could be classified by this ICD-10-CM code:

> I21 ST elevation (STEMI) and non-ST elevation (NSTEMI) myocardial infarction.

In this case, the information recorded by the physician about the patient using the SNOMED CT concept could be considered a coding for primary use, while the classification or representation of that information using the ICD-10-CM code could be considered a coding for secondary use. The primary use could be clinical care or decision making, and the secondary use could be quality or safety measurement. Multiple controlled vocabularies are used in healthcare because many were created for slightly different purposes and/or for different contexts and cultures, and no compelling reason or ability existed to develop them as a single integrated system. Now there is a reason for an integrated vocabulary, and the heterogeneity of these vocabularies is an impediment to interoperability and health information exchange. Bridging the semantic and lexical spaces among the differing vocabularies is an ongoing challenge in health informatics.

Another example of the use of a controlled vocabulary to classify or represent existing information is the representation or description of biomedical literature—for example, representing the content of reports on clinical studies. As stated, concepts from the controlled vocabulary MeSH are used in the National Library of Medicine's PubMed system to describe the subjects covered by biomedical journal articles. The article "Is sudden cardiac arrest the same as a heart attack? Johns Hopkins Med Lett Health After 50. 2011 Apr;23(2):8" is represented in PubMed by the record shown in Exhibit 2.2.

In Exhibit 2.2, the fields in boldface are the MeSH Term (MH) fields and are used to indicate the subject or topic of the article. In this case, one of the subjects or topics of the article is described using the MeSH term "myocardial infarction."

Metadata and Metadata Schema

The distinction between the two basic uses of controlled vocabulary is actually not as sharp and clear. After all, from a certain point of view, data and information are just elements (like patients, physicians, hospitals, or diseases) that may be described and about which information may be recorded. Typically, however, **metadata** refers to data about data and information and, as

EXHIBIT 2.2
Sample
PubMed Record

MID - 21523953
OWN - NLM
STAT - MEDLINE
DA - 20110329
DCOM - 20110524
IS - 1042-1882 (Print)
IS - 1042-1882 (Linking)
VI - 23
IP - 2
DP - 2011 Apr
TI - Is sudden cardiac arrest the same as a heart attack?
PG - 8
LA - eng
PT - Journal Article
PL - United States
TA - Johns Hopkins Med Lett Health After 50
JT - The Johns Hopkins medical letter health after 50
JID - 9802902
SB - K
MH - *Death, Sudden, Cardiac
MH - *Health Knowledge, Attitudes, Practice
MH - Humans
MH - *Myocardial Infarction
MH - Patient Education as Topic
MH - Risk Factors
EDAT - 2011/04/29 06:00
MHDA - 2011/05/25 06:00
CRDT - 2011/04/29 06:00
PST - ppublish
SO - Johns Hopkins Med Lett Health After 50. 2011 Apr;23(2):8.

such, has a natural affinity with the second basic use of controlled vocabulary. A controlled vocabulary may be used to record information about a patient or a journal article (primary information), while another controlled vocabulary may be used to describe facts about that information (secondary information or metadata), and further data (whether or not from a controlled vocabulary) may be used to describe facts about the metadata (meta-metadata). Such hierarchies of data and metadata are reminiscent of this oft-quoted poem from the nineteenth century (Sharp 2011):

> Big bugs have little bugs
> Upon their backs to bite them.
> Little bugs have littler bugs.
> And so, ad infinitum.

Data and metadata hierarchies, though, are typically less dramatic than the imagery in this poem.

The example PubMed record in Exhibit 2.2 demonstrates a modest hierarchy of data and metadata. The journal article is the primary object of interest; the MeSH term "myocardial infarction" is metadata about that journal article; and the definition of the PubMed fieldname MH is meta-metadata that describes it and the use, in that context, of the term "myocardial infarction."

Metadata is usually organized in the form of metadata schemas. A **metadata schema** is a collection of fields or data elements, names for the fields, definitions for the fields, and specifications of what constitute permissible values for the fields. In this sense, the fields included in a PubMed record (such as in Exhibit 2.2), together with specifications of the values allowed in those fields, constitute a metadata schema. The field MH and the specification that it has codes from MeSH as its value are part of that schema. Dublin Core (2011) is a widely used metadata schema in this sense.

Note that this general description of a metadata schema could, more or less, apply also to the specification of fields in a structured patient record—for example, patient name, patient gender, patient age, patient diagnosis, and so forth. As suggested, the distinction between data and metadata (or between the use of controlled vocabulary to record data for primary uses and the use of controlled vocabulary to record data for secondary uses) may blur somewhat. In the case of the schema for the structured patient record, the term "information model" rather than "metadata schema" (discussed later) is sometimes used. Two important web-based registries for healthcare data elements and their permissible values, which include fields such as those suggested for the structured patient record, are (1) the United States Health Information Knowledgebase (USHIK) and (2) the Cancer Data Standards Repository (caDSR) (AHRQ 2011; National Cancer Institute 2010). Both of these registries are based on the Information Technology—Metadata registries (MDR), an international standard ISO 11179 (International Organization for Standardization and the International Electrotechnical Commission 2004).

Interoperability and Vocabulary Mapping

Broadly put, the challenge to interoperability of data and information related to the vocabulary problem may be summarized as follows:

1. Different systems, individuals, or groups collect or produce data, information, and knowledge according to their needs and then represent and store the data according to their local preferences.

2. Other things being equal, the value of the data, information, and knowledge is increased to the extent that the data are available to and usable by others.

3. No given system, individual, or group is conversant with the local representation and storage preferences of every other system, individual, or group.

4. Some means for translating or mapping must be provided among different locally preferred schemes for representing and storing data, information, and knowledge.

The use of generally accepted and well-documented controlled vocabularies by different systems, individuals, or groups may facilitate interoperability. Controlled vocabularies have long been recognized as important to this end. For example, in 1963, the Group d'Etude sur l'Information Scientifique, Marseilles, proposed a system of scientific information sharing based on the idea of an "intermediate lexicon" (Coates, Lloyd, and Simandl 1979). The basic idea was that a group of scientific study centers would share information (e.g., scientific reports) by using a standard switching language or intermediate lexicon. Each study center would use a controlled vocabulary, chosen according to local preference, to represent its information (the second basic use of controlled vocabulary described earlier). The information contained in a given document or report would be represented by terms in the controlled vocabulary. For example, if the document was about possible links between obesity and heart disease, and the controlled vocabulary used was SNOMED CT, the terms used might be "obesity" and "heart disease."

Interoperability would be achieved by using an intermediate language standard that would relate terms from different local controlled vocabularies that expressed the same concept. By means of such an intermediate switching language, it would be possible for a given study center to use its customary local vocabulary to search and acquire information from the collection of another study center, even though that information was represented in the collection by a different controlled vocabulary. The key to this scheme, aside from the intermediate lexicon or switching language itself, was that each study center used a controlled vocabulary to represent the information in its collection.

A contemporary example of this switching-language solution to the interoperability problem is the Unified Medical Language System Metathesaurus (National Library of Medicine 2009). The Metathesaurus is a large database that relates terms from more than 100 controlled vocabularies, terminologies, indexing languages, and coding systems, including ICD-10-CM, MeSH, and SNOMED CT. Collectively these are referred to in the Metathesaurus documentation as *source vocabularies*. The Metathesaurus is organized by meaning; terms from different source vocabularies are linked by metaconcepts. Two terms are assigned to the same metaconcept when those terms express or share names for one concept. Thus, the Metathesaurus provides a means of translating the representation of data and information based on one source vocabulary to a representation based on another source vocabulary. For example, the Metathesaurus assigns both the SNOMED CT term "heart disease" and the ICD-10-CM term "heart disease, unspecified" to the metaconcept C0018799. Using these term-metaconcept assignments, we can translate the ICD-10-CM term "heart disease, unspecified" to SNOMED CT as "heart disease."

Typically, the **vocabulary mapping,** which supports interoperability of data and information, is a scheme for matching concept expressions among controlled vocabularies by meaning. Simply, it finds an expression in one vocabulary that has the same, or nearly the same, meaning as an expression in another vocabulary (Fung and Bodenreider 2005). However, it is possible and may be useful to have mappings between vocabularies that are not intended to preserve meaning but are instead based on some sort of associative relationships. Knowledge of ways to relate information from diverse information resources may include cross-domain integrative knowledge, such as the knowledge that the best way to interpret information on one subject is to relate it to information on some other subjects. This sort of knowledge may, for example, drive data mining using heterogeneous and cross-disciplinary data sources.

For example, a case of cross-domain integrative knowledge might be the knowledge that to understand prevention options for some particular human disease, and to further prevention and wellness programs, it may be necessary to relate information about certain animal habitats to information about certain human habitats. This might necessitate retrieving information from different sources in a coordinated manner—for example, from the bibliographic databases PubMed and AB/INFORM (ProQuest Information and Learning 2011). Consequently this coordinated retrieval may require an associative mapping between the respective controlled vocabularies—for example, between the PubMed vocabulary MeSH and the AB/INFORM vocabulary. For example, if we know that controlling mosquitoes may help prevent the spread of West Nile disease and that one method of mosquito management is to recycle abandoned tires so that they do not provide breeding grounds for mosquitoes, we may retrieve information from both PubMed and AB/INFORM based on an associative mapping between MeSH and the AB/INFORM vocabulary:

mosquito control (MeSH) → tires AND recycling (AB/INFORM).

A concept related to vocabulary mapping is that of *metadata crosswalk*. A metadata crosswalk is essentially a mapping between the fields, or data elements, included in two different metadata schema. Providing the names of the fields in the respective schema is not merely a matter of mapping between the controlled vocabularies; the permissible values for the fields and their meanings must also be considered. Numerous metadata crosswalks have been published (Day 2002; Library of Congress 2008).

Conclusion

Concept-based controlled biomedical vocabularies are used to express biomedical and health information and to serve as building blocks of information. These vocabularies are, in fact, key to effective information interoperability, information exchange, and the related goals of modern healthcare. Effective use of controlled vocabulary, however, requires the recognition of the vocabulary problem and the development of standardized expressions of information. Only by addressing the need for controlled vocabulary, as well as the emergent heterogeneity it produces, can we ensure integration and interoperability of data and information across systems, people, and organizations.

Chapter Discussion Questions

1. Evidence-based medicine might be defined as the appropriate application of the best available evidence to determine diagnosis and treatment for patients. In the spirit of evidence-based medicine, should the controlled terminology and ontology used in knowledge representation be evidence based? What would that evidence be like?
2. Describe the nature and complexity of the problem of developing a common vocabulary for clinical symptoms and services.
3. Data, information, and knowledge resources are sometimes characterized by describing their inputs and outputs. Pick one resource with which you are familiar and describe its inputs and outputs. Describe requirements for a controlled vocabulary to classify the inputs and outputs.
4. Data for public health work is often collected using structured forms such as the Acute and Communicable Disease Case Report form used by Wisconsin Department of Health Services (see www.dhs.wisconsin.gov/forms/F4/F44151.pdf). Would it be useful to use a controlled vocabulary for that form? Would MeSH be a suitable candidate?

CASE STUDY   **A Problem of Display Codes**

Timothy B. Patrick

During the course of an EMR implementation project at a large medical center, the issue of how best to design display screens for the system arises. The particular concern is what standard codes should be used for the information on the user screens. The following e-mail is a request for a consultation from an IT staff involved in the EMR project to a member of the health informatics group:

Carol,

I need your help with something, and it's a pretty big something. I wonder if you or anyone on your staff would be interested in taking this on as a project?

I'm working on the new EMR project. One of the things we're stuck on right now is standard displays of information in the EMR. Because the record is integrated (which is the good news *and* the bad news), most of the tables and code sets are shared among multiple disciplines. We need to define what we will use for our displays. For example, the code set we're working on right now is Units of Measure. Now, you wouldn't think it would be too hard to decide what the display for something like "milligrams" would be. Except the choices are MG, Mg, mg, etc.... And that's one of the easy ones.

According to the medical center's standard abbreviations, all of the above are perfectly acceptable. The problem is, to build the EMR, we have to decide on just one. So far, since we began implementing the EMR, we've included a mishmash of displays, depending on what department we were working with. Lo and behold, now we're in a real pickle, and our database is a mess. In the truly integrated EMR, there can only by one abbreviation displayed for milligrams.

Again, this is just one example out of literally hundreds (if not thousands) of pieces of information we need to standardize.

Do you have some time to help us figure out what standards are out there? We'd like to standardize on something that is nationally, if not internationally, accepted. It needs to include content for standards, definitions, and especially abbreviations for pharmacy, medicine, nursing,

(continued)

and purchasing units. We'd like to have some standards to present to the EMR Steering Committee and the Medical Records Committee for consideration.

Do you have any suggestions? I'd be happy to meet with you and discuss further if you'd like. Thanks.

Michael

Case Study Discussion Questions

1. What is the problem that needs to be addressed?
2. What solution is being considered viable?
3. How would you define (or not define) the problem differently, or define a viable solution differently?
4. What do you think is the correct solution?

SELECTION AND IMPLEMENTATION OF EMR SYSTEMS

Win Phillips

Learning Objectives

After reading this chapter, students should be able to

- List the basic steps in selecting and implementing an electronic medical record system
- Appreciate the importance of project planning, workflow analysis and optimization, and user training
- Understand the common pitfalls in system selection and implementation that could lead to project failure

---

KEY CONCEPTS

- Electronic medical records
- EMR system selection and implementation
- Project planning
- Clinical documentation workflow analysis
- EMR system user training

Introduction

The adoption of electronic medical record (EMR) systems will surely increase in the coming years. Medical practices and hospitals, however, may feel uncertain about how to best select and implement such systems. The risks of poor selection and/or implementation range from user frustration and time delays to outright abandonment of the system.

Probably most EMR implementations go through similar basic steps. A practice or hospital settles on a particular EMR for various reasons, such as the provider has other systems from the same vendor or it buys the system recommended by colleagues (Baron et al. 2005). After selection, the EMR is installed and configured, and interfaces with other systems are created. If computerized physician-order entry (CPOE) is included, order sets are obtained or created. Then, the EMR is tested and users are trained. A go-live date is set, and the system starts getting used, either gradually (a phased approach) or all at once (a "big bang" approach).

The first few days of use may be marked by unanticipated events. Users get frustrated because documentation takes longer than expected. Patients get backed up, and panic sets in. Some doctors abandon the EMR and switch back to using paper. In the succeeding months, however, as more and more users have learned to cope with the new system, patient volumes start to return. Some users may never stop complaining, but eventually widespread agreement that the organization is "not going back to paper" is reached.

A completely trouble-free selection and implementation may be nearly impossible, but careful planning can minimize the risks associated with EMR adoption. Following are our step-by-step suggestions for a smooth process:

1. Get the right people involved.
2. Develop a project plan.
3. Get acquainted with EMR systems.
4. Analyze and reengineer the workflow.
5. Develop and prioritize requirements.
6. Clarify objectives early.
7. Evaluate specific EMR systems.
8. Select a system, and negotiate the contract.
9. Learn the chosen system, and map out optimized workflows.
10. Install and configure the system.
11. Test the system.
12. Train the users.
13. Prepare for the go-live or launch date.
14. Shift into production mode.

Get the Right People Involved

Getting the right people involved in the process really goes hand-in-hand with developing an EMR project plan. It is the first step because you need people to create that plan. EMR selection and implementation should be viewed as a project that has to be planned and managed. Traditionally a project manager is put in charge of a project. The project manager directs people and tasks to make sure things get done. A small practice may not be able to devote someone to the project full-time, so a manager or clinician might have to handle the project part-time. A practice might be able to rely on the vendor for assisting with implementation, but obviously no vendor is available to help before a particular system is chosen.

For the selection process, ideally the project manager should have knowledge about the practice or hospital and its clinical processes and documentation needs. For the implementation process, ideally the project manager should have experience with systems implementation, given that software will need to be installed, systems configured, interfaces built, and training and testing conducted. Finding one individual who knows both the clinical and systems sides may be difficult, but if the selection and implementation processes were split up the implementation manager ideally should sit in on the selection process as well so that he or she could be made aware of the organization's needs and concerns. In any event, the important thing is to have a knowledgeable and experienced person be in charge of the EMR project. Running such a project effectively is difficult if a committee is in charge and impossible if no one at all is leading it.

Key clinicians, especially physicians, need to be involved in the selection process early, either by being consulted or by being invited to participate in vendor demos, site visits, requirements formulation, workflow reengineering, and vendor system scoring or evaluation. Clinician input is crucial. Physicians and nurses are the primary users of the system chosen and thus have key insights and preferences about how it should work. In addition, during and after implementation garnering support from clinicians is easier if they have a stake in the outcome, which is more likely if they have already invested time and effort early in the process. In a large practice or hospital, not every clinician (physician or nurse) can be involved, but a representative should participate from each major specialty or department that will be using the EMR.

During selection, differences of opinion may arise among clinicians and administrators about system features and functionality. The institution needs to determine whose opinion counts in the final selection decision. This disagreement can become political, so careful planning is warranted. Some large EMR projects are supported by committees that address clinical, technical, financial, and administrative needs and issues. Large hospitals and systems may even dedicate IT (information technology) project managers as well as purchasing experts, legal staff, and contract negotiators. For organizations of any size, senior leadership needs to stand behind the initiative, even if someone else is "sponsoring" the project. Computer system projects have an increased risk for failure without management support and commitment (Verner, Overmyer, and McCain 1999; Kappelman, McKeeman, and Zhang 2006; Glaser 2009; Mooney and Boyle 2011; Bernd and Fine 2011; Bebow 2011). Senior executives must make clear to the project sponsor, manager, and anyone else involved in selection and implementation that they support the project and thus will provide needed resources. If those in the trenches think that leaders are not steadfastly behind the EMR adoption, or if the selection process gets bogged down in political bickering, the project could fail.

Federal government initiatives offer incentives to healthcare organizations that adopt and use EMRs. As a result, states have established regional extension centers to aid practices and small hospitals in choosing an EMR vendor. These regional extension centers have supposedly performed evaluations and due diligence on EMR systems and vendors and thus can offer reliable recommendations. Small practices should avail themselves of such expertise. In addition, they may hire an experienced healthcare IT consultant to guide them through the process, preferably someone who has completed an EMR system implementation in the past.

Clinical staff can also be involved in later implementation, not just during selection. In training and rollout to other clinicians, they can be valuable champions, superusers, or even trainers. Having a physician champion can be important in convincing other physicians that using the system for efficient clinical documentation is feasible. For all these reasons, getting physicians and nurses on board early is important.

Develop a Project Plan

While the institution can stumble through the EMR project with only a vague idea of what steps should come next, system selection and implementation go better when planned. A plan helps those involved to control the process, anticipate needs, ensure that crucial tasks get done, manage expectations of project sponsors and other stakeholders, and guide the organization through change. During the process, the plan should be consulted and modified if needed. Details about the implementation may be further fleshed out or revised once the system is selected.

A selection and implementation plan can run from a few pages to hundreds of pages. The plan of a small practice might be simple, consisting of a list of tasks and a schedule of who will do what and when. A large organization's plan, in contrast, might include additional matters, such as specifics of communicating project progress to major stakeholders, procedures for managing risks (such as losing key personnel during the project), and detailed training and testing strategies. The vendor of the selected EMR, if it provides project management expertise, will be able to supply a basic list of tasks, a suggested schedule, and specifics about training and rollout.

The plan may use a formal process of selection, such as a request for information (RFI) and/or a request for proposal (RFP). Using an RFI/RFP is common among large institutions but is not unheard of among small practices. An RFI asks general questions about the vendor and its EMR system offerings. The organization selects the most favorable from the vendors that responded to the RFI and then sends them an RFP, which details the organization's requirements for its future EMR. When the RFP responses come back, the practice or hospital chooses the vendors to invite to make a system demonstration and arrange a site visit. These presentations help the organization decide which vendor and system best meet its needs.

In a large hospital or system, the contracts or purchasing department may handle RFIs and RFPs with assistance from the IT and clinical departments. In other institutions, selection may involve several large committees, comprising representatives of various departments, that determine needs, prepare the RFI and RFP, evaluate vendor responses and EMR offerings, arrange site visits, and score and rank the vendors and systems. A small practice may have only a few people, along with hired consultants, to create and evaluate RFIs and RFPs and to attend demos and site visits. Normally most of the clinicians and administrators involved are busy carrying out their full-time duties, so in a small practice, devoting adequate time to the selection process may be difficult. A small practice might try to streamline the process by bypassing the RFI and sending a short RFP to promising vendors and then relying on demos, site visits, and the resulting evaluation discussion as the major basis of selection. As mentioned, use of regional extension centers and consultants may be helpful.

Get Acquainted with EMR Systems

EMR systems need to be investigated at several points during the process. Unless they are already EMR experts, key personnel should develop a basic acquaintance with EMR systems early. Learning about EMRs can occur through perusing vendor websites, attending demonstrations, or visiting a nearby practice or institution that has an EMR system. While noting the capabilities of vendors and products is certainly worthwhile, finding out how an EMR works and what it can do is more important at this stage.

The reason for this preliminary investigation is that near the beginning of the selection process the practice may wish to analyze workflows with a view to reengineering documentation and certain other processes, such as ordering tests and medications, to work with an EMR (including CPOE). The idea is that rather than simply automating inefficient paper-based processes, computerization may be used to improve such processes, possibly reducing the number of steps taken to accomplish documentation and clinical tasks. However, reengineering a paper-based process through computerization is difficult without understanding what EMR and CPOE systems can do.

At this stage the investigation is preliminary, and unless the selection team has plenty of spare time, detailed vendor-sponsored site visits can be saved for later. Site visits would occur when the actual selection process is under way and the organization is trying to discern important differences between competing vendor offerings. After a system is chosen and the practice is preparing for implementation, learning even more about how the chosen EMR works and how it can best be integrated into the existing processes is important.

Analyze and Reengineer the Workflow

The term *workflow* here refers to the multiple sequences of information, communication, and decision tasks that occur during patient registration, diagnosis, treatment, and reimbursement. What flows at any given time may be data, information, forms, and patients, making "workflows" (plural) more accurate than the singular "workflow." The practice or hospital should undertake a detailed examination of its existing workflows during patient registration and scheduling, arrival and check-in, encounters, testing, diagnosis, various orders, treatment, education, and follow-up. This evaluation has three steps:

1. *Identify the current processes.* Who does what, in what order, using what information, and creating what documentation? Making a list is helpful, but using flowcharts or similar diagrams is even more beneficial. Organizations are sometimes surprised at how detailed and involved their processes are and how much variation exists among providers, offices, or departments.
2. *Determine the aspects that need modification.* This includes problems, bottlenecks, inefficiencies, and redundancies.
3. *Optimize the workflow.* This entails reengineering the flawed processes (Middleton and Janas 2008). Optimizing before steps 1 and 2 may be difficult, because the organization is still trying to determine what parts of the patient encounter and documentation involve handling paper or result in producing paper (such as in dictation, transcription, printing, faxing, writing, mailing, and so on); what parts involve communication through phone calls and conversations; and how these paper-based processes can be reduced, eliminated, or automated.

Consider, for example, a large specialist group practice that still uses paper-based records and ordering, although its registration, scheduling, billing, and reimbursement are automated or electronic. The staff should sit down and list everything that happens to a patient who moves through the practice. First, a patient calls to make an appointment. A desk staff/ receptionist then obtains basic information from the caller and enters it into the computer system, thereby putting the patient on the doctor's schedule. When the patient shows up for the appointment, the desk staff makes a copy of the patient's insurance card and requests for her to fill out a medical history form, and then another staff member leads her to the examination room to take her vital signs. These data are documented on paper. The physician then meets with the patient, performs an examination, orders tests, writes a prescription, answers questions and gives health advice, hands out educational brochures, and asks the patient to schedule a follow-up visit. A doctor's assistant may come in and administer a first dose, give a drug sample, or perform other procedures as ordered by the physician. All of these tasks, including the diagnosis and treatment plan, are documented in the patient's chart, and then the orders are manually transmitted to the lab and the pharmacy by another clinician or staff member. The lab and pharmacy then follow their separate, respective workflows.

Once all of these steps are listed, the practice may be surprised to find out the number of tasks and people involved in one patient encounter. That is, how many receptionists, techs, transcriptionists, nurses, and physicians are involved as well as how much telephoning, faxing, paper handling, and communicating occur. Consequently, how many opportunities exist for lost documents, misplaced documents, misunderstood conversations, missed telephone calls and faxes, and other communication problems? The practice may see opportunities for streamlining its processes, such as moving paper documents to an electronic record system, replacing manual (calls, faxes, paper forms) medication ordering with online ordering, and requesting lab results to be electronically transmitted. As a result, steps can be eliminated; paper messages and handoffs reduced; and communication, the speed and accuracy of decisions, patient safety, and clinical and administrative efficiency improved.

By envisioning how the practice could work when computerized, the staff can draw up an optimized workflow and identify the features and functions in an EMR that can accomplish the vision. These requirements can then be used when the practice goes shopping for an EMR.

Develop and Prioritize Requirements

Some requirements for the EMR system can be derived from what is needed to create the optimized workflow (Carter 2008). For example, if the institution plans to move from paper-based ordering, a requirement of the EMR would be CPOE capability. If the priority is to copy the contents of the previous chart note onto a newly created note, such as for managing patients with chronic diseases where much of the note is the same from visit to visit, an EMR requirement would be a capability to pull previous notes forward.

EMR feature preferences of physicians and other clinicians can be captured in surveys, discussions, and interviews. If those interviewed have earlier experience with EMRs and know what they like and didn't like, their requirements or requests may get detailed. For example, one physician might claim it important that the system allow two chart notes for the same patient to be opened at the same time—perhaps an old note and a new note, or two new notes. Not all systems can do this. Other clinician requirements are more general, such as the ability in a medication management section to enter details of current medications not prescribed by the particular provider.

Obviously the type of organization determines the desired features of an EMR. A small practice may want an EMR from the same vendor of its practice management system because the vendor likely already has built an interface that allows patient appointments and demographics created for the practice management system to be exported easily into the EMR, and clinical notes in the EMR may export information for billing (automated charge pass-through) into the practice management system. Pediatricians may want a system that tracks immunizations, while an orthopedic group may want one that easily interfaces with its PACS (picture archiving and communication system). A hospital EMR may need to interface with and be adaptable to many departmental systems, while a practice EMR may not.

In order for the best EMR to be installed and to ensure widespread acceptance of the chosen system, many voices must be heard, including the voices of administrators and clinicians. For example, administrators may desire advanced querying capabilities so that they can run management reports from clinical documentation data in the EMR rather than just from billing data in the practice management system. Such EMR reports could allow administrators to observe practice patterns previously hidden from view in billing data (ICD and CPT codes).

EMR requirements should be kept in mind during the selection process, especially when drawing up details of the RFP and when evaluating prospective systems. Personnel with decision-making power must put together a definitive list of must-have and priority features, as opposed to listing idiosyncratic features that serve only one or two clinicians or that are "nice to have." If the list is too detailed and peculiar, however, no system in existence may be able to satisfy the requirements.

The ideal product of a requirements analysis is a *requirements document*, a hierarchical or prioritized grouping of EMR needs. The requirements are specific enough to be verifiable without controversy (nothing vague like "the screens must look good") and prioritized so that the most important take precedence. Putting together a requirements document is a project in itself, so something less than this document may be adequate—as long as it gives an idea of what the organization expects of its EMR.

Federal government incentives and penalties meant to encourage **meaningful use** of EMR and CPOE systems give healthcare organizations no reason to pursue any system that is not fully certified by the **Certification Commission for Health Information Technology** (CCHIT 2011) or by other designated bodies (Ford et al. 2010). Likewise, any system chosen should have commonly available features such as the ability to create and store chart notes; manage medication, problem, and allergy lists; and store patient demographics. Various organizations have published lists of basic and enhanced standard features for EMRs. Such systems and lists do not certify usability, however, so plenty of variations exist in the way EMRs work.

One big issue to consider is the extent to which the providers will accept or reject structured data entry. Physicians are used to dictating chart notes in the form of narrative text, which a transcriptionist then types up. With an EMR, the transcriptionist could type the dictation directly into the EMR to create a note consisting of narrative text. But this misses some major advantages of an EMR. If the EMR can recognize bits of data (such as medication names), patient vitals, and standard names for diagnoses and treatments, then it can use this data in clinical decision support, such as suggesting medication dosages, pulling up relevant clinical guidelines, and issuing warnings about possible drug interactions. Later, such data can also be used for analyzing clinical outcomes and practice efficiency. By and large, however, EMRs cannot recognize such data if they are buried in chart-note text narratives. For such decision support and data analysis to work, the contents of chart notes need to be entered using special data-entry boxes, drop-down menus, and hierarchical lists and outlines that use standardized terminology and code sets (see Chapters 2, 5, and 6). To a clinician, the process of creating a chart note starts to resemble the process of booking an airline flight online. Not everyone wants to do this. Physicians who learn the specific EMR system may be able to create notes faster using structured data techniques, but others may claim it slows them down.

Many EMRs allow structured data entry, but some do not and not all that do work in the same way. They do not all use the same clinical nomenclatures (e.g., MEDCIN, SNOMED CT) (Medicomp Systems 2004; International Health Terminology Standards Development Organisation 2010). Consequently, the organization needs to consider how high a priority this functionality is and be realistic about whether many clinicians will use it. Some use of structured data entry may be needed to comply with meaningful-use requirements (ONC 2011).

Another important consideration, but one that does not concern EMR functionality, is whether to purchase a system that runs off local server computers (at the institution or its facility) or a system that stores the data and system remotely and is accessed over the Internet (through application service provider [ASP], software as a service [SaaS], or cloud computing). Small practices may find the latter model particularly attractive because it minimizes the need for maintaining technical experts on the premises.

In systems selection the typical advice is to select the software and then get the hardware needed to run it. But in EMR selection, hardware decisions may take priority over software considerations. Those who value portability may wish for touch screens, tablet computers, or personal digital assistants, so for them having an EMR system that enables such capabilities is a high priority.

Clarify Objectives Early

For many organizations EMR adoption goals are implicitly assumed and only vaguely formulated. The goals could be about the patient, such as improved outcomes and higher-quality services through clinicians' better access to records, reduced medical errors, more accurate and complete documentation, and availability of clinical decision support. Or the goals could be about the clinicians and practice, such as greater efficiency, productivity, and revenue through quicker documentation; quicker access to chart notes and guidelines; fewer lost charts; reduced costs; and meeting the government's financial incentives requirements. Of course some EMR benefits serve both goals.

Explicitly formulating such goals or more detailed objectives could occur during initial planning. Once requirements priorities have been determined, more specific quantifiable objectives in adopting the EMR can be articulated. Some believe the mark of EMR adoption success is meeting stated objectives; such success can be publicized within the organization to increase enthusiasm and support for EMR use and future healthcare IT projects. To show that objectives are met, good baseline preimplementation data are needed. Thus, early in the selection process the organization has to clarify its objectives and gather baseline data so that they can be compared with data gathered after the implementation.

EMR and CPOE systems undoubtedly bring benefits, some of which—such as improved chart access (remote access, quicker access, and multiple simultaneous access)—are easy to demonstrate. Other benefits—

such as reduced costs and fewer medical errors—are measurable but might require effort to prove. Whether information systems reduce or increase costs is a thorny issue that requires consideration of various factors. For example, one needs to take into account fewer transcriptions, less paper use, reduced medical records staff, and better care through quicker and more convenient access. These advantages are counterbalanced by higher hardware and software costs and funds spent for greater IT support. If clinicians continue dictating their chart notes to transcriptionists, and printing old notes before patient visits, some of the anticipated cost reductions cannot be realized.

Large hospitals and healthcare systems may have financial analysts and informatics specialists who can gather the data needed to show whether the implementation met the defined objectives. Small practices or facilities, however, may be hard-pressed to find sufficient time and resources to do such analyses. This may not be a crippling problem because the necessity of defining EMR adoption goals and objectives is debatable. Currently, a practice that adopts an EMR is not likely to revert to paper if goals and objectives are not met. However, formulating objectives and tracking progress can be an asset to those practices that can do it. As the saying goes, "you can't manage what you can't measure." Without stated goals, the focus can easily shift to what the EMR does not do, which is a secondary consideration, instead of what it is doing. Such information can be useful in vendor and payer contract negotiations. An EMR that is not paying off can be replaced by another one that has more potential.

Evaluate Specific EMR Systems

After the objectives are clarified, specific vendors and systems need to be investigated and evaluated. This scrutiny is more detailed than the earlier general research into EMR systems. If an RFP process is used, the EMR team has to assess the RFP responses and choose the top candidates to investigate. Site visits are common, but the team should be aware that the vendors could steer the group toward special, showcase, or model EMR sites.

Getting a real feel for the usability of a particular EMR is difficult just by watching a demo by a vendor sales representative. Even sitting down at the keyboard and trying a few tasks might not help much. With car test-drives, prospective buyers really can drive the cars because controls are standardized. Trying to test-drive an unfamiliar EMR system is like trying to test-drive a car in which all the controls have been changed—no familiar gas pedal, brake pedal, steering wheel, and so on—which would seem like a car driver trying to test-drive a motorcycle. Even with a manual in front, the driver would barely know where to start. Site visits can be more valuable than vendor demos if staff at the site (e.g., a clinician) can show how the EMR can deliver a specific, requested task and if those staff members seem honest about their system appraisal. Ideally, the team would test-drive different EMRs for many months before deciding, but that is difficult and impractical to arrange.

Some EMR teams use a scorecard approach to rate the systems on specified criteria and then tally the scores. This method may be used to assess features, functions, and usability. This approach may not be as objective or neutral as it appears, however. For example, disagreements could arise about the proper weighting among the criteria. Furthermore, not all systems may be scored by all the same evaluators. If possible, the team doing site visits and completing scorecards should remain the same from visit to visit, otherwise the reason for the difference in opinions may be hard to track—whether the system or the evaluator (but this constancy is difficult because of the time burden on the clinicians involved). The organization needs to decide not only who the real decision makers are but also what weight to give to the scorecard results in the final selection process, otherwise choosing an EMR other than the one that "won" the scorecard points may be difficult. Note, too, that criteria other than usability or other matters observable during a site visit are relevant; for example, the availability of vendor support, the business viability of the vendor, and the ease with which the EMR can interface with other systems are further considerations.

If several systems seem to be in a dead heat in the competition, and any of them would be acceptable, the team can begin pricing and contract negotiations with the respective vendors. This exercise would reveal if one vendor gives better pricing arrangements and other concessions than the others, which is much like how a car buyer plays off one dealer's price against another. Note, however, that price is typically not the only basis of the selection decision, as explained in the next section.

The organization must heed one caution about accepting vendor claims at face value. Software vendors are notorious for promising what does not yet exist but that they believe can be delivered. The vendor may assure a prospective client that interfaces are available or can be built between the vendor's EMR and other systems from that vendor or other vendors, such as the PACS, lab system, and practice management system. The institution should verify that such interfaces have already been built and are operating well at an implementation site. If this is not verified, the institution faces the risk of signing a contract now and then later spending a lot of money and time to have the interfaces built, which were initially thought to be already completed and part of the EMR package. Even if both systems adhere to standards, such as HL7 and DICOM, a smooth data exchange is not always guaranteed.

Select a System, and Negotiate the Contract

EMR selection decision should be based on many factors, including the evaluations of those who participated in the demos and site visits and the determination that the system is the one that best meets the prioritized requirements. Some compromise may be necessary, and additional information may be requested from the vendors to help the organization reach a decision. The opinions of those who know the most about EMRs, have used these systems in the past, and best understand the business and clinical processes and workflows are given great weight.

System prices are often difficult to compare because many pricing schemes exist. Pricing can be based on such factors as number of total users, number of concurrent users (licenses), volume, and transactions. In addition, there are up-front one-time fees, annual maintenance costs, additional costs for third-party software (such as databases), and expenses for building interfaces and other customization. The selection team should not base the choice of a system solely on price anyway.

Information about the vendor could be obtained by including such questions in the RFP. Vendor factors to be considered include EMR experience (i.e., number of existing installations and number of local and regional installations), availability of local support, and size and financial viability of the company (Corley 2008). An old saying about system selection was, "you'll never get fired for buying IBM," which implied a guarantee of at least keeping one's job as long as one chose a system from a major vendor. But choosing a system made and maintained by a major EMR vendor is, in fact, not an assurance that the organization and its users will be happy with the system.

Seeking an experienced legal counsel when negotiating and signing a vendor contract is wise. The vendor may insist on using its own contract form, which may seek to absolve the company from any responsibility for decisions made on the basis of information in or recommendations by the system. The contract should address multiple details, such as the following (O'Connor 2002):

- Scope of the system supplied (e.g., software, hardware, operating system, database programs, data querying, and report tools)
- Licensing
- Implementation (e.g., whether installation and training is included and at what sites, who is responsible for system backups)
- Vendor support obligations
- Pricing
- Service-level agreements (e.g., absence of downtime, system support)

Organizations should avoid signing a long-term contract with a new vendor, even for the purpose of obtaining favorable pricing. The possible consequence of such an act is having to settle or live with an undesirable, flawed EMR for many years. If no system is deemed satisfactory to the selection team, perhaps the members did not consider enough system offers initially. Another possible explanation may be that the team's requirements were too extensive, sometimes called "gold-plating the requirements." At this point, assistance from a consultant or the regional extension center is warranted; the consultant can guide or advise the team on whether to restart the process with a larger circle of vendors or to trim the requirements.

Learn the Chosen System, and Map Out Optimized Workflows

Once the contract is signed, the implementation phase can begin. At this time, implementation details of the project plan that were left to be determined should be fleshed out. Because the vendor knows the system better than anyone else and has been through many implementations, the vendor should provide advice (and possibly personnel) in planning and carrying out the implementation.

Everyone involved in implementation should learn the ins and outs of the chosen EMR. Here is where clinicians involved in the project can be an asset in guiding the system configuration and teaching other users. Furthermore, this is the time to reengineer the workflows to match or adapt to how the actual EMR works, given that the new system may come close to the requirements but is not exactly as visualized. With a vendor-supplied EMR, the organization does not get to specify every feature and function, so generally the system determines the workflow, not the other way around. However, a large hospital may require extensive custom screens and workflows from the vendor in a "build" process that can take many months.

Old diagrams and lists of the workflows should be reviewed with vendor representatives so that they can be redesigned to fit the new system. Some questions that may come up include the following:

- Who will document what, when, and where?
- Will the transcriptionist enter dictations into the EMR?
- Will speech-recognition programs be used, or will physicians use templates or point of click for structured data entry?
- What kind of computers will be used, and where will they go?
- Who will be logged into each computer and at what time to ensure a proper audit trail of user entries and to allow needed levels of access?

Redesigning workflows that have been in place for years may be one of the most difficult parts of the implementation. The vendor is not familiar enough with existing workflows, and the organization does not know enough about the new EMR (Baron et al. 2005; Spetz and Keane 2009; DeVore and Figlioli 2010). Thus, the organization must map out the new processes, conduct role plays or practices, and adjust the processes until they are optimal. The go-live day is not the time to find out the quirks, difficulties, and problems of the EMR and the new workflow.

When mapping out the new EMR-based workflows for documentation and ordering, physicians with differing work styles may have conflicting opinions. The organization needs to decide how standardized the documentation process should become. Accommodating all opinions and requests (e.g., personalized templates of chart-note structures for each physician) is unrealistic. Standardization is important to quality. For example, in an ambulatory clinic or medical office, when a patient arrives the common process is to note any changes in the patient's current medications, including those prescribed by other doctors. If one physician directs the nurse to note these medication changes on a piece of paper (which will be entered into the system later) while another physician instructs the nurse to immediately enter the note directly into the EMR, the difference in workflow can confuse nurses who work with more than one doctor. More importantly, the EMR's clinical decision support functionality that might flag possible drug-interaction problems will not work if the first doctor's workflow means the medication note is not entered until after the visit and after a new medication is prescribed. The system cannot give a warning of a conflict if it does not have pertinent, timely information. Here, the organization should step in and define a standard workflow to prevent such problems.

Install and Configure the System

Learning the system and mapping out the workflows may need to be done simultaneously with installing and configuring the EMR. If the EMR and associated database are to be installed on local servers, however, the learning may need to wait until after installation and configuration.

Installation entails physically deploying the EMR on servers, but not if an ASP/SaaS/cloud model is being used. If the system is accessed remotely, client software may still need to be installed on user computers. Configuration refers to specifications and settings that need to be made. For example, the organization may determine exactly how many and which kinds of status can apply to a chart note from initial creation to finalized or closed to history. This allows the chart note to be saved before completion and to be assigned a status that indicates how much has been completed and what else needs to be done. Types of status could include "initial," "vitals entered," "medications updated," "sent to transcription," "received from transcription," "waiting for physician review," "electronically signed," and "finalized/closed." Other types of status are as simple as "open" and "closed."

Another example of configuration is *prepopulation*, entering information into the EMR database. If physicians need their names to appear at the bottom of the chart note, someone has to populate a drop-down menu list with physician names. Likewise, if branch clinics are to have their addresses and phone numbers appear at the top of notes for patients seen at those offices, someone needs to enter the clinics' addresses and phone numbers. If physician names and office addresses must appear on prescription printouts (for patients who prefer a paper prescription), someone has to enter the information. Similarly, managers who want to create custom reports and a schedule for regular report generation will need to set up these features as well.

To run an EMR system on local servers, a small practice may need to obtain hardware and software support from a local technology services company. The EMR vendor can specify the computers to buy or may even sell servers, but the vendor may not be able to offer further tech support. Once the practice is reliant on the EMR for clinical documentation, its staff cannot afford to have unresolved computer or network problems (Baron et al. 2005; Gupta and Murtaza 2009; Ford et al. 2010).

Policies and procedures related to EMR use need to be established. For example, a backup policy must be created, and user names and passwords must be assigned. A lot of decisions need to be made, including whether and at what intervals individual users need to change their EMR password, how information from existing patient charts (notes, lab results, etc.) will be migrated into the EMR, and how much of the current charts have to be scanned. A massive scanning effort can be done up front, or the process can wait until returning patients schedule an appointment. These decisions are time consuming for busy physicians, but compounding the problem is that scanning does not populate the system in the right way. That is, medication data need to be entered in discrete form in the medication management section of the system. Such data have to be entered manually for every existing patient, because to the system each patient is a new patient (Baron et al. 2005).

Interfaces between the EMR system and other systems (e.g., practice management, registration, scheduling, billing) may need to be created or configured. If orders are supposed to go directly to labs and pharmacies, and lab results sent directly into the EMR, the lab and pharmacy interfaces have to be configured. If CPOE functionality is used, order sets need to be created to allow quick ordering of routine sets of tests. In a hospital, the EMR has to be integrated with the pharmacy, electronic medication administration, and other information systems. Radiology and/or orthopedics departments may also set up interfaces between the PACS and EMR.

Additional hardware, such as servers and user computers, may need to be purchased. The number and type of new computers may depend on workflow decisions. For example, if clinicians are to access computers in exam rooms or at the bedside, additional desktops, "dumb terminals," tablets, laptops, workstations on wheels, and personal digital assistants need to be obtained.

Test the System

The vendor has, presumably, tested and debugged the EMR before installation, but more bugs (flaws or defects) are caught and fixed during installation. With each new update, upgrade, release, or custom build, additional bugs are created. Even a well-tested, large EMR likely has many bugs, perhaps hundreds or even thousands. Some are inherent in the program and may never be found, while others could be created by incorrect configuration or sloppy interfaces.

To increase chances of catching these bugs before the go-live date, the organization and vendor together should design and carry out a thorough test plan. This plan should include scripts that require testers to go through actual scenarios of documentation. Any bugs found can be brought to the attention of the vendor, who may be able to fix them before the EMR launch or at least document them for repair in the next release of the software and suggest a temporary work-around. To be avoided is the all-too-common practice of having users unsystematically tinker around with the system before the go-live date; this is likely to catch only obvious glitches.

Unfortunately when an implementation schedule slips and time is tight, adequate testing is often one of the first areas cut short. Sooner or later many of those bugs that should have been caught will be caught, only when it happens the bug may cause a delay and frustration (such as when a clinician runs into a malfunction or roadblock when she is in the middle of something important).

Train the Users

Adequate training of EMR users before the launch is often neglected. Physicians are busy seeing patients and often find no time to attend scheduled training sessions. Nursing supervisors, meanwhile, often cannot free nurses from patient care demands to allow them to attend training. Thus, even if training sessions are planned, they may not be fully used.

Other techniques and strategies may be attempted, and they can be continued after system implementation as well. Physicians who must give up seeing patients to attend training could be compensated for attending training. Nurses, likewise, should not be expected to attend training using their own unpaid or vacation time or to come back to the same amount of work after training. Training can be offered early in the morning, late in the day, or on weekends. It can be structured so that attendees who achieve certain levels of competency after a training session get rewarded for their efforts; for example, after the first session a nurse can demonstrate competence at a certain function and thus receive an incentive—perhaps a certificate, or some other token of prestige. In one large practice, the physicians were offered the opportunity to attain competence-level designations, such as Minnow (basic), Barracuda (intermediate), and Shark (expert), through a series of training classes. It became a matter of pride and braggadocio among colleagues to reach the Shark level.

The training plan should be geared toward producing real EMR users, not passive followers. Listening to lectures or demos of the system can serve only as an introduction, never as the primary means of teaching. Clinicians need to spend hands-on time with the system, learning to accomplish specific tasks such as starting a chart note, using templates, and updating the problem list. For training documentation, pictures and step-by-step instructions may work better than the typical catalogue-like user manual that is sometimes handed out. The vendor should ask, "How familiar are the trainers with the system anyway?" Some vendors favor a "train the trainer" approach, which means the expert vendor trainers teach a few practice staff, who after their advanced introduction are then expected to function as experts and train everyone else (even though they themselves barely understand the new system). This is an additional reason that a few key personnel should become real experts before regular user training even starts. Poor training material, overreliance on classroom lectures, clinicians' absence from training, and inexperienced staff trainers could make for a perfect storm of disaster on the go-live date. A more promising training approach is to create a task-oriented training program that is hands-on, is repetitive, and uses simulated scenarios. If enough trainers are available, they should shadow physicians during the first full day after the EMR launch to look over their shoulder and offer advice. Follow-up advanced training should be scheduled weeks or months later, after users have gotten the chance to explore the new EMR.

If clinicians are documenting in a structured format, using drop-downs and lists dependent on a nomenclature such as MEDCIN or SNOMED, then training should include instructions on how the structures of the lists work and where to find specific terms. Much of the time clinicians spend creating a chart note in an EMR is wasted on searching for certain items needed to complete the note.

Some users may need basic computer training before they can be trained on using the EMR. Even in this day and age, not everyone is comfortable using a mouse or knows the difference between a "right click" and a "left click." Using an internal e-mail feature, locating and attaching files, and sorting lists are some basic EMR skills that may be covered in training. The time to find out and deliver training needs is before the go-live date, not three months later when basic tasks are not getting done.

The implementation period is sometimes viewed as the preparation for the EMR. Training is a big part of this preparation. Using an EMR, however, is a big change that requires more than training. Because some users might have trouble accepting the change, devoting time to the change management process is worthwhile (if the organization's resources allow it). A formal change management plan may be created.

Prepare for the Go-Live or Launch Date

The day of the "go live" is huge because everything seems new and different; thus, the practice or institution should seek to avoid a catastrophe. Some organizations go live all at once in a "big bang" approach, while others implement the system for selected areas or departments in phases or the organization "pilots" the system in one area first. In a phased or piloted approach, the same considerations apply—just on a smaller scale.

A large institution's plans may call for extra trainers, including the early superusers, to be available on-site to guide users when they make mistakes, forget how to do tasks, or panic. As mentioned, shadowing physicians in the beginning may be worthwhile. In addition, backup paper forms should be available in case the system gets bogged down or goes down completely. Extra IT staff should also be available to staff the help line and answer e-mails; the help-line number should be widely publicized. The IT staff should have received complete training as well, because being a network specialist does not necessarily translate to knowing how to use the EMR. The IT staff should have access to the vendor's customer support number in case the IT staff gets stumped by EMR-user questions and in case the vendor reps and tech staff are not on-site to help.

A small practice, without its own IT department, relies on the vendor and other outside tech support. Vendor communication with clinicians throughout the go-live day is crucial to keep these users informed of EMR status changes or discovery of any unanticipated problems.

In the early days of EMR use, documentation may take longer and thus fewer patients can be seen. Thus, some organizations cut back on the number of appointments scheduled for those days.

Shift into Production Mode

After the EMR has gone live and the system has been used for days, weeks, or months, the implementation phase is over. The system is now in production mode. At this point, bugs and problems continue to arise, and the internal help desk or the external vendor help desk can be contacted as needed. Third-party data in the system, such as medication names and pill doses, are periodically updated. The vendor also creates software updates and upgrades that need to be deployed.

Processes and procedures must be established for setting up new users and terminating access by users who leave the organization. A **HIPAA** security officer may need to be appointed. Technical support personnel, information system consultants, and/or the EMR vendor are retained to maintain system security, backups, and compliance with regulations. These are standard IT practices for a large hospital but may be new to a small medical office.

Plans should be made for ongoing training—for new hires and for existing staff and clinicians who need additional, review, or updates training (Goedert 2011). Periodic newsletters or e-mails with tips for optimal EMR use may be disseminated to all users. A clinician committee may be established to suggest problem fixes and system changes to the vendor.

The primary use of the EMR is to supply information to providers and others who see or take care of patients. If data are collected in a discrete, structured format, secondary analysis of the data may yield important information about practice patterns and outcomes (Glaser 2008). This would require the IT staff, administrators, vendor, and other individuals to devote at least part of their time to constructing queries of the system data or large data repositories or warehouses that are set up for **data mining** (Chapter 9). Some useful information may come from standard management reports. For example, while the billing system will report information about what was charged, comparison with information contained in EMR reports may reveal the use of supplies or provision of services that is not billed, other instances of underbilling or overbilling, or differences among physicians in examining and diagnosing similar patients.

Conclusion

The selection and implementation of an EMR system is a major undertaking. It involves not only a significant investment of people, time, and money but also a significant amount of learning new technology and changing the way information flows, is accessed, and is used. All of this cannot be effectively made through training programs alone. What is needed is an understanding of the purpose the EMR serves and its importance to the enterprise. Not everyone involved will directly benefit but nonetheless must recognize the value of the system and must commit to making the implementation or launch successful. This launch provides an opportunity for the institution to work together.

The implementation steps discussed in this chapter point out not only the complexity of launching an EMR but also the interrelationships between the steps. The goal here is to offer a practical guide through these critical steps and to warn leaders and their team about the pitfalls embedded in each step. The concepts in this chapter relate to the concepts in other chapters, particularly those that deal with the difficulty of establishing clinical vocabularies and data standards, changing the clinical decision-making process, and knowledge management.

Chapter Discussion Questions

1. Why has IT been so slow to develop in hospitals and clinics?
2. What factors should be considered when selecting a vendor, and how should each be valued?
3. Is it generally a good idea for an institution to select the system/vendor that is most prevalent in the region in order to build information exchange systems?
4. What alternative objectives exist when selecting a system, and what are the arguments for each?
5. Discuss ways in which the EMR might change workflows and the logic for why they are changed.

CASE STUDY   Zenith Internal Medicine

Win Phillips

Zenith Internal Medicine is a large multioffice practice, with 14 separate offices located in rural areas and small cities and staffed with one to three physicians and other office staff. The central office has ten physicians, and the practice's administrative, financial, and IT staff members are located at the central office. Overall, Zenith has 53 physicians, 12 nurse practitioners, 5 physician assistants, 12 registered nurses, and 18 licensed practical nurses. The full staff (a total of 300 people) includes managers, med techs, schedulers/receptionists, IT/tech support staff, and billing/coding specialists.

For a number of years, the practice has had a combined computerized scheduling and billing system from a single vendor. The CEO, Martha Lee, decides now is time to get an EMR. She calls an old college friend who works as a healthcare executive in a nearby hospital; the friend advises her to contact EMR Solutions, Inc., to see if its system might work for Zenith. Martha arranges a visit with an EMR Solutions sales rep, watches a demo of the system, and then signs a multiyear contract to have the vendor install the EMR in all Zenith offices. The price of the system is several million dollars and includes both up-front and yearly maintenance and upgrades. EMR Solutions delivers three servers to be installed on the network by Zenith's IT staff with help from the vendor's engineer. One server contains the proprietary database and the other two contain the actual EMR application.

The clinicians hear about the purchase through an announcement e-mail sent out to all staff by senior management on a Friday afternoon. According to the e-mail, the new system will be ready to use in ten business days and can be accessed through an icon that will appear on every Zenith computer. Clinicians are asked to take a 30-minute tutorial, which would be available as a menu option on opening the EMR interface. Ten days later, on a Monday morning, another e-mail announcement is sent out by senior management to inform the clinicians that they are expected to now use the EMR and can no longer carry out dictation for their chart notes.

On the go-live date, most branch offices are reluctant to use the new system. The office managers inform the nurses and med techs that they must enter the results of lab tests into the EMR. One lab is configured to send test results directly into the system, but the other labs continue to transmit results by fax, leaving the techs and nurses to manually enter the data into the EMR. This takes time. Meanwhile, many physicians completely ignore the EMR directive and continue to jot notes on paper during patient visits and dictate notes after each visit. Only a handful of physicians agree to start using the system, but they encounter problems with finding the patients they are scheduled to see. The existing scheduling system is supposed to be linked to the new EMR, so in theory the day's schedule of patients can be pulled up for easy access. That is not the case. Manual data entry and searching before each patient visit is required.

The physicians' notes-taking processes vary. Some type notes directly into the system, while others dictate to med techs during the visit and the med techs enter the notes later. Patient visits fall behind as a result, and some patients wait an hour or more to be seen. A few physicians jot down extensive handwritten chart notes during each visit and then after 5 pm enter the notes themselves by using the special templates in the EMR. But many of the templates are set up for pediatrics, not internal medicine or other specialties, making most of the categories and tabs not applicable for other physicians' purposes.

The EMR has an ordering module that allows physicians to enter prescriptions online. But the module is not populated by medication names, which forces users (specifically, the nurses) to manually enter the drug name, a practice that introduces misspellings that remain in the system for other nurses to choose inadvertently when selecting drugs from a general medication list. Prescriptions entered in the system are not transmitted electronically to any pharmacy but rather must be printed out and then either handed to the patient or faxed to the pharmacy. Finding the correct fax numbers for the pharmacies is also time consuming.

Clinicians also have trouble incorporating the EMR into their patient-visit workflow. Computers are available in exam rooms, but physicians cannot log on to use the EMR installed in these computers because the user name and password required for EMR is different from those required by the regular network. On first visit, the EMR requires the user to change his password and answer a number of security questions in case of a forgotten password. Physicians who do push through the log-on requirement encounter other problems. When they try to call up old chart notes, they (and their patients) are surprised that the EMR contains no patient records whatsoever. As a result, a mad scramble to retrieve the paper-based chart notes becomes a constant during patient visits. When

(continued)

paper charts cannot be located, the physicians have to ask patients about the history and purpose of their visit. Furthermore, the medication lists are also a source of problems. Sometimes the patient's existing medications have been entered into the EMR and are thus visible on the screen, but other times the nurse who takes the patient's vitals has to hand the physician a piece of paper that lists these drugs. Figuring out which nurse does what and how is difficult.

The EMR has a problem management module to help clinicians keep track of patient illnesses and diseases, but physicians cannot find the ICD-9 codes for diseases they do not personally manage. Some physicians enter all patient problems, while others enter just the patient-specific problems they are currently treating. Some nurses enter problems before the patient arrives, but this is not uniformly done.

Physicians are also unclear about how to handle billing. Some continue to fill out paper billing sheets, but others assume that entering ICD-9 codes into the EMR automatically sets off the billing system. However, this assumption is false, because the EMR and billing system are from two separate vendors and thus are not integrated to exchange data. When the finance department realizes this confusion during the first days of EMR implementation, they start to brainstorm solutions to the billing process.

Even before the first (go-live) day is over, the branch offices are in chaos. Someone has terminated half of the transcriptionists in anticipation of their services no longer being needed. This causes an outcry from physicians, many of whom are still dictating their notes and thus argue that the mass layoff means their notes will not be available until weeks after their patients' visits. Some clinicians, including several physicians and nurses, are openly cursing and threatening to quit. Meanwhile, Zenith's IT department is flooded with phone calls and e-mails about the problems: the system is slow or inaccessible, computers have crashed, patient records are not available or lost, user names and passwords do not work, a tech is needed immediately to fix an error or to do a quick training, and so on. One IT employee walks out for lunch and does not return.

Martha is holed up in her office, refusing to take any calls. At the end of the first week, she sends out an all-staff e-mail informing everyone to stop using the EMR until further notice and for clinicians to go back to their paper charts and dictation.

Case Study Discussion Questions

1. In this selection and implementation, what should have been done differently?
2. How can the current situation at Zenith be fixed?

EVIDENCE-BASED CLINICAL DECISION MAKING

Gordon D. Brown

Learning Objectives

After reading this chapter, students should be able to

- Understand and apply the role of health professionals in transforming clinical decision-making processes
- Conceptualize differences in the clinical encounter and in the clinical process between a traditional (micro) and a systems (macro) environment
- Justify the selective application of evidence-based medicine, and access and evaluate sources of evidence
- Conceptualize decision support systems that enable experiential knowledge to be applied in clinical decision making
- Explain the concept of community of practice

KEY CONCEPTS

- Traditional role of the health professions
- Micro and macro decision-making processes
- Evidence-based clinical practice
- Expert judgment and heuristic reasoning
- Probabilistic reasoning
- Actor–network theory
- Experiential knowledge

Introduction

Much of the literature on health informatics focuses on how information technology (IT) can be structured to enable health professionals to access and use it effectively to support and improve their decision making. Any approach to inform or alter clinical decision processes must be based on an understanding of the science of how decisions are made. IT has been applied to improve clinical decision making, but in the way that keeps IT primarily compliant with the traditional role of medicine and nursing. This use is similar to that of automating rather than transforming a process (as discussed in the banking example in Chapter 1).

The clinical decision-making process consists of both micro and macro perspectives. Micro refers to the decision process that a physician and her staff face during an encounter with a patient who presents with a symptom. The micro process might involve a single encounter, characterized by a person becoming ill, visiting a physician, receiving treatment, getting well, and leaving the system. Macro, on the other hand, refers to the clinical decision process for multiple or ongoing encounters, characterized by a person who has a chronic illness (and maybe with comorbidities) getting treatment, over time, from numerous physicians and other health professionals who are associated with different healthcare organizations. The macro process transcends time, geographic space (territory), and professional domains (technology). Instead of being viewed as a dichotomy, the micro and macro processes can be considered as belonging to the same continuum of care, along which the patient moves according to the complexity of his illness.

The paper medical record was designed to support the concept of the micro process, and it is also an underlying principle in the design of the electronic medical record (EMR). In other words, the logic of the design and application of the EMR is based on an individual clinician's micro decision-making process and, as such, supports the traditional role of the physician in the clinical process. The electronic health record (EHR) broadened the information and knowledge that physicians and staff could access, including clinical guidelines derived from data repositories and presented as decision support tools that can be applied to improve clinical decisions and patient outcomes.

The EHR, like the EMR, did not significantly alter the structure of the clinical process. Development of the EMR and EHR has not been a trivial task, and that work is evident in these systems' significance to improving decision making and quality. In addition, the EMR and EHR have changed the decision-making behaviors of health professionals, which in itself is a complex undertaking. However, decision support systems designed to fit the logic of the micro process are inconsistent with or fundamentally different from support systems based on the logic of the macro process. The micro logic is oriented toward making the existing structures and processes work better, while the macro logic is geared toward transforming the entire system. This chapter broadens the micro to the macro logic, examining how information technology (IT) enables the restructuring of the clinical decision-making process around the macro perspective.

Perspectives on Changing Health System Design

At one extreme, IT might be considered as a data-processing application (which makes what was formally presented verbally or on paper available in digital format) that presents relatively little disruption to the structure of the existing clinical process. At the other extreme, IT might be viewed as a technology that enables the substantial restructuring of the clinical process and healthcare organizations. The justification for this transformation and for selecting and applying IT is the demonstrated ability to improve clinical outcomes and patient satisfaction.

Healthcare leaders and managers must carefully consider how any technology that alters the structure of the clinical process can affect professional roles and autonomy. Such examination must include how IT enables the restructuring of the clinical process but keeps the process consistent with the essential tenets of the health professional role. To achieve this end, organization leaders, IT specialists, policymakers, and health professionals must understand the nature of the clinical decision-making process, defined in part by the role of health professionals.

Three perspectives must be considered in guiding systems (or macro) change: (1) technical perspective held by the IT specialist; (2) structural, behavioral, and financial or business perspective held by the organization leader; and (3) clinical perspective held by the health professional. Each perspective is based on a different logic, so these three inherently conflict without a clear, unifying model that optimizes their performance (see Exhibit 4.1). These three perspectives have simply coexisted in healthcare organizations over the years, and their inherent and disruptive conflicts have not been addressed except by a few integrated health systems, such as Kaiser Permanente. The technical, business, and clinical perspectives are all essential and can be mutually supportive when considered from a systems perspective.

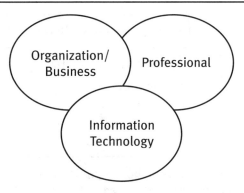

EXHIBIT 4.1
Three Disparate Perspectives in Healthcare Organizations

These essential perspectives are interrelated, but each focuses on optimizing its own function.

If a synergy among the three is not reached, the organization will be dysfunctional and performance will suffer. Synergy means integrating all three using an overall evidenced-based strategy that supports improved clinical outcomes (see Exhibit 4.2). This evidence-based solution relates clinical knowledge and the clinical function to the evidence-based knowledge about the organization's structure, behavior, and culture and shows how IT supports both the business and clinical functions. This powerful integration model results in an evidence-based decision-making process that improves clinical outcomes and patient satisfaction.

In this model, the clinical perspective is not subordinate to the business and the IT perspectives. The dominant strategy of the healthcare organization remains focused on healthcare services and clinical care. This clinical perspective, however, is broadened to include significant structural and behavioral concerns and thus takes on a systems perspective. The two important questions here are (1) how will the traditional role of health professionals change? and (2) how will professional autonomy be protected from the traditional organizational controls made in the name of improving clinical outcomes? When there is interdependency among the three perspectives, clinical outcomes are measured not only by the standard service metrics but also by the personalized care given that is considerate of an individual patient's illness and cultural, social, and religious identity. This chapter explores the concept and science that underpins evidence-based decision making from a systems perspective.

EXHIBIT 4.2
Evidence-based Model for Merging Disparate Perspectives into a System

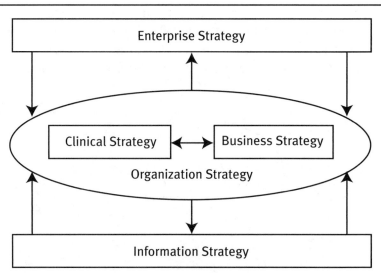

This model reflects the integration of the business and clinical functions supported by the information strategy.

Source: Figure 2.1 from Brown, Stone, and Patrick (2005). Reprinted with permission from Health Administration Press.

The Changing Role of Health Professionals

Understanding how the clinical function is fundamentally structured and how clinical work is coordinated in health systems requires an understanding of the nature of professions in society. Professions are social institutions and as such vary from society to society and change over time (Muzio and Kirkpatrick 2011). Society assigns special privileges and responsibilities to professions, giving them power and legitimacy. The role of professionals, however, changes in response to society's changing conditions, values, economics, technology (including IT), and other factors. Leaders in management, information, and clinical areas of a healthcare organization must understand this changing role of professionals, and we encourage readers of this book to explore this topic beyond the discussion in this chapter (see Muzio and Kirkpatrick 2011; Digwell 2009; Friedson 2001; Martimianakis, Maniate, and Hodges 2009).

The Traditional Role of the Health Professions

The term *professional* is often attached to jobholders in many fields, which is inappropriate because not all occupations are true professions. Professionals are those with "specialized training and knowledge, ethicality, and importance to society" (Friedson 1994, 19). Medicine, for example, is one of the most "professionalized" fields, which shows its commitment to caring for and healing patients. And society grants this profession certain privileges. In medical education, for example, universities grant physicians considerable autonomy in selecting and admitting students into medical schools, defining the curriculum, and setting educational standards. In society, physicians are given the privilege of licensing new physicians and granting board certifications. Many, if not most, medical school graduates are socialized into the profession and take an oath to society and their patients (Hippocratic Oath), which recognizes medicine as a calling. The modern Hippocratic Oath includes the following statements (Tyson 2001):

> I will remember that there is art to medicine as well as science, and that warmth, sympathy, and understanding may outweigh the surgeon's knife or the chemist's drug. . . .

> I will remember that I do not treat a fever chart, a cancerous growth, but a sick human being, whose illness may affect the person's family and economic stability. My responsibility includes these related problems, if I am to care adequately for the sick.

Likewise, the nursing profession used a modified Hippocratic Oath called the Nightingale Pledge. The Nightingale Pledge, created in 1893 to honor Florence Nightingale, the patron saint of nursing, reflected the social values and role of nurses in the last century but has fallen out of favor in modern times as the profession and social mores have changed. The pledge contains this promise from nurses (ANA 2012):

> I will do all in my power to maintain and elevate the standard of my profession, and will hold in confidence all personal matters committed to my keeping and all family affairs coming to my knowledge in the practice of my calling. With loyalty will I endeavor to aid the physician, in his work, and devote myself to the welfare of those committed to my care.

These oaths suggest that the commitment of health professionals is to the patients, whom they view as individual people with varying and unique physical conditions, social and economic status, beliefs, values, traditions, and so on. This orientation requires professionals to have autonomy—the freedom and flexibility to tailor their response according to the patient's health and social conditions, values, and other factors. This autonomy (coupled with a strong, ethical commitment to quality) manifests itself in the professional's drive to achieve high education, pursue continuing education, ensure work competency, and structure the clinical processes around the needs of individual patients. This high level of motivation and personal devotion to healing and caring are important properties of high performance, which cannot be duplicated by the traditional role of human resources in organizations (discussed in Chapter 10) and must be protected within society.[1]

The traditional role (i.e., the ability to function independently) of health professionals is based on this autonomy, personal drive, responsibility to society, and commitment to great patient outcomes. As such, health professionals tend to (and traditionally) work independently and rely on their own knowledge base to make a clinical decision. This orientation, however, presents conflicts with the standard, rule-based clinical protocols mandated by their healthcare organization, external agencies, or professional associations. The advent of IT has also challenged this traditional role and clinical processes.

The Influence of the Information Age

Information systems that are based only on the logic of IT and organizational rules and controls without regard for the clinical aspects could diminish the role of health professionals and will be, and should be, resisted by doctors, nurses, and other clinicians. However, IT and evidence-based decision guidelines are an important part of social and technological change and thus should not be undermined by professionals just so that they can protect their autonomous roles within the organization. Research has found that clinical decision support tools, such as evidence-based clinical guidelines, have been institutionalized but not yet professionalized (Audet et al. 2005). By "institutionalized," we mean that, although developed by clinicians, these tools have been implemented, mandated, and regulated primarily by the traditional organization, which follows the hierarchical, control-based, and functional structure. By "professionalized," we mean that the health professions have acknowledged the importance of these tools and have committed to using them. Thus far, that has not widely occurred.

Health professions can fulfill their social responsibility by adjusting their structure to accommodate changes in IT, systems science, and societal demographics and values. On the other hand, organizations must adjust their management structures to accommodate diversity, rapid and unpredictable change, and knowledge embedded within the institution. Hafferty and Levinson (2008) suggest that a complexity science approach could be used to recast social actors, social structures, and environmental factors to be interactive, adaptive, and interdependent. Traditional organizations are characterized by hierarchical structures, strategic plans, stable equilibrium relationships, emphasis on a common culture, and rational decision making. In contrast, *complexity science* is a systems concept that values agility of thought, creativity, risk taking, and the value of diversity. Organizations that are referred to as "learning or knowledge organizations" are nontraditional and embody the concept of complexity science. These organizations are self-organizing and able to capture and use tacit knowledge adapted to individual patients, but they are still purposeful systems in that they encourage individuals to work together to achieve extraordinary performance.

Historically, the role of health professionals was structured around the assumptions of an agrarian and industrial society, not an information-driven society. Thus, the specialized knowledge of doctors and nurses was passed from the minds of individuals; expanded by access to scientific developments and reports; and reinforced through licensure, certification, and continuing education. The health professions mandated continuing education and documenting the number of hours a professional attended classes, but this practice has moved increasingly to reexamination using problem-based instruments (American Board of Medical Specialties 2011). In the future, continuing education will likely be evidence based, linking outcomes of individual clinicians and even clinical teams to clinical decisions and decision-making processes.

In addition, the role and knowledge base of health professionals were defined primarily by professional associations. Nurses who practiced in hospitals and other highly structured organizations were more greatly influenced by organizational mandates (which conflicted with independent functioning) than were nurses in other settings. IT provides professionals the capacity to focus on complex processes and to integrate their roles to provide superior outcomes. IT enables professionals to design macro clinical processes, and IT provides decision support in the form of clinical protocols that are based on redesigned structures. Organizations must change according to the complexity and dynamics of these new structures.

The electronic information age has fundamentally changed how information is stored, processed, retrieved, and applied. If information systems are designed to serve the logic of IT or for the purpose of administrative efficiency, professionals have a right and an obligation to resist that change. The health professions also have the social obligation to recognize, accommodate, and lead the application of IT, which has considerable capacity to transform work processes and thus the traditional health professional role. IT and organization leaders must understand the privileged role of the health professions and structure systems that support that society-approved role. An example might include allowing a physician to accommodate variation in individual patient conditions and, to a degree, the personal preference of the clinician. Organizations are designed to control the terms, conditions, and content of the jobs they wish done, a structure that is inconsistent with the assumptions of the professional role. On the other hand, the health professions must recognize the value of information and knowledge embedded within systems and use them as the basis for clinical decision making. Physicians, nurses, and all other health professionals must understand the power of IT and must work as integrated teams. This, in turn, requires these professionals to fundamentally redesign the structure of their traditional roles. Such a redesign will be carried out within organized environments. When professionals resist changes merely to protect their roles, they violate their social obligation and their rights as individual professionals and as a profession in general (Currie, Finn, and Martin 2010).

The information age enables, and one might say requires, changes in how the professions function, but it does not decrease the responsibility or even autonomy of the professions in society. One such role change is that health professionals will be more integrated, working together in more structured areas in the organization. One potential advantage of the increased role of the medical profession in organizations is the increased professionalization of other workers and of the organizations themselves (Muzio and Kirkpatrick 2011). Thus, healthcare institutions could, and probably must, take on some of the qualities of the professions and in so doing transform their values, culture, and structure.

Redesigning Work Processes and Traditional Views

IT is, by nature, transformational. That means it changes not only the traditional roles of health professionals but also the structures and functions of healthcare organizations. Traditional organization structures and functions are as outdated as the roles of professionals. Leaders must work together to redesign work processes according to the clinical function and not on the basis of administrative logic inherent in functionally structured organizations. Meanwhile, physicians, nurses, and other clinicians can no longer do their jobs outside of **organized environments** (i.e., formal organizations with structure, purpose, and integrated functions), which are accountable for clinical outcomes and for structuring clinical processes.

Working together requires flexible and adaptive systems that are "less bounded" but not "boundaryless" (Friedson 2001). Such a system operates with a level of standardization—of both the clinical process and the clinical outcomes. Standardization is an inherent condition of structured work processes and is a departure from the independent or autonomous role of medical professionals. Clinical decisions are structured around clinical work processes that include the range of health professionals who have knowledge relevant to a treatment process. Leadership is shared and provided by the profession with the dominant knowledge of the case at a point in time, not by the traditional hegemony of the physician. Such approaches are evidence based, drawing on systems engineering, behavioral, and social sciences (Brown and Stone 2005). Later in the chapter we explore how clinical work might be structured within organizations, which in turn must acknowledge and respect professional roles.

Organizations and their leaders must dramatically change their view of the business function, including finance. Although still essential, the dominant structure of the organization must be designed based on the clinical function, not the other way around. Such a change in perspective requires a realignment of the values, goals, and ways of thinking by leaders as well as the redesign of the organization. If health organizations have a direct responsibility for clinical processes and outcomes, they must become a moral enterprise, taking on the values and deliberations represented by the health professions. Organizations that think like this are filled with leaders who have transitioned from "managing organizations to governing communities" (Selznick 1992, 237). In other words, the managerial role as well as the professional role are transformed in the information age.

The Structure of the Clinical Decision-Making Process

IT has considerable potential for informing clinical decision making and improving clinical outcomes (Morris 2002). Many studies of evidence-based clinical decision making have questioned this assumption, but these studies must be carefully reviewed to fully understand the measures and methods used. Horn (2006) correctly cites that the structure of the clinical process is complex and the metrics from randomized clinical trials reflect only an element of this process.

The health system has always been committed to quality and efficiency, and a number of factors (including the following) have coalesced to heighten the interest in quality and efficiency in the United States (Smith and Peck 2010):

- Increased public funding of health services demands greater accountability for quality and efficiency.
- Changing demographics (e.g., older) has dramatically increased the level of chronic care in a system that is still acute care oriented.
- Continuing advances in clinical technology enables the understanding and treatment of more complex diseases.
- Determining the sequence of chemical base pairs in the human genome project is expected to have major repercussions in the future.

In addition, patient values and patient expectations of better quality and continuity of care have changed. Perhaps the most dramatic change, however, is the explosion in information technology and its potential for (1) creating and analyzing large databases; (2) informing clinical decisions, including reporting relationships between clinical decisions and outcomes; and (3) informing customers, including patients and insurance companies.

IT has spawned an immense volume of decision support research and guidelines, but these come without sufficient explanation of the clinical decision-making process and how that process can be improved by IT. Most studies conduct "black-box testing," assuming the decision-making process and testing the impact of a decision support tool according to change in a clinical outcome. Little reporting has been done on the structure of the decision-making process and how decision support tools are designed to achieve the intended change in process (Kaplan 2001).

It is necessary to understand how physicians, nurses, and other health professionals make decisions individually and collectively and how they incorporate evidence into their decision-making process. Changes in clinical decision support systems should be based primarily on evidence-based improvement in clinical outcomes with sensitivity to acceptance and use by clinicians. Acceptance is a necessary but not a sufficient condition if the goal is to change the decision-making process (Ilie et al. 2009). Improvement must be viewed from the perspective of not only the incremental boost in outcomes but also the optimal results of transformational change.

To achieve superior outcomes, organization leaders must understand the science underpinning micro and macro clinical decision-making processes and the methods of designing decision support systems in a way that changes some essential elements but preserves others. **Clinical decision support system** (CDSS)—computer software that presents users with a knowledge base, patient-specific data, and related information at the point of care to enhance healthcare provision and management—includes not only **clinical guidelines** and **clinical protocols** but also the organization's structure, culture, and reward systems.

The Micro Clinical Decision-Making Process

The first structure of clinical decision making is the *micro process*, which involves an individual decision maker. The micro process is characterized by the clinical encounter, where one patient interacts with one clinician or one practice, is treated, exits the system, and returns to a state of health. The micro process serves the traditional role of physicians and other health professionals in acute care settings. These traditional roles were designed for maximum decision autonomy, and some degree of professional autonomy should be protected for the clinician to achieve superior outcomes. That degree of autonomy, however, should be dictated by clinical processes and outcomes, not by public policy mandates, organization rules, or professionals protecting their markets or their independence. Decisions that maximize autonomy to benefit the professionals are understandable but do not support the goal of achieving optimal patient and social benefit.

CDSS is a tool that can change the micro process. Although this system maintains and reinforces the structure of the clinical encounter, it is designed to change the decision behavior of individual health professionals. Clinical decision making is based on good scientific evidence and thus is a natural process for clinicians, who are trained in medical and nursing schools to draw from the best evidence. The gold standard of clinical decisions is evidence derived from closed clinical trials and sound statistical analysis. Typically, the evidence and recommendations presented by the CDSS to inform or guide clinical decisions are accompanied by statements of the level of research support (AHRQ 2012). The intent of a CDSS is to offer the best available evidence at the point of clinical encounter, and that evidence is generated by seasoned researchers in respected health centers.

Sound arguments can be made to support the use of clinical guidelines (Farand and Arocha 2004). The effectiveness of applying evidence-based clinical guidelines has been questioned by a number of researchers, who argue that there is a difference between evidence-based medicine and evidence-based practice. Duggal and Menkes (2011, 639) state that evidence-based medicine is defined as "the conscientious and judicious use of current best evidence from clinical care research in the management of individual patients." They draw on the work of Sackett and colleagues (1996), who recommend that research-derived evidence must be combined with clinical expertise to arrive at evidence-based practice. Evidence-based practice, in turn, derives information from both clinical research and medical practice

PROFESSIONAL VERSUS INDIVIDUAL AUTONOMY

Note that a difference exists between professional and individual autonomy. Professional autonomy is the freedom of the profession (as opposed to policymakers, boards of directors, financial managers, and other organizational mandates) to derive evidence and develop guidelines and protocols to be used by professionals in a specific field. Individual autonomy, on the other hand, is the freedom of the individual professional to use or follow the guidelines. The issue here is degree; at one extreme, an individual professional has discretion to deviate from the guideline if an individual patient condition merits that deviation. At the other extreme, a physician has the discretion not to use clinical guidelines and protocols in his or her practice.

(Sackett et al. 1996). This concept considers factors such as expert opinion, patient experience, clinician experience, and peer review. Duggle and Menkes do not include the organization as a factor of evidence-based practice, but the organization is an important variable in evidence-based practice (see Chapter 7).

The Institute of Medicine's report *To Err Is Human* notes that 15 years elapsed between the time professional associations accepted the idea that clinical decisions must be supported by good science and the time that idea was widely applied within the health professions (Kohn, Corrigan, and Donaldson 2000). A strong support for electronic information systems is that such technological capability could have reduced this time frame from 15 years to several months or even days, enabling organizations and clinicians to enhance clinical performance earlier. *To Err Is Human* also cites the power of electronic information systems to bring information and evidence to guide clinical decisions. Clinicians have countered with valid arguments that clinical guidelines frequently become absolute standards, reinforced by external financing agencies and healthcare organizations, that do not recognize the need for variability in clinical decisions as a result of variability in patient conditions and treatment desires or preferences. This inflexibility is a failure of organizations and regulating agencies.

Embedding clinical guidelines into the EHR requires standardization of clinical outcomes and decision processes. Standardization and formalization increase the level of institutionalization of the clinical process and alter the traditional concept of professional autonomy. This loss of decision-making autonomy has been met with resistance by the health professions. Some loss of individual autonomy, however, does not necessarily mean loss of professional autonomy.

Health professionals who retain individual autonomy in making clinical decisions and coordinating the clinical function go against the transforming power of information technology and the demands of their patients. Information systems (e.g., CDSS) bring accumulated scientific and experiential knowledge, including collegial consultation, to the point of clinical decision making. Collegial consultation entails the sharing of information among all professionals involved in a case. This decision-making structure transforms professionals from individual and independent agents to members of an integrated, corporate work unit. "Corporate" here does not mean finance or business. In this context, it refers to the working together of various individuals, which IT not only makes possible but also assumes, within organized environments (Muzio and Kirkpatrick 2011). The coming of the corporation is discussed in Chapter 7, but suffice to say here that clinicians are needed to lead the organization's movement to evidence-based decision making. To fulfill that role, clinicians must gain a good understanding of organization and systems design and behavior and the transforming power of IT.

Interactions within the micro process have received much attention in recent years, as medicine, nursing, and other health professions have increasingly focused on patient-centered care (Hudon et al. 2011; Frampton and Guastello 2010; Enes 2011; Kaba and Sooriakumaran 2007). This care entails, among other things, communicating with patients; showing empathy and compassion; and being willing to consider the broader social and psychological factors that could affect a patient's illness, diagnosis, and treatment. In a micro process, the patient is the center of the clinical decision—but only for a specific encounter within the setting of that encounter. When the patient gets treatment from multiple health professionals, goes to other doctor offices or organizations, or sees the same primary clinician over time, the clinical decision making becomes a macro process. That is, all the people (including the patient and family) and settings involved in providing health-care services work together and interdependently to make clinical decisions.

The Macro Clinical Decision-Making Process

The *macro process* is a systems view of clinical decision making. It involves all health professionals, health institutions, and patients and families in the entire clinical process. The chronic care clinical process, the primary application of the macro process, frequently transcends social sectors, which involves social work, education, housing, and many other services. The macro perspective views the design of work processes by health organizations and professionals as a complex adaptive system. **Complex adaptive system** is an organization with a large number of interdependent parts or agents that have their own schemata (pattern relationships), present interaction complexity, and are self-organizing but can adapt to their environments and help create those environments (coevolution) (Tan, Wen, and Awad 2005; Bergeson and Dean 2006). Such organizations are different from traditional organization and management models, which have stated missions, goals, authority structures, structured work processes, and bureaucratic rules and regulations. Complex adaptive systems comprise many interconnected components that work together to adapt to and match the complexity of the environment. Such assumptions are consistent with patient care and the role of health professions in a system.

Often, clinical processes go beyond a single encounter and can be characterized by a patient with a comorbidity and thus visits many health professionals for treatment over a span of time. This patient makes repeat visits and receives care or services from multiple clinicians, institutions, and offices. A chronic illness such as Type 2 diabetes, for example, might require the patient to see a primary care physician, endocrinologist, ophthalmologist, nutritionist, and social worker, each of whom is located in a different office. Those afflicted with a chronic illness might never return to a state of complete wellness, and thus they need to be involved in managing their health rather than simply be compliant with doctor orders and recommendations. Chronic care is rapidly increasing in many countries as their populations age, in part because of better management of acute conditions through early detection and more effective therapeutic interventions.

From a systems standpoint, even short-term or acute illness (which typically is treated as a micro process) requires a macro process because the patient who gets better still needs preventive and maintenance services and thus should not exit the healthcare system. Good health is a chronic condition itself and should be the main focus of an effective health provider. Managing chronic good health is complex and more challenging to health professionals and organizations than clinical encounters related to treating a disease or illness. For good-health clinical processes, the traditional professional role (micro)—functioning as an independent decision maker—may not be the most effective. In contrast, a systems or macro process—decision making involving all the actors over a period and across geographic areas—is more appropriate to ensure coordination of care, communication among multiple professionals, access to services, evidence-based practice, information sharing, and so on. IT that goes beyond automating processes (or is transformative) enables both the clinical process and the clinical outcomes because it overcomes the time, space, and profession boundaries inherent in the treatment of chronic conditions.

Chronic care services have not been well integrated and have been difficult to coordinate, but IT has been changing that. Integrating and coordinating activities over time, territory, and technology are core qualities of information systems (Charns and Young 2010). Health informatics enables health organizations and professionals to structure the clinical decision-making process around patients, transcending individual professionals and organizations to provide continuity and avoid duplication and gaps. This macro view, which also includes the patient as co-producer of care, is structured to enhance the entire care delivery process. It addresses the errors that occur during handoffs from one individual or organization to another, the inefficiencies of duplication of tests and services, and the gaps as a result of breakdowns in clinical processes. As chronic illness and emphasis on chronic good health grow, so will the importance and expectation of managing the entire clinical process with the macro approach.

The reengineering of clinical processes and decision-making behavior must draw on an understanding of the role of professionals, organizations as complex adaptive systems, and the transforming power of information technology. IT can become the superstructure that supports the management of clinical processes. This superstructure, however, must be based on the science of clinical decision making, not on traditional professional practices or roles that focus on the individual rather than the system and that use IT to automate rather than transform. This science anchors the design and provides the evidence for clinical processes.

The Science of Clinical Decision Making

IOM reports and other research have found considerable variation in clinical decision-making behavior and outcomes, including how scientific evidence informs the decision process (Kaplan and Frosch 2005). Examining what knowledge is and how it is acquired, transmitted, and applied in decision making is an age-old philosophical pursuit (Geisler and Wickramasinghe 2009). While no consensus has been reached on how knowledge is acquired, transmitted, and used, enough information about this topic is available to guide the development of decision support systems. Some scholars have critically addressed this important area of inquiry, but further work is needed (Lemieux-Charles and Champagne 2004). Here, we present the existing assumptions about the science of clinical decision making; then later, we address the art of clinical decision making and how it can be informed by experiential knowledge.

Arguments for Using Science-based Guidelines

The application of science to clinical decision making raises two questions: (1) how are clinical decisions made? and (2) how is clinical evidence used to improve the process? Decision making draws on cognitive sciences, which recognize multiple perspectives depending on the nature of the decision being made and the decision maker's level of expertise. Highly complex decisions made by highly trained domain experts draw from the science of expert reasoning. Decisions made by those without a high level of expertise or those who make routine decisions draw from the science of probability theory (Farand and Arocha 2004; Geisler and Wickramasinghe 2009).

Expert reasoning defines knowledge as learning how to compose increasingly complex concepts, an exercise that results in a higher level of expertise. This category of decision makers includes clinicians in academic medical centers who conduct clinical trials. *Probabilistic reasoning*, on the other hand, examines decision models that are data driven and believes that decisions are improved by the introduction of decision support, such as clinical guidelines and protocols (Cohen and Neumann 2008). Another scientific base of clinical decision making is the actor–network theory (Greenhalgh and Stones 2010). This theory focuses on the complex process of individual decision making (actor) within the total milieu (network) in which decisions are made and examines the contribution of team members and the total setting to the decision. *Actor–network theory* is particularly important for understanding decision making within communities of practice (examined later in this chapter).

Another perspective that must be considered, although it is focused on *ex post facto* decision making, is accountability for clinical decisions and outcomes. Under accountable decision making, clinical evidence is used as the basis for evaluating the effectiveness and efficiency of clinical decisions as well as a prompt to improve the decision process. The evaluation function has gained importance in the United States because increasingly the payment for services is made from public funds, although this is also of interest to private payers. Such an accountability mechanism might seem intrusive to expert clinicians whose practices represent the highest levels of clinical practice, but institutional and social accountability is not a selective process that distinguishes between experts and novices. For clinicians who are unaware that their skills do not reflect the best scientific knowledge or those who choose not to improve, such an accountability mechanism can be justified.

Clinicians are trained to draw scientific knowledge from laboratory findings and clinical trials to support their clinical decisions. As new scientific findings are generated, they are distributed, interpreted, selected, and applied. Using evidence in decision making is based on empirical approaches to decision support. For example, Grant and colleagues (2004) describe various decision support systems on the basis of concepts such as Bayesian reasoning and fuzzy sets and describe the application of computers to calculate probabilities on the basis of observations of patient-specific parameters. Such approaches draw on the traditional strength of computers to gather, analyze, and report information from large data sets. The question is how consistent this logic is with the structure of the clinical decision-making process and how this information actually improves decisions. Few would argue that the traditional approach of waiting many years to put evidence-based clinical decisions into general practice is not an acceptable standard. According to probabilistic reasoning, bringing the accumulated body of scientific knowledge to practicing clinicians is logical for decision support systems, and it demonstrates the power of electronic information systems.

Health informatics has enhanced the use of scientific information as the basis of evidence in clinical decisions. In fact, accessing and displaying clinical evidence serves as the primary logic of the design of CDSSs. Probabilistic reasoning draws on the power of computers to gather and analyze large data sets and is a logical response to the increasing interest to improve clinical outcomes and provide greater accountability of health systems. Using scientific information as a basis of clinical guidelines and protocols is logical from the perspective of basic scientists, information scientists, and policymakers, but it might engender faulty assumptions about how clinicians make decisions. Probabilistic reasoning should be viewed as one form of examining and using evidence but not as the sole logic that underpins the entire decision-making process. To do so would make complex clinical decision processes mechanistic, which is inappropriate for most but not all clinical decision contexts.

Does using scientific information actually improve clinical outcomes? Study findings report that clinical guidelines (based on scientific evidence) result in outcomes improvements, although the types and quality of guidelines frequently make generalizations difficult (Latoszek-Berendsen et al. 2010; Hoomans et al. 2011). Studies of the effect of clinical guidelines tend to focus on specific specialties and diseases and caution against overgeneralization. Much attention also has been given to the quality of evidence reported in the guidelines, physician acceptance of such evidence, and its effect on quality (Tricoci et al. 2009; Alonso-Coello et al. 2010). In addition, decision support tools have focused heavily on decision making by physicians and, to a lesser extent, by nurses and other health professionals. Overall, research consistently shows the positive relationship between the use of decision support tools and improved clinical outcomes.

Are these outcomes improvements incremental or optimal? Most studies report on improved clinical outcomes as a result of incremental change to use better information to support the decisions, but they do not address changes in the structure of the clinical process itself. Few studies explore the transformation to macro clinical process. Such studies would require drawing on the science of dynamic systems, which deals with organizational structure, behavior, and culture, and developing a set of conceptual and computational tools to explore new approaches to modeling nonlinear interactions among health professionals. Optimization modeling is explored in greater depth in Chapter 9.

Clinical guidelines tend to be developed by a clinical specialty and thus might not be accepted by other specialties; this raises the question of the nature and level of the science presented as evidence. The science might be designed to support a preconceived assumption about what services should be delivered by what specialties. Guidelines based on the best science should be developed by multidisciplinary teams and thus should be independent from government, industry, and special interest. Guidelines developed by multispecialty teams are based on a systems view (actor–network theory) oriented on the macro process. The ongoing argument is that guidelines based on good science have universal application when adjusted to fit local values and capability. As in industry, the science and technology of organizing and efficiently delivering high quality and personalized healthcare and medical services could reach a global market (this is explored further in Chapter 14). Future research is needed, however, to refine the understanding of the design and management of integrated health systems that produce exceptional levels of clinical quality and efficiency.

Cautions on Using Science-based Guidelines

Failure to use probabilistic reasoning–based guidelines might be due to the absence of recognized guidelines founded on sound, multivariate statistical analyses in a specific clinical area. Resistance to using guidelines might also result from the manner in which the guidelines are presented (e.g., computer–user interface) or the nature of the clinical decision being made. The operative question is how information is represented with regard to data aggregation, data relationships and trends, information display, processing speed, and the relationship between the level of science that supports findings and its acceptance by health professionals (Balas et al. 1996).

While decision makers share common traits, they vary by profession, specialty, practice principles, and so on. The challenge then for information systems is to be adaptable to the variations related to or affecting clinical outcomes. Decision support systems structured around the logic of IT and not the clinical decision process are flawed and have limited effectiveness. As stated in Chapter 3, with a vendor-supplied EMR system, you do not get to choose everything about how the system is going to work; rather, the system determines how you are going to work. This requires a fundamental understanding of electronic systems and their capability to adapt to, dictate, or transform the structure of the clinical decision-making process. When physicians' performance is measured by their compliance with prescribed metrics, the organization might select metrics that support an existing decision process. This approach has the effect of moving the target to catch the arrows.

Failure to use evidence-based decision guidelines could lead to the organization's enforcement of rules-based decision guidelines. The assumption behind these decision rules is that clinical decisions are mechanistic and thus institutionalize the decision process on the basis of distorted scientific evidence. Such attempts are likely to be resisted by clinicians. The danger here is that organizations and policymakers will turn probabilistic decision tools into decision rules reinforced by financial or some other punitive measures. Legislative mandates might be based on a similar assumption, establishing incentives that are based on selected decision rules. The Patient Protection and Affordable Care Act (ACA) of 2010 (Public Law 111-148) and the rules for implementing it take on many prescriptive elements (US Congress 2010).

There are several explanations for why clinicians do not generally use decision support systems. However, resistance to accepting probabilistic reasoning—because of clinicians' reluctance to use electronic information systems or their assumption that decision tools intrude on the clinical decision-making process or that they are inconsistent with the personal utility function of clinicians—cannot be justified in an accountable health system.

Experiential Knowledge and Clinical Decision Making

Researchers argue that clinical decision making is not only a science but also an art, with the art component derived from experience and human reasoning (Geisler and Wickramasinghe 2009). A person's experience in framing and making decisions draws on his own intuition, rules of thumb, heuristics, and reminders (Farand and Arocha 2004). Because of the complexity, variability, and personal nature of clinical decision making, it is unclear to what degree individual autonomy influences these decisions, because the clinical sciences and the reporting of clinical evidence have not matured to the level of the "harder" sciences (Farand and Arocha 2004).

The art of clinical decision making is based on a structured decision-making process and the rigor of heuristic reasoning. *Heuristic reasoning* (a structured way of thinking, including introspection, conceptualization, and sudden insight, that leads to problem solving that is interrupted and discontinuous) is not fully consistent with mathematical representation and cannot be standardized. The empirical evidence that validates the concept and its contribution to clinical outcomes is limited, and the related studies available need further testing but do guide how and when heuristic reasoning is applied and how it incorporates clinical evidence. Support for heuristic decisions comes from introspection, assumptions about overt behavior, or simulations. Heuristics provides rigor to decisions that cannot or are not probabilistic or nonprogrammable. In this way, it reflects how clinicians make decisions and thus should be incorporated in the design of CDSSs (Grant et al. 2004).

Beyond the experiential knowledge that informs individual clinical decision making is the clinical milieu in which the decision-making process takes place. Actor–network theory, as mentioned, includes the entire clinical setting in developing clinical guidelines and protocols, emphasizing the tacit knowledge generated through group interaction. Considerations such as team composition and interaction, culture, information systems support, and the care setting all affect decision making and contribute to improved outcomes (Real 2010). As such, according to actor–network theory, the use of experiential knowledge balances the use of rules-based clinical guidelines. This is particularly true in that clinical guidelines are designed around the work of individual professions and specialties. More and more tests of naturalistic designs are available that present information about the network of care, including patients. (*Naturalistic design* is a research method that involves observing subjects in their natural environment. Such a design can serve several purposes, but here it refers to making observations without disrupting the behavior of the clinician or patient.) Thus, a need exists for clinical teams themselves to develop and apply guidelines based on the best available evidence and the collective knowledge and experience of the team. These team-designed guidelines can greatly contribute to improving the decision-making process. (Knowledge-based decision making is explored in Chapter 8.)

A Systems View of the Clinical Process

All IT interventions exact some form of change—whether cognitively, behaviorally, structurally, or all three. Behavioral change is sometimes reported in terms of whether or not professionals use a computer in some way in their practice (meaningful use), but such measures are of limited value in themselves. Using the computer as a data processor might represent a significant "behavior change" for clinicians but provides little meaning as a measure of change in the decision-making process, and by itself is spurious. As cognition increases, the easy assumption is that a corresponding change in decision making (which then leads to improved outcomes) would follow. The relationship among information use, increased cognition, behavior change, and improved outcomes underpins the "meaningful use" rubric of the ACA.

Human decision making is complex, and organizational leaders, IT specialists, and clinicians must have an appreciation for this complexity when considering evidence-based decision making and designing CDSSs. Simplistic assumptions do not make designing decision tools easy nor serve health informatics well. There is variability among the health professions, within any given specialty, and among individuals in clinical roles. Many CDSSs are based on a rationalist perspective that excludes contextual issues. These perspectives evolve from traditional values and practices, but they themselves pose limitations on the science that informs the clinical decision-making process.

The design of current decision support systems, in general, is based on a specific unit of analysis—for example, a clinic or hospital. When a patient is discharged from a hospital or referred to another provider, there is a need to continue the coordination of care through information exchange. In the past, information exchange was accomplished by fax or other paper transfers; today, it is increasingly done electronically by linking EMRs. In the future, patient information will likely be stored in a data vault or on the web using advanced storage technology. The structure of the information exchange will likely affect the level of cognition and/or change the behavior of those involved in the exchange, but it will not necessarily alter the unit of analysis. Typically, information exchange systems are assessed on their speed of transfer, data configuration, and security, but not their impact on clinical decision making. Simply, information exchange allows health professionals to gather information on patients from multiple institutions and, in so doing, can better inform a decision and potentially prevent duplicate tests. However, in itself information exchange does not fundamentally alter the structure of the macro clinical decision process.

To change behaviors and processes, the type of change desired must be defined first. The structure of the decision-making process can be viewed as a continuum—from getting clinicians to use the computer as a data processor, to changing their decision-making behaviors by embedding decision tools such as alerts and reminders, to making the clinical process as the unit of analysis. Decision making based on the structure of the clinical process includes determining which professionals should be involved, how they relate to each other, how evidence is introduced to inform their decisions, how clinical team members interact during the decision-making process, and what information is needed by the decision support. As one progresses along the continuum, the degree of structural change increases, which in turn requires more collective activity. Collective activity might include shared data systems, communications networks, clinical outcomes reporting, a reimbursement mechanism, and shared culture and values. These functions need corporate involvement, which might discourage many health professionals. To make this work, new corporate structures that use evidence-based clinical outcomes must be created, and experts in medicine, nursing, allied health, systems engineering, health informatics, and organization theory must be involved in this undertaking (Muzio and Kirkpatrick 2011). The unit of analysis might be an integrated team that transcends professions, clinics, and hospitals. Such a team might be conceptualized as a community of practice, a concept further developed in Chapters 7 and 8.

Changing the clinical decision-making process is inherently a systems campaign, requiring an understanding of clinical and IT sciences and their effects on user cognition and behavior. The transformation to a systems perspective changes the organization structure, its culture, clinical processes, and service financing.

Conclusion

The process by which physicians, nurses, and other health professionals make decisions raises important questions for organizations. Is the decision-making structure the same for all decisions and health professionals? Should the decision unit of analysis be the individual professional or the community of practice? How should professionals be structured and interact, and how does that level of interaction relate to outcomes, including clinical outcomes, patient involvement and satisfaction, and continuity of care? What evidence exists to support types of intervention processes? How does the degree of professional integration relate to clinical outcomes?

A rich and growing science provides evidence on clinical decisions and processes. This evidence can serve as a basis for designing clinical work processes and the architecture on which decision support systems are built. This science must be carefully examined. Healthcare organizations have a mission of providing clinical services but were structured (and most currently function) according to the logic of business, which is inconsistent with the tenets of the clinical function. Adopting a systems view of healthcare organizations does not imply changing the clinical perspective to fit the existing organization logic. Rather, new evidence from the science of both clinical decision making and information systems must be derived to support the restructuring of organizations. This interdisciplinary perspective will change the traditional assumptions of clinical decision making, organization design, and health informatics. Chapter 7 presents a framework for this integration. An information system designed on the logic of information technology (e.g., automating paper-based medical records) but lacking an understanding of clinical decision processes has limited potential; in many cases, such systems cannot justify the financial investment.

Regulating and rewarding the meaningful use of IT by physicians are appropriate, but that threshold for meaningful use is minimal. The effective use of IT likely cannot be realized from regulations and financial incentive programs. Health informatics must include the study of complex systems and its power to transform the structure of clinical decision-making processes into the macro perspective. If not, IT that is applied in the clinical areas has a limited purpose—that of automating instead of transforming.

Chapter Discussion Questions

1. Name the changes in roles of health professionals in the health field.
2. Why might evidence-based clinical practice expressed as clinical guidelines not achieve an optimal outcome?
3. What are dangers of institutionalizing clinical guidelines and protocols given the traditional structure of organizations?
4. If expert reasoning can be justified as a legitimate basis for clinical decision making, how can evidence-based solutions be justified?
5. Discuss the concept of community of practice as it relates to the structure of the clinical decision process.

Note

1. The dominant recognition and protection of individual perceptions and needs is not inherently true in all societies, such as those that have highly socialized and nationalized health systems (such as the United Kingdom) where the public good might override individual needs and expectations. To some degree this is true even in private, market-based systems (such as in the United States) where public funding might override some individual consumption desires. The assumption in pure market-based systems is that the public good should not override individual clinical needs, but that too might change. Such a change does not inherently negate the assumptions of market-driven health systems but should be purposeful and not inadvertent.

CASE STUDY   Developing a Rapid Response Team at University Hospital

Karen R. Cox

In 2008, The Joint Commission added rapid-response capability to its National Patient Safety Goals on the basis of evidence, although contradictory in nature, that rapid-response teams (RRTs) could reduce the incidence of cardiac arrest and pulmonary failure of patients on acute care floors. The Joint Commission initiative followed the Institute for Healthcare Improvement (IHI) 100,000 Lives Campaign, which set as one of its six quality-improvement measures the establishment of RRTs (IHI 2006).

RRT is a specialized trauma care unit considered as a key component of acute inpatient care. The RRT concept was created as a result of evidence that staff nurses' "failure to rescue" led to serious adverse events (Halvorsen et al. 2007). A serious adverse event may be defined as an unintended injury that results, in part, from delayed or incorrect medical management that exposes the patient to an increased risk of death or measurable disability (IHI 2006). RRTs, then, aim to improve the safety of a hospital-ward patient whose condition is deteriorating. In addition,

> [RRTs] are based on identification of patients at risk, early notification of an identified set of responders, rapid intervention by the response team, and ongoing evaluation of the system's performance and hospital-wide processes of care. (Halvorsen et al. 2007)

The Setting

The Center for Patient Safety (CPS) at University Hospital, a 450-bed teaching hospital that is part of the University of Missouri Health Care, is active in the IHI and gathers baseline data on the number of codes, hospital deaths due to respiratory or cardiac failure, and the level of patient deterioration. Through the Patient Safety Network (PSN) database developed by CPS, the hospital is able to provide the following baseline assessment.

The current response protocol is in effect for floor nurses, who became concerned about an acute deterioration of a patient. The nurses are instructed to first call the attending physician to seek advice on the course of action to take, but they report that the attending does not respond to calls; this results in the continued deterioration of the patient. The other recourse by nurses is to initiate a Code Blue, but they are reluctant to do so, particularly early in the episode. When a patient is "coded" but not in failure, the nurses frequently perceive or actually receive negative comments or sanctions from the code team. This information circulates to the charge nurse and other nursing staffs and is perceived as a question or doubt of the competence of the nurses involved. The comments further scatter throughout the PSN but do not constitute any statistically significant finding or even a basis for data; nonetheless, they are thought by the CPS team to be a coherent set of observations. The question now is whether CPS would go forward with such information as evidence for initiating an RRT or some other intervention.

Problem Identification

CPS is faced with the challenge of extracting existing knowledge embedded within the hospital to determine if the care process needs to be restructured and, if so, how to do that while still providing appropriate continuity. The acute inpatient setting is one of the most structured care environments, along with the intensive care unit (ICU) and surgical unit. By the time a patient lands in acute care, a diagnosis has been made, physician orders have been completed, and the care turns to a charge nurse and a nursing team. The physicians' orders might call for other clinicians, such as respiratory and physical therapists, but the care process here is highly structured with each health professional bringing his or her technical skills appropriate for the patient's condition. Some patient conditions, however, can deteriorate unexpectedly, which rapidly negates the highly structured process and existing treatment protocols.

CPS organizes an interdisciplinary planning team to gather recommendations on how the hospital might improve care for patients who exhibit early stages of distress. The planning team consists of a CPS representative, a hospitalist, two ICU nurses, and a senior respiratory therapist. Together, the team discusses these questions:

- Is there a problem, and what evidence exists to support that finding?
- What are the implications of initiating an RRT on the design of current clinical practice?
- What professional skills are needed on an RRT?

(continued)

- How should the RRT be structured?
- What conditions would warrant calling the RRT?
- How would the RRT differ from the current code team?
- How many calls might the RRT expect per shift, and how long is an average response time?

The ICU nurses raise concern about how conditions could be identified and how informed responses could be made on patient care floors without the benefit of electronic monitoring devices and other information technology employed only in the ICU.

The Design

The first decision the interdisciplinary team addresses is the composition of the RRT. Considerable discussion time is spent on the membership of the RRT. The team wonders, "Does RRT composition make a difference, and what is the correct structure for the hospital?" Different institutions take different approaches, and the IHI identifies a range of RRT membership possibilities, such as the following:

The Best Structure for the RRT[1]
- ICU registered nurse (RN), respiratory therapist (RT), intensivist, or hospitalist
- ICU RN and RT
- ICU RN, RT, intensivist, and resident
- ICU RN, RT, and physician assistant
- Emergency department RN or ICU RN

The current code team at the hospital includes a hospitalist, an ICU RN, and an RT. How would the RRT differ from the code team in composition and response threshold? The hospitalist thinks he should be on the RRT, a position strongly supported by the medical staff, in case clinician orders need to be changed and because he has responsibility for the clinical quality in the institution. His concern is the frequency of RRT calls and the time demands of this additional responsibility. He favors the restrictive use of the RRT and developing response guidelines for floor nurses. In his discussions with the medical staff, he knows that the physicians stress that the protocol should require the attending physician be notified before the RRT is called. Meanwhile, one of the two ICU nurses favors an RRT that includes a senior critical care nurse to ensure the highest level of technical quality, a respiratory therapist, and a liberal call policy. She envisions the RRT as an extension of the ICU to the nursing floors. The tradeoffs of team composition seem to be the level of technical expertise versus how early the RRT should be called for a potential rescue.

The CPS representative supports having redundant membership (e.g., both critical care nurses and respiratory therapists) to ensure that the RRT is still able to fully respond even if one member is occupied. She recommends two critical care nurses and three respiratory therapists. She also suggests that selection of RRT members be based on their people skills and not only clinical competency. The rest of the interdisciplinary team view this as an interesting thought.

Guiding the team's decisions are other institutions' RRT structures as well as IHI's recommendations for early warning systems. Exhibits CS4.1 and CS4.2 are IHI guidelines for initiating an RRT response. The team knows that one significant asset it has is the availability of a standardized database (from the hospital's electronic medical record), which identifies diagnostic and treatment data on conditions preceding the crisis situation. Could these data be usable to prevent future failures to rescue and also calls on false-positive cases? The team is concerned about the lack of scientific evidence that serves as guidelines appropriate for comparable hospitals. The team then decides to develop a standard clinical protocol that the charge nurse could use to alert or inform the RRT about a patient's condition. The team also considers adopting the SBAR (Situation Background Assessment Recommendation) protocol to provide structured documentation for alerting members of the RRT about the patient's condition.

Exhibit CS4.1

- Staff member is worried about the patient
- Acute change in heart rate <40 or >130 bpm
- Acute change in systolic blood pressure <90 mmHg
- Acute change in respiratory rate <8 or >28 per min or threatened airway
- Acute change in saturation <90% despite O2
- Acute change in conscious state
- Acute change in urine output to <50 ml in 4 hours

Source: Reprinted with permission from *How to Guide. Getting Started Kit: Rapid Response Teams.* Cambridge, Massachusetts: Institute for Healthcare Improvement; 2009. (Available on www.IHI.org).

(continued)

Exhibit CS4.2

- Systolic blood pressure   <101   >200
- Respiratory rate   <9   >20
- Heart rate   <51   >110
- Saturation (room air)   <90%
- Urine output   <1ml/kg/2 hours
- Conscious level   Not fully alert

- If a patient fulfills <u>two or more</u> of the above criteria <u>OR</u> you are worried about his/her condition, page the resident from the admitting team and the Rapid Response Team.
- These two parties MUST review the patient <u>within thirty minutes.</u>

Source: Reprinted with permission from *How to Guide. Getting Started Kit: Rapid Response Teams.* Cambridge, Massachusetts: Institute for Healthcare Improvement; 2009. (Available on www.IHI.org).

The Implementation

Department directors are kept fully informed at executive meetings about the RRT planning and progress, and the information is repeated at various staff meetings. Senior managers want to make sure that everyone is informed.

At one meeting, the head of the ICU expresses a concern that with the liberal use of the RRT, the ICU nurse on the team might become overextended. Formal and informal meetings of staff nurses are much more animated. Much of their discussions include the subtle negative feelings that a code generates and the code team's feelings of resentment if the patient does not suffer a cardiac or respiratory arrest. The nurses announce that nursing directors caution them against calling external support as doing so reflects poorly on the nurses' performance reviews and could be used as a basis for the floor not receiving a number-1 rating.

One idea initiated by nursing is the development of guidelines that indicate when RRT alerts should be given and what protocols to follow before alerting the RRT or before the RRT's arrival. Such guidelines, along with briefings at shift changes, could support the team-nursing concept. One young clinical nurse specialist, a recent graduate, argues that with such guidelines even the patient's family could be included among those who are informed about identifying risks and who are enabled to initiate an RRT call. This suggestion is discouraged by members of the nursing staff who feel that families lack sufficient training to initiate such a response and that such actions need to be first reviewed by the clinical ethics committee.

Administrative management does not participate in the implementation discussion because "this is a clinical not an administrative issue" but does ask how much the RRT will cost and if the expense can be reimbursed. The IT department, meanwhile, is concerned about how to develop rapid-response guidelines for nurses within the existing EMR framework. Besides, IT's priority is currently focused on CPOE and on improving the human–computer interface in primary care. CPS thinks that a database on the rapid response by nurses and the RRT would be valuable. It could be mined (1) to see what combination of factors related to cardiac or pulmonary distress in hospitalized patients causes their conditions to rapidly deteriorate and (2) to generate alerts to staff nurses and attending physicians. Such an information system could monitor the clinical progress of patients and generate information on conditions related to potential distress. Staff also suggests that these data could be used to design a realistic simulation training program featuring the newly acquired medical mannequins.

Note
1. This list is reprinted with permission from *How to Guide. Getting Started Kit: Rapid Response Teams.* Cambridge, Massachusetts: Institute for Healthcare Improvement; 2009. (Available on www .IHI.org).

Case Study Discussion Questions

1. Why had hospitals not initiated an inquiry into the deaths of patients from respiratory or cardiac failure before the IHI initiative, given the level of clinical expertise and the institutional commitment to quality?
2. Critically assess the process of determining the composition of an RRT. What professional skills should be always present for any call? Should RRT members be selected based on their people skills or technical competency?
3. How does the RRT relate to the entire caregiving team at University Hospital? Based on the team caregiving concept, who would you include on an RRT for a given episode?

(continued)

4. Why do nurses call physicians when patients are in distress, and why do physicians frequently not respond? Why do nursing directors caution nurses against calling the code team?

5. Critically analyze the structure of communications to inform and enlist members of the nursing and other departments.

6. Give examples of the application of expert reasoning, probabilistic reasoning, and actor–network reasoning in this case. What are sources of knowledge, and how are they accumulated and used?

CLINICAL DECISION SUPPORT IN MEDICINE

Yang Gong

Learning Objectives

After reading this chapter, students should be able to

- Understand the impact of scientific evidence and its acceptance and use in clinical medical practice
- Learn to identify areas that might benefit from a decision support system, and evaluate the challenges surrounding developing and implementing such a system
- Discuss the human-centered approach in clinical decision support systems
- Develop a sufficient knowledge of decision support systems to make an intelligent purchase suitable to your company's needs from a decision support vendor

---

KEY CONCEPTS

- Clinical decision support systems
- Design, implementation, and maintenance
- Human factors in computer and decision support system use
- Understandability, usability, and functionality
- Human diagnostic reasoning

Introduction

The history of the clinical decision support system (CDSS) can be traced back to some of the earliest development of technology in medicine, including the 1890 US Census when punch cards were used to collect data (Shortliffe and Sondik 2006). From there, technology advanced into the business world, where decision support system was first developed for financial and strategic planning purposes. CDSS was not even mentioned as a possibility until the 1950s, when in 1959 a well-known seminal paper discussed reasoning foundations of medical diagnosis in terms of probability and logic (Ledley and Lusted 1959a; 1959b).

Health information technology is continuously evolving to aid the healthcare community in providing the highest quality and safest care. Quality and patient safety are important parts of healthcare that are becoming essential to an organization's success. Much of the potential value of electronic health record (EHR) systems comes from the CDSS components that assist clinicians in making care safer, more efficient, and more cost effective. Some examples are health maintenance reminders, drug–drug interaction checking, dose adjustment, and order sets (Wright et al. 2011).

Definition and Types of Clinical Decision Support Systems

Clinical decision support system can be defined as computer software that presents users with a knowledge base, patient-specific data, and related information at the point of care to enhance healthcare provision and management. Users of CDSSs are clinical decision makers, which refer not only to physicians and nurses but also pharmacists, medical technologists, and other health professionals. A CDSS is a valuable tool because it offers individualized or patient-specific recommendations and options for diagnosis, treatment, and medication. This capability, in turn, enhances healthcare quality, patient safety, and efficiency of care delivery. In addition, CDSS allows clinicians to access medical information in a timely manner. Other benefits of this tool include helping to reduce adverse drug events, such as drug–drug interactions and drug–allergy interactions (Wright and Sittig 2008), and to reduce the total charges per admission and overall hospital costs (Kinney 2003). Additional analysis is needed to realize the scope of benefits possible with CDSSs.

Although CDSSs are excellent tools for improving patient care, they are just that—tools. Humans are still in charge of interpreting the information presented and applying it to a given clinical encounter. Computers and information software are not decision makers and thus cannot override human decision and diagnosis. This is especially true in a clinical setting where organizational factors or clinical flow are outdated and/or not integrated into the decision support system. Thus, humans should always use the available CDSS information with discretion. Clinical decision makers must also keep in mind that CDSS is an assistive technology, offering reminders and alerts but relying on the clinicians themselves to act within the scope of their expertise.

CDSS comes in two types—knowledge-based or non–knowledge-based—and may be used for clinical intent, mechanisms of intervention, and methods of reasoning. **Knowledge-based CDSS** is loaded with and offers recommendations from a large body of expert and science-based information, including best practice and evidence-based medicine, and thus may be used for every clinical decision. A classic example of a knowledge-based CDSS is MYCIN, developed by Shortliffe in the 1970s (Shortliffe 1976). MYCIN is an expert system that uses **production rules** (e.g., IF some condition is true, THEN the following inference can be made or some action taken) to recommend appropriate therapy for patients with blood infections. However, MYCIN was used only in a research setting but not in real practice.

Non–knowledge-based CDSS is developed by learning from experiences of clinical decision makers and/or by finding patterns out of this learning to make recommendations. This type of CDSS functions as an artificial neural network (ANN), which is inspired by the way the biological nervous system processes information. ANN is an interesting approach that has been tested in the process of data mining and knowledge discovery. The principal tasks of ANN are to identify key features that are important for the classification or prediction of a problem and to determine the way in which these features should be combined to create an output variable representing the classification or prediction. At present, non–knowledge-based CDSS is used in an experimental way, and use of knowledge-based systems is more common.

Basic Components of Knowledge-based CDSS

Globally, healthcare organizations are striving to improve healthcare quality and patient safety. To achieve this goal, scientific discoveries and knowledge must be translated into practical applications. Basic scientists provide clinicians with new tools for patient care and for assessing these tools' impact, and clinical researchers make novel observations about the nature and progression of disease that often stimulate basic investigations. The medical knowledge should be translated from "bench" to "clinics," and then that information should be turned into a computerized format that presents the medical knowledge base. A **medical knowledge base** is a systematically organized collection of medical knowledge that is accessible electronically and interpretable by computer.

A knowledge-based CDSS typically has three components: knowledge base, inference engine, and communication mechanism or interface. The knowledge base contains the rules and associations of the compiled data. The **inference engine** combines the rules with patient-specific information. The **communication mechanism or interface** allows decision makers to see the computational results and supports data input through direct or indirect methods.

Challenges of CDSSs

CDSS is used for a range of purposes (from quality and safety to efficiency) and across multiple clinical domains (such as screening, diagnosis, and therapy). Despite its great potential, CDSS is not commonly used outside of a small group of mostly academic medical centers. According to Wright and Sittig (2008), one reason for this limited appeal is the relative difficulty of integrating CDSS into clinical workflows and computer systems. The CDSS component should be embedded in a larger health information system, which is already part of many health professionals' work practices. For example, in a knowledge-based nursing initiative (see Chapter 6 for the full discussion), logic for clinical alerts specialized to a particular problem (e.g., risk of falls) is added "behind the scenes" to clinical assessments that already are included in the information system. Clinical alerts and assessments have to be coordinated to fit into the workflow.

Some CDSSs suffer from the issues of human–computer interaction. Many enthusiastic users of CDSSs have found that some programs are cumbersome to access, slow to perform, and difficult to learn. Users are likely to be frustrated if the CDSS requires the manual reentry of information available in other computers or systems. An interoperable CDSS that helps reduce manual data entry is critical to user acceptance. In the early stages, most CDSSs were standalone and did not support data sharing with other systems. As the Internet becomes a pervasive tool in many service industries, CDSSs continue to evolve in sophistication, levels of integration, and user friendliness.

A small number of institutions have had great success with CDSSs, but that success has not been replicated in community settings (Wright and Sittig 2008). The need for "robust methods to identify, describe, evaluate, collect, catalog, synthesize and disseminate best practices for CDSS design, development, implementation, maintenance, and evaluation" is one of the challenges that faces clinical decision support. As a core component of CDSS, diagnostic decision support software enhances the performance of many image and signal devices in narrowly defined clinical domains (e.g., automated arterial blood gas interpretation, protein electrophoresis reports, automated differential blood cell counters, electrocardiograms [EKGs]).

As mentioned, CDSS is just a tool that leaves the interpretation and application tasks to humans decision makers. These clinicians take the information from the CDSS and combine it with information they have gathered from a patient encounter, fit the information into their clinical workflow, and apply all this knowledge to the situation at hand. In the foreseeable future, CDSSs cannot supplant but can enhance human decision makers (Berner 2007).

Design and Implementation Challenges: Human Factors

CDSS is designed to assist clinicians within the scope of their expertise. It can be used for clinical intent (e.g., diagnosis, therapy, prevention), mechanisms of intervention (e.g., alerts, reminders, critiquing), and methods of reasoning (e.g., probabilistic, forward chaining, backward chaining, rule based, case based). When used effectively, the system can increase efficiency and decrease medical errors (Sittig et al. 2008, 3020).

Many human factors are involved in CDSSs. These factors come into play in three phases: development, implementation, and utilization. During CDSS development, factors such as the gap between developers and end users can affect the outcomes. For example, users' expectation may be different from the system's capability. Understanding users' information needs and cognitive characteristics is essential in designing a human-centered information system (Gong and Zhang 2005). A human-centered theoretical framework called TURF (task, user, representation, and function) has been proposed for the design and evaluation of a CDSS (Zhang and Walji 2011).

Human factors during implementation can hinder a system from being used to its full potential, and there might not be an optimal solution for all of them. Training, however, is deemed essential for preventing user confusion and unrealistic expectations and for facilitating implementation and user acceptance. Reluctance to change, lack of incentives, and administrative burdens should be minimized during implementation.

Even after implementation, utilization and usability issues can still limit the effectiveness and efficiency of a CDSS. Sometimes clinicians do not trust the system and thus do not trust its outcome. In response, the organization should assign a physician champion to promote the benefits of a CDSS. Other times clinicians find that the information is difficult to access (Trivedi et al. 2009). In such a case, human-centered design should be further reinforced, highlighting the features that make utilization and access as unencumbered as possible. Alert fatigue also can affect physician usage; clinicians tend to ignore too many alerts (Grizzle et al. 2007). Human-factors researchers indicate that involving clinicians in usability studies at all stages of the CDSS development is critical. Seeking frontline-users' feedback contributes to successful system utilization and compliance, particularly because the system changes the users' existing decision process.

Free Text Technology

Free text is a method of entering or reporting data and information into the CDSS using natural language. In contrast to predefined menus or drop-down lists, free text does not allow the computer to automatically extract properties and relationships for the data found in the EHR. According to Sittig and colleagues (2008), 50 percent of the information entered by a clinician about a patient's health condition is done in free text, and the use of free text to drive clinical decision support is one of the top-ten challenges in CDSS design and development. Among the data and information entered into the system in free text are x-ray reports, discharge summaries, clinician notes, medical history, physical examination, and sign-out notes (Demner-Fushman, Chapman, and McDonald 2009).

Several technologies are used to manage free text within a CDSS, and these technologies come in two types: natural language processing (NLP) and artificial intelligence (AI). Each has programs that serve a multitude of purposes. In general, NLP converts information from an unstructured into a structured format. MedLEE is an example of an NLP that captures data from narratives and then creates structured reports for further computing process (Bakken et al. 2004). AI, on the other hand, is a cognitive model that relies on human reasoning, which proves to be useful in non–knowledge-based CDSS. One example is Project ISABEL, an AI inference engine. Project ISABEL extracts from and structures information for medical textbooks, and the program generates diagnostic reminders from this knowledge base in response to the unstructured or free-text clinical information (Suntharalingam et al. 2005).

Interoperability

One of the challenges in health information technology today is the integration and interoperability of provider and organizational systems, including EHR, CPOE, and CDSS. Interoperability focuses on linking all providers to the same patient information to enable better decisions and increase patient safety and quality. Fragmentation of patient information can cause medical and administrative errors and miscommunications.

Computerized physician-order entry (CPOE) enables clinicians to electronically enter orders for inpatients' treatment. These orders are then transmitted through computers to the clinical staff or to the relevant departments, such as the pharmacy and/or laboratory, for fulfillment. CPOE provides real-time clinical decision support, such as dosage and alternative medication suggestions, duplicate therapy warnings, and drug–drug and drug–allergy interaction checking. CPOE is replacing the conventional methods of order entry, enabling clinicians to immediately send, receive, and respond to analytical and treatment-specific requests. Benefits of CPOE include decreased delay in order completion, reduced errors related to handwriting or transcription, order entry at the point of care or off-site, error-checking for duplicate or incorrect doses or tests, and simplified inventory and posting of charges.

Interoperability among EHR, CPOE, and CDSS delivers many advantages, including more reliable and timely information about a patient's health status, fewer errors, increased public reporting, and availability of alternate or backup systems in case of a system failure. To realize these benefits, however, healthcare organizations must settle interoperability issues, including standardizing computer languages and system designs. Despite institution's efforts to develop and implement CDSS, widespread adoption and acceptance has still not been achieved. A large roadblock to acceptance is workflow integration. A viable CDSS has to cover all aspects of clinical tasks within complex workflows. If a CDSS is not properly integrated, users have to take extra steps to gather needed information, which causes disruptions and frustrations.

CDSS Application to Medical Domains

Before CDSS development occurs, developers should assess the information needs in a specific medical domain. A medical domain generally refers to structured knowledge within a specified diagnostic category, using a common language classification, such as the Unified Medical Language System or UMLS. Medical domains provide clinicians a common classification for expressing diagnoses and related clinical interventions. As discussed in Chapter 2, medicine lacked the development of a classification language for expressing the elements of diagnosis, treatments, and outcomes corresponding to the rapid development of computer-processing capacity. Domain knowledge is structured by and around medical specialties, which leads to acceptance by the profession but contributes to the difficulty of developing a common language system. A patient with multiple problems, in effect, exists in multiple medical domains (considered as abstract constructs to simplify how we think about objectives of practice). Each of these domains corresponds to a discipline, hence the need for interdisciplinary teams to care for the patient.

Understanding the three kinds of information needs is essential to the process of selecting a domain (Osheroff et al. 1991):

1. *Currently satisfied information needs:* information recognized and known by the decision maker as relevant to the problem
2. *Consciously recognized information needs:* information recognized yet not known by the decision maker as necessary to solve the problem
3. *Unrecognized information needs:* information necessary to solve the problem yet not recognized as important by the decision maker

Each domain has unique information needs, and its clinicians may have different kinds of information needs. Thus, domain selection must be a thoughtful exercise (not done simply to test a computer algorithm) to ensure that the resulting CDSS is worth everyone's time.

Clinical-Domain CDSS Examples

This section discusses some CDSSs used routinely in the clinical setting or that laid the groundwork for modern systems. Developed for narrowly defined clinical domains, such as diagnosing acute abdominal pain and interpreting acid-base disorders, these CDSSs include AAPHelp, MYCIN, DxPlain, ABEL, GermWatcher, and ISABEL.

AAPHelp

Acute abdominal pain (AAP) is the United Kingdom's most common surgical emergency. Appendectomy, specifically, is the most common abdominal emergency operation. Diagnosis of AAP, particularly in the early stages of presentation, is difficult, and only around 50 percent of people who come to the hospital with AAP are correctly diagnosed (AAPHelp 2011). This leads to unnecessary admissions, investigations, and interventions. The negative appendectomy rate is still between 20 and 30 percent and as high as 50 percent in young women (AAPHelp 2011).

AAPHelp is based on clinical evidence and best practice from the United Kingdom and Europe. This CDSS contains information collected for 15 years from more than 100 UK and European hospitals that treated patients with AAP (Horrocks et al. 1972). Developed in the early 1970s by Professor Tim de Dombal, AAPHelp is used to support clinical assessment and decision making and as a tool in clinical practice and education.

Clinical assessment is critical for AAP. When a new patient's medical history is entered into the electronic clinical-assessment protocol, the relevant database is automatically selected. A Bayesian statistical analysis is carried out, comparing the new patient's history with the information in the database. This, in turn, generates a probability of the most likely diagnosis. This probability is then used to identify patients in the database with a similar clinical presentation as the new patient.

MYCIN

MYCIN is an artificial intelligence (AI) program developed by Edward Shortliffe in early 1976 at Stanford University. It is written in LISP programming language, a widely used language in AI applications. The name MYCIN is derived from the common suffix of many antibiotics (e.g., Gentamycin, Erythromycin, Vancomycin). MYCIN is a backward-chaining, rule-based decision support system designed primarily to identify bacterial infections and to recommend antibiotics dosage according to patient's body weight. MYCIN consists of three subcomponents: consultation system, explanation system, and rule-acquisition system. As a consultation system, MYCIN asks questions, draws conclusions, and gives advice. The explanation system translates rules to English before the information is displayed. The rule-acquisition/modification system allows domain experts to enter and change rules. MYCIN had about 200 rules in 1976 (Shortliffe 1976).

DxPlain

DxPlain is a decision support system developed in 1984 in the Laboratory of Computer Science at Massachusetts General Hospital and acts as both an electronic medical textbook and a medical reference system. DxPlain uses a modified form of Bayesian logic and, through an interactive collection of clinical information from the user, is able to provide clinical interpretations. In its original version, DxPlain contained information on approximately 500 diseases. In 1987, DxPlain was distributed nationally through a dial-up network and provided information on nearly 2,000 diseases (Barnett et al. 1987). A standalone version was used in the mid-1990s. The advent of the Internet brought DxPlain to the web; the web-based version has replaced all other versions.

Currently, DxPlain offers information on more than 2,400 diseases and more than 5,000 clinical findings and averages 53 findings per disease description. To further enhance the utility of DxPlain, each disease-finding pair has two associated numbers; the frequency-specific findings occur in the disease and probability that a finding suggests the disease. Finally, DxPlain provides the user with a "crude approximation" of the disease prevalence (very common, common, rare, or very rare) as well as a ranking (1 to 5) on the impact of not considering the disease if it is present.

Massachusetts General Hospital still owns DxPlain; however, it is available to other hospitals, medical schools, and healthcare organizations. Institutions can obtain an Institutional Evaluation License, which allows the organization to evaluate the system for free for one month. The organization may then obtain an annual license agreement after the trial period.

ABEL

ABEL (acid base and electrolytes) was developed at the Massachusetts Institute of Technology in 1981 as a doctoral memory by Ramesh Patil. It was the first expert system using causal reasoning to manage a specific disorder (acid-base metabolism and hydroelectrolytic disturbances). ABEL's premise was that in order for a consultation program to be acceptable, its essential capability must be to understand the illness. Before ABEL, the first generation expert systems were based on a phenomenological approach, which is the description of associations among different phenomena without the knowledge of the underlying causal mechanisms. Therefore, the causal process was represented just by linear associations among different acid-base metabolism conditions.

ABEL's purpose was to emulate the clinicians' process of diagnosis, where alternative hypotheses are developed after an analytic observation of different variables from the patient's illness. In this way, ABEL achieved an understanding of the disease and provided a coherent interpretation of the collected data. This is possible because the knowledge network was organized into three levels: (1) anatomical: the organs and its systems, (2) physiological: the normal function of the organs and systems, and (3) pathophysiological: failures in the normal function during disease and its manifestations. Although ABEL did not find a real clinical application, it represents a historic turning point in the development of CDSS. In Patil's words, it was "a small step in the right direction" (Patil 1981).

GermWatcher

GermWatcher was developed by Washington University in St. Louis, Missouri. It belongs to the clinical domain of infection control in hospitals. A rule-based alert system, GermWatcher was commissioned in February 1993 at Barnes-Jewish Hospital (BJC) in St. Louis and has been in routine clinical use since then (Kahn et al. 1993). The GermWatcher/GermAlert family of expert systems is designed to support infection control specialists in detecting, tracking, and investigating infections in hospitalized patients. The National Nosocomial Infection Surveillance System provides a set of national standards for nosocomial infections to monitor and minimize infection rates in the United States. An enterprise infection control application system based on GermWatcher was attempted in 2006.

ISABEL

ISABEL is a web-based CDSS that can be used as a standalone application or can be integrated into an existing electronic medical record (EMR). ISABEL uses a patient's demographic information and clinical features to produce a list of possible diagnoses, flagging important, time-sensitive "don't miss diagnoses."

ISABEL was created after Jason and Charlotte Maude's daughter (Isabel) was inaccurately diagnosed. The system went through two years of research and development before a pediatric version was launched in 2002, followed by an adult version in 2005 (Ramnarayan et al. 2004). In 2009, the American Medical Association selected ISABEL as the CDSS tool for its physician portal. Because ISABEL was designed for clinicians with diagnostic doubt, the system guides the user through the diagnosis process, rapidly providing a structure of where to start looking and what specific questions to ask. The system minimizes risk at most important decision point-in-care processes, offering diagnosis-driven knowledge from "gold standard" sources such as textbooks, journal abstracts, web resources, and hospital-specific protocols.

As mentioned, ISABEL can be fully integrated into an EMR. In this capacity it can provide a one-click, seamless diagnosis support with no additional data entry. If not integrated with an EMR, ISABEL can easily be integrated into the normal workflow—accepting data as free text or in a structured format as a standalone system but requiring separate data entry. ISABEL is not intended to replace a physician but rather to enhance the diagnostic-determination process by complementing the expertise of the clinician.

Conclusion

CDSS is becoming an essential component of healthcare information systems. The timely supports provided by CDSS hold promise in reducing medical errors and improving healthcare quality. In early CDSSs, knowledge acquired directly from medical experts was represented by rules, probabilities, or cases. Current CDSSs do not learn from data and rely heavily on knowledge-based and rule-based reasoning. Two factors may prevent non–knowledge-based systems to be used in healthcare: (1) Data are not adequately structured and thus might be unavailable to generate knowledge and learning, and (2) non–knowledge-based approaches are not well disseminated or evaluated in the healthcare field. The core of knowledge-based CDSS is expert and science-based information on the various diseases under consideration and the set of findings that might occur in patients with those diseases.

Chapter Discussion Questions

1. What are the basic components of a typical knowledge-based CDSS?
2. How can CDSS help reduce medical errors and near misses?
3. What is the biggest barrier for CDSS implementation in healthcare?
4. Why is a human-centered approach critical in CDSS development, implementation, and utilization?
5. Discuss and compare some CDSS examples in terms of reasoning approach, application scope, and practical utility.

Project IMPACT: Clinical Decision Support in Critical Care

Gordon D. Brown

The Setting

Leaders of the critical care unit at Western Metropolitan Medical Center recommend to the executive staff to acquire access to Project IMPACT, a database that contains descriptions of intensive care unit (ICU) patients, their care, and outcomes. This recommendation is appropriate for the institution's commitment to quality of patient care and is championed by the director of the critical care unit, who holds a national leadership position at the Society of Critical Care Medicine. The critical care unit's physicians also support Project IMPACT and are similarly involved with the Society of Critical Care Medicine, which developed the database for Tri-Analytics (see www.trianalytics.com/programs_pi.html).

Project IMPACT was acquired by the Cerner Corporation as a strategy for collaborating with physician groups. Other products of the company include the following:

- IMPACTessentialT, a registry that includes data elements that describe patient demographics, admitting diagnoses, condition and acuity, lengths of stay in ICU and hospital, and condition on discharge
- IMPACTsepsisT, a registry for severe sepsis in ICUs

The goal of Project IMPACT is to provide a database for monitoring and reporting critical care treatment and outcomes for subscribing institutions. The database provides a centralized, efficient, and consistent means for collecting and analyzing data on ICU patients. A better understanding of these occurrences and the performance of each center and physician will enable staff to evaluate equipment and training, improve practices, and ultimately improve outcomes. More efficient treatment of critical care patients is needed given that their care represents 14 percent of acute care costs annually.

Western takes the recommendation and subscribes to Project IMPACT as a strategy to boost clinical quality. Subscription enables the institution to access software that establishes data standards, checks for data quality, and automatically prepares data for submission to the central

IMPACT database. Critical care nurses enter data from the clinical records into IMPACT, which, in turn, supports ICU research and quality improvement by generating 21 reports and providing an ad hoc querying capability.

The Problem and Solution

From the IMPACT reports on outcomes and quality the critical care leaders learn that patient outcomes are at about industry averages, with some variation among clinical staff. The reports are discussed during clinical rounds and at staff case conferences. Staff members are receptive to the reports and conclude that much of the variance is the result of the differences in severity among patients and IMPACT outcomes are not severity-adjusted. Western encourages all staff to review the reports and explore ways of improving outcomes, but staff members are not clear on what specifically needs to be improved to achieve higher scores. The differences in treatment processes raise the question of whether systematic variations in clinical processes lead to the variations in outcomes.

Western has two separate quality groups: the clinical quality committee and the critical care quality committee. The two groups meet and observe that Western's average performance does not live up to its goal to be one of the top quality institutions in the Midwest. In addition, they discuss that the literature on quality improvement suggests that providing outcome information is not sufficient to transform processes and that specific interventions should be explored.

The critical care staff, after seeking advice from the clinical quality committee, decides to develop clinical guidelines as a basis for linking clinical processes with clinical outcomes; the guidelines would complement the IMPACT database. Some critical care physicians resist the idea and restate their concern that participating in Project IMPACT would lead to further institutional interference—namely, new guidelines and standardization on clinical practice. The physicians argue that in critical care units the knowledge of highly trained specialists is the gold standard for decision support and is disseminated through grand rounds and educational meetings.

In response, the director of critical care forms an interdisciplinary team to examine the establishment of clinical protocols. The team includes the medical director of the ICU, the nursing director, two nurse

(continued)

managers, an IT representative, and a secretary. Western believes that its own professional staff should establish the guidelines so that the protocols reflect local practices and patient conditions and gain acceptance from other professional staff.

The Implementation

The interdisciplinary team consults the clinical quality committee, which fully supports the development of clinical guidelines. The team is happy with the science that supports the guidelines and the contribution of the IMPACT database to validate the protocols and to systematically reduce errors, improve efficiency, and increase patient satisfaction. The team learns that research studies indicate that a project such as theirs can increase ICU productivity by up to 50 percent, significantly reduce severity control, and raise survival rates. The interdisciplinary team and management have high expectations for the clinical guidelines. The guidelines are developed as paper-based physician order charts and made available for easy access.

Western's executive and management team recognize the need to carefully implement the guidelines. A full orientation is scheduled for all health professionals to train them on how to follow the new protocols. This includes the following:

* Classes and educational materials are provided to all nursing staff, and all ICU nurses are required to demonstrate competency with using the guidelines.
* ICU's medical director acts as the instructor to physicians in all clinical units.
* Protocols are introduced as paper documents, which are supposed to be entered into the EHR as physician orders.

After the extensive training, the expectation for improvement is even higher.

The Results

The results after the first month of implementation show little improvement, but management and staff alike realize that true improvement would take time. After three months of no significant change in outcomes, an analysis of the charts reveals that many physicians still are not using the new guidelines. When asked, these physicians cite their reasons: forgetting to use the guidelines, disagreeing with some protocols, and dismay that Western is interfering with the clinical process.

The interdisciplinary management team reviews the development and implementation of the guidelines. The members realize that organization-wide use is not driven by training and administrative mandates alone. They made these false assumptions:

- Nurses are involved at the start of the clinical process when the patient arrived, so they would initiate the use of guidelines as the basis for taking physicians' orders.
- Structured interaction would strengthen the team-oriented approach developed in the critical care unit to improve quality and outcomes.

Instead, the reaction from many physicians is immediate and strong resistance, general discontent, and refusal to collaborate despite the presence of scientific evidence. Management is perplexed that the level of evidence supporting the guidelines is not enough to change physicians' behavior. The leaders initiate a recognition and reward program for units that meet a target of 90 percent compliance. Rewards include a recognition banquet, which honors the unit as a team.

When other units begin to demonstrate that their use of the guidelines led to improved outcomes, physician reluctance and resistance start to dissolve and turn to determination to incorporate the guidelines into the clinical practice. Two months later, compliance increases from 45 percent to 85 percent, and within four months the number goes up to 90 percent. Some physicians even propose innovative ideas on how the guidelines can be effectively incorporated into the clinical process, including embedding the protocols into Western's EHR. The concern here is that withdrawing the recognition and rewards banquets might result in recidivism to previous levels, but 6- and 12-month analyses of medical records reveal that compliance is maintained at more than 90 percent. Physicians and their teams who use the guidelines and elicit input from critical care nurses are not only raising the compliance rate but also achieving consistent improvement in clinical outcomes.

The sustaining force behind this project is Western's commitment to quality. The director of the critical care unit believes that clinical teamwork and the organizational culture of caring have improved as a result of this undertaking.

(continued)

Resource

Plost, G., and D. P. Melson. 2007. "Empowering Critical Care Nurses to Improve Compliance with Protocols in the Intensive Care Unit." *American Journal of Critical Care* 16 (2): 153–57.

Case Study Discussion Questions

1. Differentiate clinical registries or databases from clinical guidelines/protocols.
2. Discuss the legacy of a clinical specialty developing clinical outcomes guidelines and forming its own quality improvement committee that is separate from the institution's quality improvement committee.
3. What effect does reporting Project IMPACT data have on improved outcomes without relating the outcomes to an intervention?
4. Why are the IMPACT database and the clinical guidelines separated from the institutional EHR?
5. What knowledge is contained in the guidelines that complement the Project IMPACT database? How is knowledge embedded within the guidelines?
6. How is the clinical process changed? What are the factors involved in a change in clinical process?
7. What are indicators of a strong leadership and culture within the ICU at Western? What knowledge do the critical care nurses bring to implementation of clinical protocols at Western?
8. If you were at Western, would you support sharing the clinical protocols with other institutions within the Western system? With competitors in the region? Nationally? What is your commitment to quality improvement in the community related to proprietary knowledge?

CLINICAL DECISION SUPPORT IN NURSING

Norma M. Lang and Timothy B. Patrick

Learning Objectives

After reading this chapter, students should be able to

- Understand the unique features of nursing practice
- Explain nursing clinical decision support in the context of translational research
- Articulate the importance of standardized terminology to clinical decision support systems
- Name the key players in developing a nursing clinical decision support system
- Describe the steps in developing a nursing clinical decision support system

---

KEY CONCEPTS

- Nursing clinical decision support
- Standardized terminology
- Standards versus local context

Introduction

A clinical decision support system (CDSS) provides clinicians, staff, patients, and other individuals with knowledge and person-specific information, intelligently filtered or presented at appropriate times, to enhance health and healthcare. CDSS encompasses computerized alerts and reminders to care providers and patients, clinical guidelines, condition-focused medical and nursing order sets, patient-data feedback, summaries, reports, and other decision making in the clinical workflow (President's Council of Advisors on Science and Technology 2010). Multiple national and regional activities are under way to enhance health information technology and health information exchange (HIE), clinical decision support, and quality e-measures and improvement. Each of these efforts is dependent on (1) the use of standard-ized terminology or controlled vocabulary and (2) the effectiveness and efficiency of translational research.

From the point of view of nursing, the patient's reality is character-ized by a nexus of conditions. A patient with a hip fracture, for example, is hospitalized for a hip replacement or hip-pinning surgical procedure. How-ever, this person might well be confused or depressed; suffer from urinary incontinence, sleep deprivation, unmanaged pain, immobility, delirium, or dehydration; or have Parkinson's disease. Furthermore, nursing concerns the patient, who participates in the continuum of care, including the home and community. Data and information systems focus primarily on medical ele-ments related to the ICD-10-CM (International Classification of Diseases) and CPT (Current Procedural Terminology) categories, terminologies, and codes (NCHS 2011; American Medical Association 2011). Administrative data usually receive greater attention than clinical data because of interest in reimbursement and regulation requirements. However, if additional clini-cal conditions are not identified and interventions are not put in place and recorded, the patient can receive inadequate care and be transitioned to inap-propriate care venues, which could result in death.

The practice of nursing is based on science and knowledge of how to assess and intervene to resolve clinical patient problems (Hagle and Senk 2009). Research that informs nursing practice has dramatically increased, but bringing that evidence to the bedside or the site of patient care is a continuing challenge. Adding to that challenge is that nurses must consider medical knowledge as they implement physician-directed care. Nurses are also required to understand pharmacology and to make medication-related decisions on their own, such as whether a patient needs medicine. Physical therapists and dietitians have to make similar clinical decisions and thus must also grasp both medical and pharmacology concepts.

Significant research has explored nurse-identified problems and interventions for which nurses are required to develop patient-centered care plans. The 24/7 integration and application of nursing, medical, and pharmacological knowledge is unique to hospital nursing. While informa-tion systems can track the multitude of data associated with concurrent and interrelated patient conditions, they are no panacea. In fact, serious questions remain about the ability of these systems to assist nurses in applying the data and information to real-time clinical practice. Unless integrated and defrag-mented, the enormous amount of data may become a barrier to the effec-tive management of the patient's health needs. The sine qua non of patient care is to transcend, interpret, and synthesize information silos (or isolated, department-specific thinking) so that they can be integrated and prioritized and thus can present a complete view of the patient's condition, her plan of care, and her health behavior. Such a view of the patient, congruent to the practical reality of day-to-day nursing care, is a fundamental challenge in developing clinical decision support and documentation systems for nursing (Lang 2008).

Integrated Example: Knowledge-based Nursing Initiative

The knowledge-based nursing initiative (KBNI) is one example of an initiative that transforms research into practice—that is, it brings integrated knowledge to the bedside or the site of patient care (Elsa, Lang, and Lundeen 2006; Lang et al. 2006). KBNI, a partnership of Aurora Health Care, Cerner Corporation, and the University of Wisconsin-Milwaukee College of Nursing, was designed and implemented to synthesize the available research on a specific phenomenon of concern; to make that referential knowledge actionable for clinical decision support and documentation by embedding it in an electronic system; to test the use of the system in a hospital; and to acquire, analyze, and report clinical data from the hospital's clinical repository and data warehouse (Hook, Burke, and Murphy 2009; Kim et al. 2007; Lang 2008; Lundeen, Harper, and Kerfoot 2009; Murphy et al. 2010).

KBNI is a reference model for those developing CDSS using standardized terminology (a set of multiword terms and relationships purposely selected to express thematically related concepts and the associations between them). Note that KBNI is not representative of all the specific details of all nursing CDSSs that address all other contexts of nursing care; it is one example that has affinities with those other contexts. The development of a nursing CDSS as illustrated by KBNI involves a partnership among researchers, health organizations, health professionals, IT experts, and an IT vendor that designs and builds information systems. While KBNI's setting does not characterize that of all or even most healthcare organizations, we selected this initiative to systematically describe the broader complexities of the design as well as the implementation and adoption of clinical decision support and documentation systems. These complexities result from the assumptions embedded in commercial decision support systems (Karsh et al. 2010). For example, as part of the structure of the KBNI initiative, the vendor partner produces a CDSS. The vendor may then sell that system (which was created for the exact purpose and specifications of the partnership) to other customers (which may in turn not have the resources to carry out the expensive and extensive process the system requires).

The steps followed by the KBNI are presented here not only to help healthcare organizations improve their CDSS development efforts but also to inform them of the problems that could arise in the course of system development and implementation, including and especially the challenge of using standardized terminology. Specifically, in this chapter we discuss the basic steps for identifying the content of nursing CDSS and its relationship to translational research. These steps may be separated into two groups: (1) The first steps are based on science and applicable to all healthcare organizations and system developers, and (2) the second steps trace where the science in the first group meets the local organization and practice. The commercial CDSS product design might determine to what degree this second group is enabled and should be a consideration in product selection (see Chapter 3). The interaction between science-based standards and local context leads to three fundamental problems: (1) the system documentation problem, (2) the vocabulary problem, and (3) the system drift problem. We discuss these three problems and their interrelations. The chapter concludes with a discussion of our main thesis: the need for a CDSS that provides an integrated, prioritized, and evidence-based view of the whole patient.

A Model of Developing CDSS with the Use of Standardized Terminology

Developing an evidence-based nursing CDSS entails gathering and then translating scientific research into the day-to-day nursing practice. This translation of evidence to practice involves both Type 2 and Type 3 translational research (Institute of Translational Health Sciences 2010). Type 2 is the development of practice guidelines or recommendations based on health discoveries, and Type 3 is the integration of these guidelines or recommendations into the CDSS. Notwithstanding the neat division of development into Type 2 and Type 3, the fundamental lesson here is that the CDSS should not be implemented *de novo*—that is, without regard to existing operational processes, especially the workflow of clinicians. Although the implementation is most likely to alter the decision-making and care processes, it must give due consideration to the current approaches in place. Thus, the CDSS may need to be retrofitted, to some degree, to the organizational culture, practice, information systems, and management strategies. Retrofitting is a challenge to standardization and interoperability. The more local customization and changes are made, the more risk is presented to the validity and reliability of the data in relationship to the research-based practice recommendation.

Development Steps

Exhibit 6.1 depicts the steps in developing a nursing CDSS and documentation system to address a specific problem domain—fall risk (Hook, Devine, and Lang 2008; Hook and Winchel 2006).

In Step 1, the demographic for the population of interest is determined; in this case, the demographic of risk for falls with injury consists

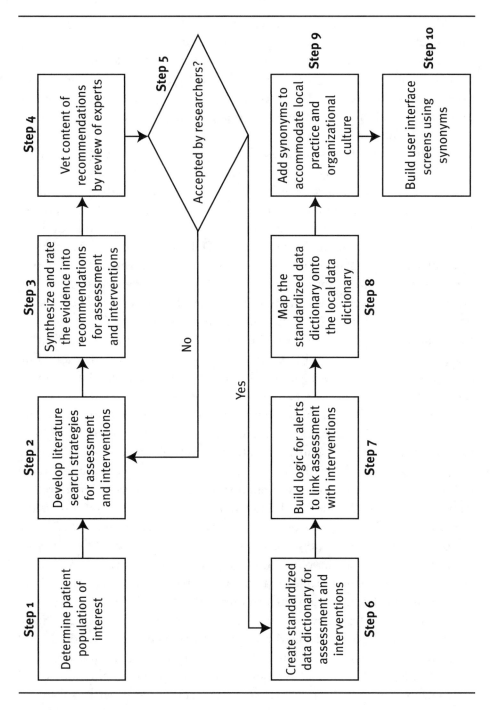

EXHIBIT 6.1
Steps in
Developing
a Nursing
CDSS and
Documentation
System

of hospitalized patients in general medical-surgical units. At this point, a researcher is assigned to be responsible for knowledge development or gathering pertinent and quality information for inclusion in the CDSS. The clinical phenomenon of concern (PoC) is coded to standardized terminology and is described in detail, including the population of interest. This is a critical step because the standardized data results guide the literature search for studies on specific populations. If the population of interest is elderly, female, and inpatient, the evidence gathered should be relevant to the risk factors and interventions for that particular demographic, not for the general population. Likewise, the risk factors identified in a specific type of hospital unit (the venue) differ from those factors at home, nursing home, or in the general community.

The choice of standardized terminologies to use in coding the PoC is critical. The field of nursing is huge; more than 3 million nurses work in the United States, providing care in a range of venues in healthcare organizations and at home. In addition, nursing is as complex as the health problems and needs of patients and their families. Medicine has a long history of using standardized terminologies, such as the ICD-10-CM and CPT. Yet the use of controlled vocabulary in nursing is fairly recent, occurring in just the past three decades. Current nursing terminologies include the North American Nursing Diagnosis Association (NANDA), the Nursing Intervention Classification (NIC), Nursing Outcome Classification (NOC), the Omaha System, the Clinical Care Classification (CCC), and the International Classification for Nursing Practice (ICNP) (Coenan and Bartz 2010; Coenan and Kim 2010). A complete list of recognized nursing vocabularies can be found on the website of the American Nurses Association (see ANA 2010).

In Step 2, the search for relevant research and preexisting guidelines is launched. The KBNI work, for example, is built on a synthesis of original research and published guidelines. The research librarian plays a key role and becomes a partner of the knowledge developer. Librarians are experts in indexing policies and correlative search strategies for different bibliographic databases, such as PubMed and Cinhal, and journal indexes related to the nursing PoC. Experts in evidence-based clinical practice and statistics are important here, as they know the study design features (e.g., different types of "blinding," such as the blinding of subjects as to whether they are in the control or experimental group) that produce strong or weak evidence. They also document the fit of individual studies with the PoC.

In Step 3, the collected evidence for the specific PoC is summarized, synthesized, and combined in the form of assessments, interventions, and outcomes. Step 3 is a highly collaborative step in the translation process.

In Step 4, the evidence synthesized into assessment, interventions, and outcomes is reviewed by the partners—particularly, the experienced health professionals, IT experts, and experts in evidence-based clinical practice and statistics. As mentioned, the end goal of the translation is a CDSS and documentation system implemented in an existing local environment. Thus, some of the experts may be representatives of the local environment. Another essential partner is the IT vendor. This partnership is important if the content is to be designed and built into a useful decision support system (Lang 2008; Lang et al. 2006; Kerfoot et al. 2010). The ideal implementation is dependent on the interrelationships among researchers, clinicians, IT experts, and vendor's design and building experts (Kerfoot et al. 2010).

In Step 5, the decision to accept the evidence from Step 4 is made. If the assessment and interventions are not affirmed by research and clinical experts, then further evidence collection and synthesis may be necessary. If affirmed, then the process of codification and implementation begins.

In Step 6, a data dictionary (also known as metadata schema) is created to codify the assessment, interventions, and outcomes recommendations. A data dictionary consists of data elements and permissible value sets, which are sometimes referred to as "questions and permissible answer sets." A value set for a given data element may be enumerated or nonenumerated. In an enumerated value set, the permissible values are listed, while in a nonenumerated value set, the permissible values are described. Exhibit 6.2 is an example of a data element with an enumerated permissible value set. In the exhibit, the data element "changes in voiding habits, details" is part of the assessment for a fall risk CDSS. Its permissible values are aspects of changes in voiding habits that are, according to evidence, associated with risk factors for falls. Here are the "should-haves" for the data dictionary:

- Should be developed according to an established standard such as ISO 11179 (International Organization for Standardization and the International Electrotechnical Commission 2004).
- Should use standardized terminology for the data element and permissible value concepts and should include definitions of the terminology. (The definitions of the permissible value concepts are not included in Exhibit 6.2 for the sake of brevity.)
- Should include specification of the evidence supporting the association of permissible values with a given data element. (The specifications of supporting evidence are not included in Exhibit 6.2 for the sake of brevity.)[1]

EXHIBIT 6.2
Data Element with an Enumerated Permissible Value Set

Data Element	Permissible Values
Changes in voiding habits, details	Urgency
	Frequency
	Incontinent
	Nocturia
	Polyuria

In Step 7, the system logic associated with assessment and interventions for alerts and other actions is created. For example, conditional logic may be constructed to indicate a risk of falling, such as the following:

The patient is at risk of falling if the patient's Morse Fall Scale total >= 45.

Outcomes are typically included and are usually represented by a maintenance, prevention, reduction, or elimination of the problem. One example is reduction in falls. Sometimes intermediate outcomes are used, such as "the patient and family verbalize the steps they will take to reduce falls."

Steps 1 through 7 (marked in boldface in Exhibit 6.1) should apply to all healthcare organizations and information system developers. The process of embedding the results of steps 1 through 7 in a specific local operational context is carried out in steps 8 through 10. Here, careful consideration and evaluation must be given to the existing operational context. Again, note that the nursing CDSS should not be implemented de novo; rather, it should be implemented in an existing operational context. Thus, the standard practice might be for all patients to be assessed for "changes in voiding habits," and the existing value set for that data element might be more extensive than the value set strictly relevant to "fall risk" decision support.

Steps 8 through 10 are the province of the local organization and CDSS developers. A working partnership with the researchers is highly desirable and valuable. Thus, the local organization likely wants to avoid the best evidence and to continue its current practices, in spite of the science-based recommendations; such unrestricted localization must be prevented. Localization must always be tempered by comparison to the current science. This is often a point of contention and angst in translational research. Exhibit 6.3 depicts the data element "changes in voiding habits" with the subset (marked in boldface) of the value set that is relevant to fall risk according to the best available evidence (steps 1 through 7). Changes in the science-based recommendations (delivered by steps 1 through 7) need to be noted, as such changes may affect the strength of the recommendations when locally implemented. Local changes in terminology may, for example, result in questions about interoperability and comparative analysis among different local implementations of science-based recommendations.

In Step 8, a detailed mapping and reconciliation is created between the standardized data dictionary (created in Step 6) and the data dictionary or dictionaries that characterize the local system. Often the data dictionary that characterizes the local system may be underdocumented, and sometimes it consists largely of the names of database fields and the data type (e.g., integer) of those fields. The potential for sparse documentation of the local

Data Element	Permissible Values
Changes in voiding habits, details	**Urgency**
	Frequency
	Incontinent
	Nocturia
	Polyuria
	Burning
	Anuria
	Dysuria
	Oliguria
	Catheter
	Distended
	Unable to void

EXHIBIT 6.3
Data Element
with a Full
Permissible
Value Set

system is more reason that the standardized data elements and values should be clearly defined.

In Step 9, more controlled localization is performed. Neither the standardized terminology in the data dictionary nor the terminology in the data dictionary of the local information system may be language normally used or preferred by the local organization's nurses who will use the CDSS. Terminology that is foreign to a given user's understanding may be an impediment to his or her use of the decision support system. Thus, **locally preferred synonyms** for the standard names of data elements and value concepts must be collected and available for the user interfaces of the CDSS. Note, however, that the use of such local synonyms must be carefully controlled and carefully linked to the standardized terminology. Again, localization must always be tempered by comparison to the current science, paying close attention to the tension between local needs and the rigors of the science-based recommendations.

In Step 10, locally preferred synonyms are used to construct the user interfaces—particularly the screens for data entry and reporting—of the CDSS. Again, note that while the names of data elements and values that appear on the user interface screens may be different from the standardized names in the data dictionary, they may be mapped or linked to those standardized terms as synonyms. This allows the data from assessments to be captured, behind the scenes, in a standardized form to facilitate interoperability and compatibility with other data sets, perhaps from other institutions. Considering the value of such standardized data, the risk (or the opportunity cost) associated with the common practice of including an "other" choice in an enumerated value set should be noted. For example, in addition to the five explicitly specified values for the permissible value set shown in Exhibit 6.2, an "other" choice may be included to allow the specification of a natural language or essentially nonstandardized description of a value for the data element, in case one of the listed values did not suit the user. It is important to consider that including an "other" choice may bring the risk of a kind of *semantic leak*, whereby a user unfamiliar with the value choices as enumerated, specifies a natural language expression that is essentially a synonym for the specified term, though not one that is explicitly linked to the standardized term. Such cases may lead to a failure of the CDSS in the case of specific patients because the recommendations for interventions based on the assessment of the patient may not be presented to the nurse as a result of the fact that the natural language expression in the "other" field (though a synonym of the enumerated value, at least in a natural language or practical sense) may not be logically linked in the CDSS to those recommended interventions.

Three Problems in Development and Management

The problems in developing and managing a nursing CDSS and documentation system result from the interaction between science-based standards and local context. These interrelated problems are (1) system documentation problem, (2) vocabulary problem, and (3) system drift problem.

System Documentation Problem

In every step of development and management all aspects of the CDSS must be adequately described. Lack of documentation causes a **system documentation problem**. System developers appear to instinctively *not* document (or at least underdocument) their work. Part of the reason may be that much of the work is done by operational staff members, who are more goal driven to complete the specific deliverables and meet the "go-live" deadline than focused on documenting the process. Exhibit 6.4 relates a case that illustrates a system documentation problem. Any local modifications of the science-based recommendations, either in content or expression, should be well-documented. Recording changes in expression prevents the vocabulary problem.

As part of an organization's project to build an EHR for its hospital and clinics, a core database group meets weekly to discuss issues related to basic data elements and their display counterparts. During a meeting, one member, Mr. Johnson, urges the group to record every decision and change made. To emphasize his point, he relates a cautionary tale.

Several years earlier, the hospital faced a system security audit. In the course of preparing for the audit, staff discovered a series of medical record numbers that were not in use and whose purpose was not documented. After much consternation and digging through old files, staff determined that the numbers belonged to patients of an old mental health services unit, which was now separate from the hospital and clinics.

Mr. Johnson tells the group that lack or poor documentation could put the organization in the same predicament. Much time and effort were expended, and much anguish created, to trail the origins of an ultimately trivial series of numbers.

EXHIBIT 6.4
Illustration of a System Documentation Problem

Vocabulary Problem

Not only is nursing care complex, it also uses complex terminology. Standardized terminology can help achieve the goal of improved healthcare by supporting greater efficiencies and effectiveness for translational research. Nursing science or research, however, is not reported using standardized terminology. Thus, a vocabulary problem exists even at the point of synthesis. (See Chapter 2 for a more general account of the vocabulary problem, particularly as it relates to interoperability.) The localization of the science-based recommendations (as delivered by steps 1 through 7), including the terminology with which they are coded, is inevitable. Such localization is appropriate, given the retrofitting of the CDSS implementation, and likely involves the localization of the terminology used to express data elements and their values in the system. Yet without the clear reference point of standardized terminology used to express the science-based recommendations, the link between the local system and the recommendations may be strained or at least unclear, resulting in the system drift problem.

System Drift Problem

The children's game of "telephone" produces a surprising, and sometimes amusing, conclusion. The game starts with one person whispering a message or story to another, and then that second person whispers it to another, and so on. When the initial message is relayed to the last person in the chain of receivers, the details have changed—both in content and expression. The essence of the telephone game can be applied to a nursing CDSS; that is, the changes that occur from the science-based recommendation to practical implementation in the local environment may be the result of a cascade of (seemingly) minor adjustments to the content and expression of the original evidence during the development process. These modifications represent the **system drift problem**. Another complicating factor here is that scientists do not always agree even on the common intervention problems that nurses face. In fact, the steps in the translation may involve a mediating step of implementation of the science-based recommendations in the vendor-built CDSS, which is then localized to the customer's environment. Because of such system drift, the recommendations as implemented in the CDSS are based more on local practices than on scientific evidence.

Conclusion

From the point of view of nursing, patient reality is often characterized by a nexus of interrelated and complicating conditions. As such, a decision support and documentation system that provides an integrated, prioritized, and evidence-based view of the patient is needed. To develop such a nursing CDSS, strict attention should be paid to the steps necessary to produce science-based practice recommendations that may be shared across institutions. The translation of evidence into practice *never* has a clean slate. Developing science-based recommendations is important and so is implementing those standard recommendations into the local, existing, and actual working healthcare environment.

Chapter Discussion Questions

1. Explain why the implementation of a nursing CDSS must take into account the local operational environment.
2. What is the role of the IT vendor in the development and implementation of a nursing CDSS?
3. What is an information silo? How may information silos be avoided?

Note

1. The work reported here was supported in part by AHRQ grant number 290-06-0016-2 ("Using Evidence-based Practices and Electronic Health Record Decision Support to Reduce Fall-related Injuries in Acute Care"), in particular the coding of the risk for falls content and the inclusion of selected content in the AHRQ United States Health Information Knowledgebase (USHIK). This work was also supported in part by National Science Foundation Partnerships

for Innovation grant award 0650323, which advanced team science among several scientists from multiple schools in the University of Wisconsin-Milwaukee.

CASE STUDY   Questions of Evidence

Timothy B. Patrick and Norma M. Lang

Chris, an academic health informatics specialist; Parker, a registered nurse; and Alex, a hospital clinical IT manager and strong proponent of electronic health records (EHRs), are discussing the virtues of EHRs for managing nursing care data and information and the obstacles to EHR-based clinical decision support.

Parker: To show you that EHR can't handle complex situations, listen to this case. Selina Jones is 80 years old. She is admitted to the hospital medical-surgical unit after a fall. It appears she has sustained an injury to her hip that requires a surgical intervention. She is in moderate pain but has difficulty moving, nauseated, calling for her dead husband, very anxious, and not understanding what happened to her—let alone the diagnostic tests, surgical plan, and other treatments she is and will be receiving.

Selina's daughter has assigned herself the authority to make healthcare decisions for her mom. The daughter agrees to have the surgeon do a surgical pinning of Selina's hip. The registered nurse is responsible for doing the patient assessment and making the decisions on how best to prepare the patient for surgery, so the nurse has to communicate these decisions to other members of the clinical team. The surgeon and registered nurse are also responsible for creating the postsurgical plans, which include visits to a physical therapist and a social worker.

Surgery is complete. Selina is sent home, but she continues to have unmanaged pain, confusion, anxiety, no ability to participate in her own treatment or therapies, and no understanding of the risk for falls. She can't sleep well, has acquired pressure ulcers during the hospital stay, and suffers from urinary incontinence.

Chris: Her family situation and medical issues do sound complicated. Alex, you must admit that your EHR is no panacea for this.

(continued)

Alex: Of course it's no panacea—nothing is. The golden rule in IT is good data in, good information out. If you enter inadequate data, you can't expect complete results.

Chris: Good data in, good information out certainly requires more than the usual ICD and CPT codes entered into the EHR. But let's back up and focus on decision support. At the university hospital, we designed a set of standard nursing practice recommendations for assessment and interventions related to fall risks. So how could we determine whether nursing practice in your hospital conforms to our practice recommendations?

Alex: The data fields in our EHR database have to match the key concepts in your practice recommendations.

Parker: A standard approach matches both sides to a reference vocabulary, like SNOMED CT.

Chris: Suppose your EHR used SNOMED CT or some other standard vocabulary in the first place? Then you really could achieve good data in, good information out.

Alex: Yes, but not everything's perfect. Besides, operations has its own pressures. As Shakespeare wrote, "There are more things in heaven and earth, Horatio, than are dreamt of in your philosophy."

Chris: Is matching of data and concepts enough? It seems that your data have to show that the right (according to *our* recommendations) assessments and interventions were taken. For example, according to our recommendations, incontinence is a risk factor for falls, so if the patient assessment included that, a protocol for fall prevention is implemented.

Alex: Good example—and you could find that in our data.

Chris: Always? And why would you find that?

Parker: Because that protocol for that assessment is common practice?

Alex: Our clinicians are experts and follow good practice in their care plans.

Chris: In our recommendations we cite clinical studies that provide evidence for incontinence as a risk for falls.

Alex: Isn't it enough if our practice and your recommendations agree on what ought to be done even if the reasons are not strictly the same?

Chris: I don't think so. Maybe it would be in a simple or an isolated case, but I'm not comfortable with that position in general—and certainly not in a complicated case like that of Selina Jones.

Case Study Discussion Questions

1. Can the case of Selina Jones be managed by dealing with each of her problems separately? If not, how can an EHR keep track of her case?
2. Alex's statement "operations has its own pressures" implies a conflict between informatics and operations. Do you agree? Why, or why not?
3. Describe a procedure for matching the EHR data fields to the practice recommendation assessment and intervention concepts.
4. What is Chris's concern at the end? Do you agree or disagree? Why, or why not?

THE COMING OF THE CORPORATION: TRANSFORMING CLINICAL WORK PROCESSES

Gordon D. Brown

Learning Objectives

After reading this chapter, students should be able to

- Assess how the traditional structure of healthcare organizations defines the design of the information system and the clinical function
- Understand how healthcare financing has affected clinical decision making specifically and the clinical function as a whole
- Conceptualize the role of information technology in supporting integrated clinical work processes within healthcare organizations
- Apply the concept of standardization and coordination of work
- Conceptualize the design of an organization as a system to achieve optimum clinical outcomes and with an increasing focus on the patient
- Explain how structuring around the clinical function transcends professional boundaries and enables the creation of a community of practice

---

KEY CONCEPTS

- Organization structure
- Community of practice
- DRG-based financing
- Jobs, tasks, and work processes
- Coordination of work
- Transforming power of IT
- Business versus clinical function

Introduction

The phrase "the coming of the corporation" is the title of the last chapter in Paul Starr's Pulitzer Prize–winning work *The Social Transformation of American Medicine,* which explores the increased size and power of organizations in the health system. Starr (1984) concludes that the growth of corporate presence results from the creation of larger hospitals; the advent of integrated health systems; the market influence of suppliers, including pharmaceutical companies; and the likelihood that a greater number of physicians would become employees. An even more profound change is occurring today: More work of the medical and other health professions is being carried out in organized environments, making the organization directly accountable for clinical outcomes and thus the clinical processes (Muzio and Kirkpatrick 2011). This phenomenon has nothing to do with whether or not physicians are employees of the organization, because it affects the medical staff regardless of institutional affiliation. Many other factors contribute to the coming of the corporation, including shifts in the socioeconomic landscape of the health system, such as an increase in chronic care; changing patient values; and advancements in clinical science and information technology (IT). IT enables the transformation but, as in other sectors, does not create it (Maiga and Jacobs 2009; Nakata, Zhu, and Kraimer 2009).

The Patient Protection and Affordable Care Act (ACA) of 2010 mandates healthcare institutions to purchase a computerized information system and to demonstrate its "meaningful use." The term *meaningful use* refers to the level with which the acquired IT is available and used to support clinical decision making; it does not concern the transformation of the clinical process. Note that healthcare is one of the few sectors in which federal mandates and direct financial incentives are deemed necessary to motivate clinics, hospitals, and other healthcare organizations to invest in basic IT (US Congress 2010). In this chapter, we examine why organization leaders undervalue and seem to have a limited vision of the transforming power of IT. (This transforming power has been explored since 1980, with the publication of *The Third Wave* by Alvin Toffler.)

The Traditional Structure of the Healthcare Organization

The structure of hospitals, nursing homes, and clinics is based on the logic of the business function, the dominant and default function of an organization (Brown and Stone 2005). Traditionally, the corporation does not assume responsibility for clinical processes or outcomes, and it attempts to avoid interfering with physicians' clinical decision making (see Chapter 5). Its primary role has been to provide the clinical function with support and resources, including capital, facility construction and maintenance, personnel administration, billing and collections, legal, and so on.

Meanwhile, the traditional structure of clinical services in most hospitals is based on medical specialty and nursing services. In hospitals, this structure consists of pediatrics, surgery, internal medicine, among others, and is organized by hierarchy within clinical departments. These departments have dual accountability—first to the attending physicians and the orders of those physicians (clinical) and second to the corporation (administrative), specifically the department director, chief executive officer, and governing board. In hospitals, the clinical structure also includes clinical support departments, such as radiology, laboratory, and pharmacy. Clinical departments are structured under an associate administrator, who has management training, years of experience, and diplomacy to maintain the delicate balance between organizational and clinical accountability. For example, the director of nursing possesses a high level of clinical expertise as well as organizational seasoning and savvy. The laboratory, pharmacy, and radiology operate as somewhat autonomous "clinical" units under the direction of a pathologist, pharmacist, or radiologist working in an administrative structure of the department. (See Exhibit 7.1 for an example of the traditional structure of the organization.)

These traditional, autonomous, and hierarchical structures are incompatible with the design of electronic information systems (even the electronic medical record [EMR]), whose logic is based on total institutional integration. Implementing an EMR does present technical challenges, such as standardization, but it transforms the orientation of clinical information from clinician and department to institution (see Chapter 3). As discussed later in the chapter, once the integration of information is achieved, it has the power to enable the transformation of the clinical function itself.

The dominant organization structures are hierarchical in nature, with each department led by a series of managers and directors who, in turn, report to higher-level leaders. Known as a vertical structure, this organizational design is believed to provide stability and enable the efficient use of specialized equipment and staff to support the rapidly expanding medical technology. In a vertical structure, information, communications, decisions, resources, and plans flow between frontline workers, middle managers, and senior managers.

As mentioned, the business function became the primary logic for the structure of the traditional organization. This business-function structure included departments such as finance, personnel, housekeeping, food service, maintenance, and public relations, to name a few. The business side (or corporate) became dominant in healthcare because of several factors, such as most chief executive officers and chief operating officers had a business, not clinical, orientation; the principal responsibility of governing boards was to oversee finances and prevent legal trouble; and accreditation agencies based performance on input measures, such as the percentage of the medical staff who were board certified. In addition, financial performance was easier to measure and interpret than clinical processes and outcomes. This hierarchical

EXHIBIT 7.1
Traditional
Structure of
a Healthcare
Organization

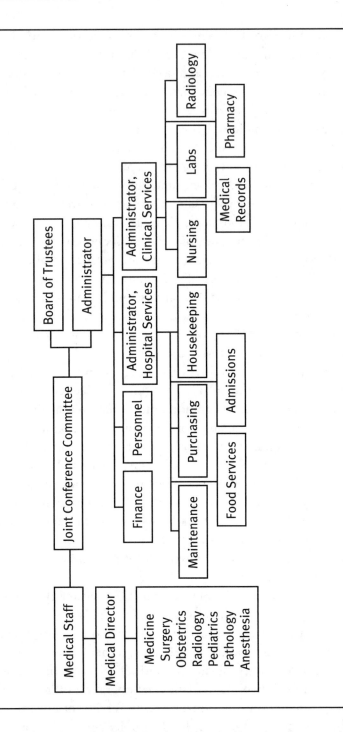

mindset has been strongly embedded in the organizational culture and has been difficult to change.

Hierarchical functional structures offer some advantages but are poorly designed for rapid change, flexibility in coordinating highly integrated work processes, empowering frontline workers, and innovation. The assumptions and limitations of functional structures are in direct contradiction to the enabling qualities of advanced IT and to the structure of the clinical process, which is examined later in this chapter. (The term *advanced IT* does not refer to the technology per se but to how IT is applied to enable the transformation of clinical work processes.) Although hierarchical functional structures continue to dominate the healthcare field, they are increasingly considered ineffective by information-driven environments (Tseng 2011). The early architecture of health information systems was designed according to functional structures and automating existing processes. This architecture lives on today and causes incompatibility problems in daily clinical operations, which require and demand integrated (not silo) information. In this chapter, we present the history and the future of health IT.

Evolution of the Clinical Function

The corporation has had varying and increasing influence on the clinical function over the past century. The primary impact has been on healthcare financing, which, in turn, changed how and which healthcare services are delivered. This section summarizes the major factors that have shaped the evolution of the clinical function.

Health Insurance

In the 1920s the first private health insurance plans altered the clinical process by identifying the specific services that would be covered and the setting in which these services would be provided. Insurance primarily paid for high-cost surgeries and other complex interventions provided in hospitals. The cost of these services was spread among everyone enrolled in the plan. This method of financing limited how and where physicians treated patients and thus altered the doctor–patient relationship. Known as the "third party," insurance was widely disliked by physicians and other clinicians but was reluctantly accepted nonetheless because of the financial reality that patients and families needed help to pay for rising healthcare costs.

In addition, insurance contributed to making organizations larger and more complex. Insurance companies needed a standardized system for paying the healthcare bills the plan enrollees incurred. Healthcare organizations responded by developing a financing function based on a new classification of clinical services called *medical procedures code* (MPC), which was developed by the American Medical Association. In theory, MPC was a way of standardizing measures of clinical services for the purpose of scheduling, coding, billing, accounts receivable, and collections. In practice, MPC contributed to the long and controversial process of standardizing clinical vocabularies, diagnoses, and units of service; later, it became the basis for measuring clinical outcomes, developing clinical decision support, and transforming clinical processes. The finance department became the initial locus of development of electronic information systems. It was a natural beginning for an information system because the department could draw on standardized terms and measures (used for accounting, financial, and insurance transactions) to enter into the system. As emphasized throughout this book, standardization is an essential requirement of computer applications.

Managed Care

The managed care movement grew rapidly in the 1970s. It shifted the framework of healthcare financing from an illness-based model to a population and wellness-based model. Such a model required providers (both hospitals and clinicians) to share risks for a defined patient population and offered incentives for health maintenance and for efficient and effective healthcare delivery. At the time, hospitals and clinics were not structured for capitation payments, except for a few plans such as Kaiser Permanente, which can serve as models for future change (Halvorson 2007). More significantly, healthcare providers did not desire to make a radical shift from illness-based insurance models on which they had become oriented and dependent. Capitation financing heightened the role of health provider and financing corporations and reduced the individual clinician's decision-making autonomy, a radical change that was not popular with most physicians or hospitals. Being accountable collectively for a population's health, clinical quality, and operational efficiency required focusing on health outcomes, process–outcome relationships, and the coordination of care, which were feasible only through restructuring the health system.

Standardization and measurement of clinical process and outcomes became the nemesis of the health professions and healthcare organizations, and so did accountability for outcomes and coordination of clinical processes. Providers' reluctance to take on these tasks resulted in insurance companies as external agencies to, again, step in and introduce control mechanisms (e.g., preadmission and preauthorization procedures, clinical gatekeepers) to enable them to manage the providers' risk. Healthcare organizations, such as Kaiser Permanente, that did embrace the assumptions of capitation demonstrated a workable solution, by standardizing and measuring population-based healthcare services and their outcomes and designing clinical processes across specialties, institutions, and practice locations on the basis of the outcomes measures (Scott et al. 2000). Advanced IT (or information systems) was the enabling force behind the transformation of clinical processes, developing measures of clinical outcome and structuring processes on the basis of outcome measures. Such a demonstration caught the attention of policymakers and increased the dissonance within the healthcare system. Demonstrations showed that the evidence/knowledge base made possible by IT could result in improved clinical outcomes; only the lack of provider will and powerful self-interests impeded change. Similar payment mechanisms have emerged, such as bundled payments by the Centers for Medicare and Medicaid Services (CMS), but they are focused on micro processes and identified with a politically palatable phrase as "bundled payments" rather than managed care (RAND Compare 2012).

Diagnosis-Related Group

In the early 1980s, reimbursement strategies led by CMS changed from a cost-based scheme to the case-based diagnosis-related groups (DRGs), forcing healthcare organizations to redesign their cost measurement and information structure to assign costs by diagnosis (e.g., normal vaginal delivery) rather than by functions (e.g., nursing). To develop case-based measures of cost, hospitals had to persuade reluctant health professionals that clinical services could be sufficiently standardized to enable institutions to assign a valid cost figure. This was not a trivial task given that few hospitals had adequate accounting systems to allocate cost by clinical service. In addition, hospitals measured cost on the basis of reimbursement logic and not activity (actual factor inputs), so measurement was done with a "rubber ruler" (i.e., costs based on reimbursement rate not true costs). Thus, the controversial concept of standardization was again raised; this time, the resisters argued that DRG is a further invasion of the clinical process and questioned the degree to which clinical services could be standardized and measured. The use of federal funds in purchasing medical services became the financial impetus that moved the healthcare system toward standardizing services on the basis of DRGs.

Under DRG financing, MPC was integrated into other coding and classification schemes, such as the International Classification of Diseases and the Medical Diagnostic Codes. Healthcare administrators were inclined to assure their medical and nursing staffs that the standardization of clinical services under DRG was for financial purposes only, would not intrude into clinical decision making, and would not interfere with caregiving. Such promises by management were either naive or intentionally deceptive. If the cost of services provided within a given DRG were in excess of what was included in the DRG reimbursement algorithm, there was a financial loss on that service, and institutions had limited ability to "subsidize" the DRGs that lost money. Thus, healthcare organizations had to develop a process to measure, monitor, and manage the services provided within a DRG. This resulted in the incremental increase of the corporation's responsibility for and involvement in structuring the clinical function, and a new equilibrium was reached between individual decision-making autonomy and corporate guidelines and rules.

Institute of Medicine Reports

In the 1990s the Institute of Medicine (IOM) report *To Err Is Human* garnered much attention. The public discussions about the report revolved around the estimated 100,000 people dying in hospitals every year as the result of medical errors (Kohn, Corrigan, and Donaldson 2000). The report framed clinical quality and safety as a public health concern and called for increased accountability for the public monies being spent on healthcare services. Federal financing of healthcare services became the justification for the American public, government, and employers to take greater interest in improving quality and safety for everyone who uses the healthcare system. Another IOM report, *Crossing the Quality Chasm,* recognized the ability and legitimacy of measuring and comparing clinical outcomes and called for the application of well-known quality improvement methods, such as root cause analysis (IOM 2001).

The IOM reports acknowledged the power of information systems (and supported such investments) to improve the clinical function and increase accountability. Multiple evidence shows that healthcare organizations can achieve superior outcomes and elevate their clinical performance with the help of IT (Dewett and Jones 2001). IOM viewed IT primarily as it applies to *medical informatics*, which includes CDSS and computerized physician-order entry or CPOE. Nonetheless, IOM's recommendation to apply IT to healthcare gave rise to the federal mandate to adopt electronic information systems in healthcare operations and thus greater standardization of clinical outcomes. Not only did the IOM reports generate dialogue about quality and safety of healthcare delivery, but they also raised the visibility and adoption of health IT. IT applied to the clinical function created a dialectic process that is grounded in quality and safety. Everyone in the health system can commit to clinical quality and safety, but achieving them requires change that is quite disruptive.

The IOM reports probably overstated the assumption that advanced IT would cause, as opposed to enable, fundamental change in clinical processes. The importance and complexity of making fundamental changes in clinical processes and the organizational structure and behavior is understated in the IOM reports. The committee that produced the reports is partly responsible for this perspective, but what may be true as well is that the reports were viewed as the first phase of a complex change process, with subsequent reports addressing how informatics can play a role in transforming healthcare. In any event, the reports do raise a dialectic that can encourage healthcare leaders to take advantage of available evidence from the clinical and information decision sciences, engineering, management, and social sciences to transform the system of care. It is incumbent on leaders to design such systems and not wait for the public sector to mandate change through regulation and controls. Creating a high-performance health system through regulation and control is the ultimate oxymoron.

The Integrated, Systems Perspective

The integrated perspective is based on complex adaptive systems. As discussed in Chapter 4, complex adaptive systems are characterized by a large number of interdependent parts or agents that have pattern relationships and interaction complexity, are self-organizing, and adapt to and create their environments (coevolution) (Tan, Wen, and Awad 2005; Bergeson and Dean 2006). Such systems are, by nature, transformational in that they call for new delivery models and new organizational designs. As such, in order for a healthcare organization to support an integrated clinical function, it must undergo change. This change must be led by leadership teams, whose members have a mastery of clinical science, organization and systems theory, and IT. IT is considered within a systems perspective and may be the most significant development in the healthcare system since the Flexner Report, which set the scientific and educational standards for medical education in the twentieth century (Flexner 1910).

Transforming the Corporate Work Processes

Most work related to clinical care is performed by people, not machines. The job is seen as the culmination of how tasks are organized and coordinated and how responsibilities are assigned to individuals. Responsibilities are accomplished by performing tasks, and the tasks make up a job. Jobs are then linked to form the work process. This is the work structure.

Much discussion occurs about adopting robotics and other machine-driven work processes, which eliminate the "job" as the unit of analysis. While robotics is increasingly applied in medicine (such as robotic wheelchairs; robotic dispensing of medication; and surgery assistance, such as the Da Vinci Surgical System), especially for procedures that are well suited to the assumptions of machines, healthcare as a whole will always remain a people-intensive industry. Most work in healthcare organizations is carried out by a range of health professionals, who are interdependent and hold interactions with patients. The question becomes, how can these complex human work processes be standardized but still allow professionals an appropriate amount of decision-making autonomy?

The logic of jobs and work processes is based on many factors, including the nature of the work, the technology that supports the work, and the value of the work's outcomes. Service industries (such as healthcare) differ from product industries (such as car manufacturing) in that in service the value accrues from the work process and the outcome. As healthcare becomes more consumer oriented, the value derived from the clinical process in which the patient is a co-producer is likely to increase. Financing and regulatory mandates are incongruent with this value-enhancing trend of true patient involvement. Patients as co-producers of health will demand that electronic health records become personal health records, which will give patients access to information on health and wellness, their individual DNA profile, and clinical information such as guidelines and level of evidence; it will also enable patients to form social networks around shared medical conditions and experiences. This demand for greater access will outpace the development of such a system, not because of technical limitations but because of the failure to envision and design systems for the future.

Healthcare organizations' accountability for clinical outcomes entails accountability for clinical work processes as well. The focus of process improvement should extend beyond the traditionally structured departments and caregiving units and encompass the entire structure of the clinical process. The phrase "managing the clinical process" is used here with reservation because it is viewed as synonymous with management by departments or by insurance companies and thus raises concerns among health professionals, who have been acculturated in these traditional organizational structures. In fact, many healthcare leaders hold the same outdated view. However, the phrase as applied here points to the design of the clinical process by the clinical teams.

Profound restructuring should be viewed as good news by clinical professionals, but it will be resisted by those who continue to maintain an allegiance to the independent functioning of individual health professionals (Muzio and Kirkpatrick 2011). Nurses and physicians who work in highly structured institutions, such as hospitals, should welcome the change because it is based on the logic of the clinical function and should decrease the tension between the business and patient care sides. Corporate accountability for clinical outcomes should not be viewed as a diabolical scheme of chief executive officers (or left-wing politicians), as many healthcare executives are admittedly similarly unaware of the significance of this transformation and challenged by their ability to lead it. IT enables profound changes in almost every sector of society, such as communications, finance, transportation, corporate collaborations, and global systems. The health system will not be immune from this transforming technology.

In Chapter 4, we discuss changes in the traditional role of health professionals. This role served as the logic for the design of accessing services, receiving and coordinating care, paying for services, and accessing medical information. It is also embedded in the design of formal organizations, health policies, and the extensive regulatory and accreditation systems. In traditional organizations, decisions may be assigned on the basis of the professional's "authority of imputed expertise" (Friedson 1994, 64) or may come from the formal line of authority. Neither form of decision making is totally compatible with patient values and wants. Consequently, when IT follows the same logic, its transforming power is negated.

Research into the effect of health professionals' roles and relationships in the new environment (in the study's case, genomic medicine) has found that competition (likely brought on by traditional views of professional role and identities) between and among professionals negates or neutralizes the advantages offered by this "less-bounded" clinical environment (Currie, Finn, and Martin 2010). This finding highlights the complexity of transforming corporate work processes. That endeavor will almost always encounter or uncover ingrained systems inadequacies and interdisciplinary conflicts and behaviors, which only a full alignment of the organization, clinical, and IT functions may fix. In other words, you cannot reconcile one or two of the components and then ignore the rest.

Work Design Models

Many approaches to designing and coordinating jobs exist, depending on the tasks involved and the technology available to support those tasks. Work design draws on a rich body of evidence (see Ackoff, Magidson, and Addison 2006; Bøllingtoft et al. 2009; Mahesh and Suresh 2009). In his classic book *The Structuring of Organizations*, for example, Henry Mintzberg (1979) offers five approaches to coordinating work—(1) direct supervision, (2) mutual adjustment, (3) standardization of skills, (4) standardization of work processes, and (5) standardization of outcomes. Direct supervision is self-explanatory, and mutual adjustment and standardization are discussed in the next section.

The Industrial Revolution introduced the world to mass production. This industrial work design was characterized by highly structured tasks and coordinated work processes—all performed on assembly lines. Standardization was the key to this efficiency and effectiveness. Worker skills, jobs, work processes, and quality were standardized to ensure consistent outcomes and impose tighter company control. The management structure was hierarchical. Many of the approaches of mass production were effectively applied to the business side of healthcare, including purchasing, maintenance, finance, and human resources. The clinical side, however, have called for less industrialized and mechanistic tactics and more personalized approaches. This has been the clinical function's basis for resisting standardization.

Professional Autonomy Versus Standardization

Clinical decision making and the clinical work process evolved outside the direct purview of the organized environment, and they have been (and continue to be) based on the clinical or health professions logic, not on the business or formal organization logic. As such, individual health professionals have driven the clinical encounter, making medical decisions for the patients and then handing them off to the care of other professionals (either through external referrals or internal handoffs to the next provider in the healthcare continuum). This structure of the clinical encounter has defined how IT systems are designed and function, how providers (hospitals and doctors) are reimbursed for healthcare services, and how other components of the organization work. This clinical work process supports and protects the autonomy of health professionals and their decision making. Thus, clinical process has been separated from the business work processes and the traditional, hierarchical structure of hospitals and clinics.

Healthcare organizations continue to recognize the high degree of autonomy among physicians and other clinicians (as it has been defined and structured traditionally in medicine) and, to a lesser degree, among nurses and allied health professionals. The clinical process has evolved. It now primarily uses two approaches to the coordination of work—standardization of skills and mutual adjustment, both of which are compatible with the professional's autonomy. One needs only to walk into a healthcare facility to observe that standardization of skills is everywhere. Name badges, dress codes, or uniforms visually represent the standard expectations from healthcare workers. Academic degrees, licenses, certifications, credentials, skills, and specialized training are just some of the standard requirements from health professionals who seek employment or medical staff privileges. Work coordination occurs between people on the basis of standardized skill sets.

At the core of this work coordination is mutual adjustment, one of Mintzberg's (1979) approaches. *Mutual adjustment* is the direct interaction through structured communication between two or more people who are trying to accomplish the same goal. In the emergency department (ED), for example, mutual adjustment may occur between the ED doctor and the nurses, the nurses and medical technicians or allied health staff, and the ED doctor and a physician specialist. This communication (which could take place person to person, by telephone, by chart notes, and by secure e-mail) allows parties to exchange explicit as well as tacit knowledge and thus gain mutual understanding on how to approach or solve a problem. Organization theory recognizes the inherent limitation in mutual adjustment—namely, it is very complex to carry out the work process in different locations; across time, such as shift changes and repeat visits; and by workers or professionals with dissimilar skill sets and competencies (Charns and Young 2010). In fact, *To Err Is Human* indicates that handoffs over time, space, and specialty are the most vulnerable points for errors (Kohn, Corrigan, and Donaldson 2000). The reason for this vulnerability is that clinical work processes are defined by the health professionals who perform the tasks, not by the logic of the clinical process itself.

Professional autonomy is based on the assumption that clinical outcomes and processes cannot be standardized. However, this assumption frequently conflicts with the reality of clinical work. This assumption has been increasingly refuted by research studies, policy analyses, and data-intensive reports (see Kohn, Corrigan, and Donaldson 2000; Dartmouth Atlas of Health Care 2012). Professional autonomy also fails to recognize the interdependencies between clinical work and other jobs, many of which have nothing to do with direct caregiving or medical interventions. For example, the tasks of medical coding and revenue cycle management affect the clinical process and rely on standardized reporting. Functions such as housekeeping are part of the process. If rooms and patient-care areas are not cleaned, patient treatment and recuperation are compromised. The case study for this chapter demonstrates this reality.

The structure of the clinical encounter has defined the design and function of the IT system, the reimbursement of hospitals and doctors, and other elements of the healthcare organization. Simply, this historic structure serves as the DNA of the organization and process design and thus its information systems architecture.

Clinical Protocols and Advanced IT

The EMR was designed to improve communications between and among health professionals. As such, the EMR was an automating technology, converting paper medical charts into electronic information and making them easy to store, recall, analyze, and transmit. Designing information strategy around existing clinical decision processes was probably wise for vendors selling IT systems and CEOs trying to implement them because the strategy was minimally intrusive of the professional's decision process. Even with the addition of decision support tools, the EMR was still structured around the traditional role of health professionals. This IT strategy can inhibit innovation in the structure of clinical decision making and reflects a lack of understanding of the transforming power of IT (Zammuto et al. 2007). The delay in applying advanced IT is the result of (1) the complexity of developing essential clinical vocabularies, data standards, and evidence needed for electronic communication of clinical information (see Chapter

2) as well as (2) the failure to view IT as a transforming and not an automating technology.

Information technology has enabled innovation in caregiving. For example, healthcare professionals, working as an integrated team, developed and applied clinical protocols as a guide in postsurgical cases and demonstrated improved clinical outcomes (Zander 1992). These efforts are commendable, given that using standardized work processes, such as clinical protocols, in a traditional institution is difficult in itself. Protocol development and use was facilitated by the protocols' application to surgery, a complex but highly procedural clinical service. Medically complex diseases, such as Type 2 diabetes, are less procedural and rely on multiple health professionals, services, and specialties that one institution alone may not be able to provide. Here, standardization offers the opportunity for work coordination (allowing the disparate processes to synchronize) and for informed clinical decisions (based on the patient's needs and available scientific evidence).

A caveat is in order here. While standardization is necessary, its implementation must be carefully done. Few clinical processes are mechanistic in nature, unlike industrial processes as described earlier. As such, the population-based clinical guidelines and protocols embedded in the decision support system of an EHR cannot be applied in a mechanistic manner. Applying clinical guidelines and protocols within current hierarchical, functional structures increases the risk that decision support systems will be based on overly strict rules, controls, and standard procedures that are mandated by the organization and reinforced by a culture of blame. That is the nature of hierarchical organizations (which are themselves a contrast to organizations in the information age), particularly those with complex work environments and a highly professionalized workforce. If these guidelines and protocols become "institutionalized" (absorbed into the operation as the rigid standards of practice), contextual information, such as unique patient conditions and tacit knowledge shared during team interaction, might be lost. Strictly enforced standardization not only undermines professional autonomy but may also compromise clinical quality. As a result, professional staff will and should resist them—either directly or indirectly. Leadership in transforming clinical processes must come from health professionals who understand the transforming power of IT and the structures required to support that transformation. Such structures will allow clinical decision makers a degree of autonomy in situations where clinical judgment is needed and where the use of advanced IT and standardization can lead to quantifiable improvements.

Knowledge-based Organization

Healthcare leaders must understand that structuring the IT (the decision support system) according to the clinical function entails providing frontline workers with technical training and authority to coordinate work and adapt to changes in the clinical process. In many instances, coordination of work transcends time, location, and profession and is enhanced by the use of an interactive communications system, similar to IBM Dialogue. Informal discussions among professionals and with the patient about diagnosis, treatment, prognosis, and prevention strategies are important for capturing latent and tacit information and converting that information into valuable enterprise knowledge. (This concept is explored in Chapter 8.) Informal communications as the basis for clinical decision support and knowledge-based IT is a fundamental premise of health informatics. As such, work design is flexible, is dynamic, and mimics the health professions' approach to coordinating work rather than the rigid industrial model.[1] The results are dynamic interpretation of clinical outcomes and processes and work carried out by a team of multiple professionals. Some level of decision-making autonomy is possible, but that autonomy comes with expectations of corporate (shared) responsibility and accountability for clinical practices and outcomes.

Healthcare organizations must change their structure and culture to enable knowledge workers (health professionals) to have the motivation, freedom, and skills to coordinate their work; propose innovation; and adapt to change. Rewards for excellent team performance must be given as well. The health system has always recognized that it is a people-intensive industry but did so primarily by concentrating on the number, specialization, and salary and other financial rewards of the professional and nonprofessional staff. A knowledge-based organization, in contrast, increasingly draws on principles of organization behavior to create work environments in which workers are committed, empowered by IT, and part of multidisciplinary teams. (Such environments are discussed in Chapter 10.) In addition, a knowledge-based organization discovers new areas of specialized labor and gives these workers a level of autonomy and freedom to innovate as they work within the organized environment (Muzio, Ackroyd, and Chanlat 2008).

Integrating the Triad: IT, Organizations, and Professions

One might speak of "balancing the triad" when referring to the relationships among IT, organizations, and the health professions, but that phrase casts these three as competing perspectives, where each does not reach an optimum condition. The phrase "integrating the triad" might be more appropriate as it refers to the interdependencies among the three perspectives, where each complements the others and together they elevate the system to a higher level of performance. (*Troika* might be a better term given the Russian origins of the science of informatics.)

Societal change and complex markets have created the necessity for healthcare organizations to develop innovative structures that can be tailored to specific operational demands. Hierarchical functional structures are not well suited for this purpose, and organizations in other sectors have adopted more decentralized, loosely coupled, and self-organizing models (Bushe and Marshak 2009; Yeager and Sorensen 2006). IT played a major transformational role in other industries such as banking, transportation, communications, and supply chain management and achieved much better internal integration than occurred in healthcare. In other chapters we review the evolution of biomedical, nursing, pharmacoinformatics, and other informatics threads and management information systems as separate disciplines. The business side of the health enterprise has adopted IT applications from other sectors, such as supply chain management (Dilts and Zhang 2004; Avery and Swafford 2009; Smith, Nachtmann, and Pohl 2011). Other business areas, such as the revenue cycle, have been slower to innovate, probably because of the traditional perception that measuring costs and managing the revenue cycle and accounts receivable in healthcare do not follow standard accounting principles and financial procedures as other industries do. Why innovation has lagged in healthcare is unclear, although part of the reason may be that the health system is highly professionalized, highly regulated, and heavily subsidized, which tend to favor the status quo. However, recent initiatives to manage the revenue cycle by linking clinical, financial, and insurance data systems do reflect systemic change (Hagland 2011; Gale 2009; Russell 2010). The interdependencies among IT, organizations, and professions are demonstrated by the growing evidence that business functions, such as supply chain management, stimulate change in other areas, including the structure of the clinical function (Sear 2011; Kubick 2009).

As mentioned, significant structural changes are occurring in the clinical function, but much of this transformation is driven by financing, accreditation, and patient demands—not by health professionals. The danger is that restructuring based on the business logic will not optimize clinical performance. Many healthcare leaders continue to view the business and clinical functions separately, even as the two sides have become more interdependent (Brown and Stone 2005; Potash 2011; Banaszak-Holl, Nembhard, and Bradley 2012; Miles 2011). Unilateral change results in retrofitting other areas using faulty logic. For example, the healthcare software company IDX Systems (2012) created software that was based on business logic but detached from IT that was based on clinical logic. With such a system, basic units of analysis such as "Who is the patient?" created confusion because the "patient" from a business perspective was frequently a spouse, parent, or legal guardian who owns the insurance or is responsible for paying the bill; from a clinical perspective, the "patient" is the person who actually receives the service. Early efforts at an "integrated IT" occasionally generated reports that named males as patients in maternity wards because the male was the insured person. This is but one example of the difficulty of integrating two (or more) information systems designed on the basis of conflicting logic.

Community of Practice

Organizations and information systems that follow the logic of clinical protocols shift the structure of the clinical process from individual practitioners to teams. Teams have been traditionally used in healthcare but formed within a given organization or even a clinical department; this is the logic used in establishing medical homes. The development of clinical teams within institutions is an important precursor to redesigning organizations themselves, based on the logic of the clinical process (Borghoff and Schlichter 2000; Faulconbridge et al. 2011). Team membership and function are based on clinical evidence and inherently transform traditional clinical and organization designs.

With the increase in chronic care, the clinical process will continue to transcend organization boundaries. For example, a patient with Type 2 diabetes may require an endocrinologist, family practitioner, advanced practice nurse, social worker, health educator, and a nutritionist. This collection of health professionals constitutes a community of practice. A community of practice is different from a provider-based team in that the community is defined by the nature of the illness and the scientific evidence to treat it, not by professional or organization boundaries. At the center of this community is the patient, and as such, the clinical process is oriented around patient satisfaction and thus high-quality, integrated caregiving (Zoe and Court 2010). Customer satisfaction is a core principle of Deming's work on quality improvement (Alomaim, Sihini Tunca, and Zairi 2003). The community of practice is the unit of analysis and serves as the framework for applying guidelines and protocols for cognitive and behavioral change. The independent variable then is the community of practice, while the dependent variables are patient outcomes, satisfaction, and the efficiency of the clinical process.

With advanced IT, the community of practice can be distributed organizationally and geographically as well as temporally and has demonstrated positive results (Rothschild et al. 2004). A community of practice is a multi-professional team formed according to the clinical process and not dictated by professions or the organization; both the profession and organization then adapt to support this structure. The community is versatile because its membership composition is tailored to meet individual patient needs. Such a structure allows the infusion of the maximum degree of team-based scientific evidence and collective experiential knowledge into the decision-making process. Patients are co-producers, able to participate and bring their input into the decision-making process. Although they do not control the decisions, patients are given the chance to weigh the medical evidence during team interaction and thus are well-informed about changing their own behavior (Kahn, Aulakh, and Bosworth 2009). Here, "patient compliance" is transformed to "patient participation."

Information Architecture

The framework of information systems based on enterprise strategy—that is designed according to the logic of the clinical function—becomes the superstructure that supports both organization and professional IT. "Superstructure" does not mean an imposing, monolithic power; rather, it refers to a solid IT foundation that makes loosely configured but tailored and dynamic information systems work seamlessly and in unison. This requires health professionals to come together to define clinical protocols for treating complex clinical cases. Professionals who practice in teams, working beyond individual professional boundaries, must adopt new behaviors that are often different from those they learned from and fostered by their profession's socialization (Friedson 1994; Muzio and Kirkpatrick 2011; Zoe and Court 2010; Noordegraff 2011; Anderson et al. 2011). In addition, organizations must avoid the danger of replacing behavior by eliminating professional autonomy and mandating rules and regulations (Timmons 2011).

The ACA might provide the opportunity to create interorganizational communities of practice (US Congress 2010). Specifically, the legislation calls for the creation of accountable care organizations, which are essential for managing the care processes. The question is whether new corporate designs will emerge or if old structures, values, and philosophies will simply be linked together and repurposed as new, to which we caution, "you can't build a skyscraper by nailing together doghouses." Building new organizational models requires innovation, risk taking, and a systems perspective. The ACA sets forth a plethora of rules and regulations, many of which could negate the potential of these new corporate entities.

Currently, the US healthcare system is at a confluence of poorly designed clinical processes and poorly structured organizations and financing systems. Compounding this problem is the overlay of information systems designed on the logic of dysfunctional and disparate perspectives. It is little wonder that conflict, stress, poor quality, and lack of continuity exist. The good news is that both knowledge and technology exist to help leaders make needed improvements in all areas—from quality, safety, and patient satisfaction to financing, accreditation, and regulation and beyond. Maintaining and improving old structures are simply inadequate for current and future demands.

Conclusion

The dominant organizational structure continues to be based on the logic of the traditional, hierarchical business function, although many organizations have begun the complex work of restructuring.

The healthcare sector differs from the product industry and, to some degree, from other entities in the service industry. Patient care is highly personal and is imbued by many disciplines such as medicine, finance and economics, organizational science, religion, and sociology. Because illness and health needs are different from one person to the next, the responsibility for caregiving has been assigned to health professionals, who are trained to manage the variation and provide highly personalized care. This factor remains an important consideration in the design of future systems. However, the chronic nature of diseases coupled with the power of advanced IT provides healthcare organizations an opportunity to expand this caregiving approach to a systems-based structure in which the business, clinical, and IT functions are integrated to enable better work coordination and thus better patient outcomes. The field of medical informatics supports the traditional structure of clinical decision making and work processes (Stead 2005). This is a complex and important science that serves as a foundation for further healthcare system transformation. Health informatics extends medical IT to include clinical and organization IT systems. In doing so, it transforms clinical and public health informatics and helps achieve optimal systems outcomes.

Chapter Discussion Questions

1. Give some examples of the increased presence and influence of corporations on clinical practice in the US healthcare system.
2. What has been the dominant organizational structure in healthcare, and how has it affected how clinical services are delivered within organizations and/or across the healthcare system?
3. How did IT facilitate the federal policy shift to hold healthcare organizations accountable for clinical outcomes and thus clinical processes?
4. How did payment by DRG alter the organizational accountability for clinical outcomes and the way cost information in hospitals was gathered and analyzed?
5. What is a community of practice? How might it be structured, including the role of IT, to manage chronic care?

Note

1. Rigid production models have also given way to dynamic models of production and distribution.

> **CASE STUDY** | **Transforming the Clinical Process at Farmington Endoscopy Center**

William C. Kinney

Transforming the clinical work process in healthcare is not going to be a simple task, as many of today's work solutions are rooted in decades-long and even century-old autonomous and hierarchical structures. As mentioned in the chapter, Paul Starr's *The Social Transformation of American Medicine* explained how US healthcare evolved into a system that separates the business side and clinical side of care delivery. Separating the two functions ultimately created two diverging approaches, leaving the patient caught in the middle. Regulations from both the insurance industry and federal government are trying to bring the two sides together in the interest of what is best for the healthcare system as a whole. The IOM's reports on medical quality highlighted the inefficiencies and mistakes that resulted from the increased complexity of healthcare. Although IT exists to change the system, it has lacked the leadership and skills needed to bring about a redesign that, in turn, could transform existing processes and structures.

The IOM reports and subsequent analyses have highlighted IT as a tool to improve quality and efficiency. Clinical decision support system (CDSS), in particular, has been identified as a priority health IT, as it pushes evidence-based health recommendations that lead not only to better clinical processes, quality, and outcomes but also to lower healthcare costs. The challenge in adopting CDSS is determining where and how to apply the evidence.

This case highlights the use of health IT to transform the clinical and business processes. Readers should take note of who the relevant players are, the information needs in care delivery, and the method of leveraging information to make care delivery more efficient and effective.

Farmington Endoscopy Center

Farmington is a Midwest college town with a population of more than 100,000 and a large and productive medical community supported by a local medical school. The medical community serves not only the residents of Farmington but also the residents of the surrounding rural communities, some of whom drive more than two hours to get to their respective clinic or hospital. The limited number of primary care physicians who work in rural settings, lack of supporting facilities, and varying socioeconomic backgrounds all add to the complexities of rural medicine. Rural communities also have few manufacturers and corporations that hire employees and provide employer-sponsored, private health insurance. This leaves many rural patients no choice but to enroll in government-supported healthcare programs.

Farmington Endoscopy Center (FEC) is a freestanding, physician-owned endoscopy facility that serves both adult and pediatric patients. The main procedures—esophagogastroduodenoscopy (EGD) and colonoscopy—are performed by six gastroenterologist (the owners). Last year, it completed almost 5,000 cases, and this year it is anticipating a 5 percent growth in volume by adding a new physician. FEC is owned and managed by the physicians, but a full-time administrator is in charge of day-to-day operations, compliance with state and federal safety/accountability standards, billing and collections, and staffing. Rounding out the staff are eight nurses, four receptionists, one billing specialist, and one certified registered nurse anesthetist (CRNA).

Patients are referred to FEC for an endoscopy procedure by the six physicians, each of whom runs a separate outpatient clinic, or by independent primary care or specialty physicians. The independent primary or specialty care physician assumes patient-management responsibilities for the results of the endoscopy, so the gastroenterologist who performs the procedure is essentially a technician whose responsibility to the patient ends at the completion of the procedure. Both EGD and colonoscopy are not painful, but they are uncomfortable and thus require sedation. Administered by the CRNA, sedation techniques range from applying topical anesthetic to running an intravenous line of light anesthesia (where the patient stays awake and can communicate) or a heavy dose of anesthesia (where the patient is unconscious and could stop breathing and may need respiratory support). The CRNA is licensed by the state but cannot act as an independent provider and must be under the close supervision of the gastroenterologist. Throughout the procedure, the gastroenterologist is ultimately responsible for the patient's well-being.

Areas of Improvement

Susan Michaels, the FEC administrator, is reviewing last year's reports to find ways to increase volume. Both private and public insurance have changed their rules, resulting in lower reimbursements. Meanwhile, healthcare costs continue to rise, further cutting into profits. Needless to say, the FEC physician owners are concerned. Susan identifies two problem areas in the reports:

(continued)

1. The center has a day-of-procedure cancellation rate of 8 to 12 percent. These patients show up for their scheduled procedure only to be cancelled by the clinic because of some factors that were not known before their arrival. The top-five factors are blood-thinner usage, unidentified cardiovascular risk, failure to adhere to NPO (latin for "nil per os," which means no food or drink hours before a procedure), improper guardianship, and lack of bowel prep.

2. Regulations have doubled the amount of required paperwork to be completed for each patient. Explanation of patient rights and privacy policies, medication-reconciliation process, deep venous thrombosis evaluation, and complication reporting are just some of the tasks or forms that must be completed before a case can be closed. The planned addition of another physician to the practice would increase the number of cases, exacerbating the paperwork problem. Susan is considering hiring another nurse to help the existing staff with the workload, a move that would enable the FEC to accommodate more patients and complete the paperwork quicker.

Fortunately, Susan just returned from a health IT workshop that presented a new logic and tools for how to define the dimensions of a problem and derive workable solutions.

Information Needs

Evaluating and managing patient health needs is about acquiring information and making a decision based on that information. A wise physician once stated that 90 percent of the information a physician consults to arrive at a diagnosis is contained in the patient's medical history. Much of today's health IT efforts pay attention to the physician's information needs for two reasons: (1) The doctor is ultimately responsible for healthcare evaluation and management, and (2) the doctor gets paid based on a certain level of information she gathers. A careful review of current EMRs shows that information is maintained in vertical silos or "buckets" and based on billing and collection needs. Information is compartmentalized and cannot be shared easily among all players in the care delivery process. Compartmentalization also hinders the use of the information and masks the time-sensitive value of that information. Time, in this case, is chronologic and pertains to information that must be gathered and acted upon before an event.

In the case of scheduled procedures, decisions need to be made days before the encounter. Anticoagulation therapy, for example, is information that must be relayed before a patient's appointed surgery or intervention. Appropriately managing anticoagulation is not necessarily straightforward, and a new healthcare player (e.g., a cardiologist) may need more information or guidance. CDSS can ensure that relevant patient information, research evidence, and best practice are available at the right time, a system that is infinitely valuable to a freestanding endoscopy center or ambulatory surgery center.

Information Gathering Process for an Integrated IT

Susan decides to use IT to address FEC's two problems. She identifies the information needs of each player (i.e., physicians, CRNA, and nurses), and then she breaks down the problems into components to better understand the clinical processes and find ways to integrate them to improve efficiencies and patient satisfaction. The ultimate goal is to create a sophisticated data-capture and management IT with an integrated CDSS. The steps she takes are as follows:

1. List each team member involved in an endoscopy procedure. Does the team composition change according to who initiated the patient referral? What steps do the physicians follow to refer patients to FEC? The referring physicians' information needs must be considered so that a better request-for-procedure ordering process can be developed.

2. List the information needs of each team member, including the supporting players who perform billing, collections, and other administrative tasks. Here are a few examples of these needs:

   • The gastroenterologist needs to know why the patient is there. Is this a screening colonoscopy because of a family history of colon cancer? Is this a patient with anemia and guaiac-positive stools?
   • The nurse needs to know if the patient had surgery in the last 30 days, as this increases the patient's risk of deep venous thrombosis. The nurse also needs a current list of medications to complete the medication-reconciliation process.
   • The CRNA needs to know if the patient is taking an angiotensin-converting enzyme inhibitor. Current recommendations are for patients to not take this medication on the morning of a procedure. The CRNA must know the patient's cardiac history and be

(continued)

able to identify potential risk factors that would affect the patient's choice of sedation.

- The referring physician needs a system for telling the FEC gastroenterologist, nurses, and CRNA information on the patient, including tests, medications, and risk factors, that could affect the patient's ability to receive the procedure on the day it is scheduled.
- Scheduling needs to know which patients are scheduled for what procedure and how long the procedure is estimated to take. Scheduling staff is responsible for reminding the patient of the appointment time, date, and any preparation (such as the NPO).
- Registration needs to know the patient's demographic and social status. Is the patient a minor? Who will be present to sign the consent? If the child is in foster care, does FEC need to obtain a court order to do the procedure? If the patient is an adult, is he of sound mind and body, or does he have a legal guardian?
- Procedure room nurses need to know the capability of supplies and equipment to meet the needs of the patient. Is the patient wheelchair bound, and if so, should more time be added to the schedule? Does the patient have an artificial joint, as this will affect where the electrocautery grounding pad is placed?

3. Construct a timeline of the information needs across the encounter.
4. Identify overlapping information needs between players.

As a final step, Susan determines the time component of each information need to ensure that it is available at the appropriate time, which could reduce cancellations. Susan considers available consumer technology, such as the Internet, smart phones, and apps, to enhance the IT option. Susan also looks into outsourcing.

A successful health IT solution for FEC results in a significant reduction in cancellation rates and in a faster or same-day completion of the administrative, regulatory, and nursing paperwork. Such improvements enable FEC to schedule more patients and complete more procedures.

Case Study Discussion Questions

1. Assume the role of Susan Michaels. Follow the steps she has laid out to identify FEC's areas of concern and the information needs of every player in the clinic.
2. What other information needs can you think of that may be entered into a CDSS?
3. Develop a model for reducing the cancelation rate for FEC procedures.

KNOWLEDGE-BASED CLINICAL DECISION MAKING

8

Gordon D. Brown, Kalyan S. Pasupathy, and Mihail Popescu

Learning Objectives

After reading this chapter, students should be able to

- Identify the four types of knowledge, and apply them to the clinical decision process
- Describe and apply the principles of knowledge management to the clinical decision process
- Define the essential features of knowledge-based decision support systems
- Apply levels of knowledge related to different types of knowledge-based decision support
- Articulate the influence of different types or levels of health system transformation on the structure of the clinical function

---

KEY CONCEPTS

- Knowledge management
- Explicit, implicit, latent, and tacit knowledge
- Evidence-based clinical decisions
- Knowledge socialization
- Innovation and system transformation
- Translational and transformational research

Introduction

Several forces contribute to the dynamics and complexity of health information systems. Basic and clinical sciences that inform clinical decisions have
exponentially grown. Equally, advances in the information, systems, and
social sciences are revealing the interdependencies among clinicians, institutions, and social sectors and the ways to manage these interdependencies.
Meanwhile, the complexity and dynamics of the healthcare environment itself
makes capturing and presenting all available knowledge difficult (Geisler and

Wickramasinghe 2009). This knowledge, which informs clinical and organizational decisions, consists of both scientific and experiential or judgment knowledge. Evidence-based knowledge is derived from scientific analysis, while experiential knowledge or judgment comes from interactions about and within a given work process. Judgments here are based on values and accumulated experience of the decision makers. Information technology (IT) enables knowledge capture and management but does not create knowledge on its own. Knowledge generation and application in clinical decision making should serve as the logic for designing IT systems.

The typical strategy of a well-led healthcare organization is to enlist all available assets to improve its competitive positioning and achieve excellence. One of these assets is the institutional knowledge detailed in documents, rules, policies, processes, and the like along with the specialties, inarticulated wisdom, and experiences of health professionals and high-performing employees. This knowledge asset, particularly in highly professionalized service sectors such as healthcare, complements and potentially outweighs other assets, such as land, labor, and capital (Isaac, Herremans, and Kline 2009; Carlucci and Schiuma 2007). Information and knowledge, unlike all other assets, is not depleted as it is consumed but instead increases in value and can be leveraged.

The information age requires leaders to adopt new assumptions about how professionals and organizations function. When considering the value of IT, leaders must look at its fluidity, which enables the knowledge assets of multiple organizations to be strategically aligned. Multiorganization collaboration is possible with formal but loosely configured IT systems that are flexible enough to be tailored to fit different situations. Information-enabled systems have considerable potential to improve healthcare services and bring about superior outcomes because they are highly integrated, tailored to individual patient conditions, and efficient. These characteristics are reflected in the language of the Patient Protection and Affordable Care Act (US Congress 2010).

This chapter discusses knowledge management within organizations and in communities of practice. Knowledge-based IT transcends organizational boundaries by enabling the formation of loosely configured multiprofessional teams and multi-institutional systems.

Definition and Use of Knowledge in Decision Making

Knowledge management is broadly applied in several fields, and its definition varies depending on how it is applied. In this chapter, we use the context of clinical and managerial decision making and thus use this definition by Lee (2000):

A discipline that promotes an integrated approach to identifying, managing, and sharing all of an enterprise's information needs. These information assets may include data bases, documents, policies, and procedures as well as previously unarticulated expertise and experience resident in individual workers.

Harnessing all of the knowledge assets of an organization requires the deployment of advanced IT and constitutes a core function of health informatics. As discussed in Chapter 1, health informatics comprises information derived from bioinformatics as well as imaging, clinical, and public health informatics—all of which are incorporated with the concepts of open systems, organization theory, and engineering and behavioral sciences. Each science brings knowledge, whose application is altered and enhanced by advanced IT. Health informatics then adds to an organization's knowledge management, enabling the transformation of clinical work processes by helping professionals use clinical and biological knowledge more effectively. The measure of the effective utilization of existing knowledge is outcomes, including patient wellness, service coordination, clinical quality and safety, and system efficiency.

Knowledge Organization

Knowledge organizations are information-oriented organizations that focus on creating change through innovation, not on adapting to change. This concept was introduced by Senge (1990, 14) as an organization involved in "generative learning" and not "adaptive learning," saying that through learning "we expand our capacity to create, to be part of the generative process of life." The knowledge organization concept was broadly applied and institutionalized in the 1990s. Such wide adoptions of the concept suggest a tendency of institutions to adopt because of external pressures (e.g., accreditation or regulation) or because of a desire to be trendy by self-identifying as a knowledge organization without understanding its basic principles (Arndt and Bigelow 2000). Regardless of adopters' reasoning, knowledge is a powerful strategic asset in an environment that ceaselessly demands clinical quality and accountability but has limited resources (Brown, Stone, and Patrick 2005).

A knowledge organization is characterized by a culture and management structure that is different from those of traditional, hierarchical institutions. In a knowledge organization, senior executives engage in more innovative and creative pursuits, involving health professionals and other knowledge workers. Health professionals are highly valued, but their level of individual independence is subsumed by collaborative work, structured as loosely configured, adaptable, tailored, and creative work teams. In this era of rapid knowledge generation, new health professions (such as genetics nurses) will be spawned and must become effective members of the team. The health professions alone tend to be protective of knowledge domains and to be reluctant to accept new professionals coming in as colleagues (Muzio, Ack-royd, and Chanlat 2008).

A control-oriented organization that pursues a knowledge strategy must first understand the power of a committed culture and then be able to create it (Khatri et al. 2006). Many leaders may conclude that culture does not make a difference, but in fact these leaders lack an understanding of this complex concept and how to forge it (see Chapter 10). Multiple and interrelated dimensions of knowledge management make it complex to understand and apply. Thus, there is a need to understand how decision processes, particularly clinical decision support, are contained in knowledge-based systems, but a more pertinent concern may be how current decision processes can be changed by these systems.

Knowledge organizations recognize the power of IT as they seek to transform their mission, structure, processes, and culture. Becoming a knowledge organization is not the end point, however; rather, it is an aspiration on a journey that may never really be completed, as new technologies and approaches emerge all the time. Healthcare organizations that are implementing an electronic medical record (EMR), electronic health record (EHR), or information exchange without recognizing and committing to the transforming power of IT have not yet started on this journey.

The Principles of Knowledge Management

Considerable exploration and evidence are available that support the application of knowledge management (see Robey, Boudreau, and Rose 2000; Lemieux-Charles and Champagne 2004; Carlucci and Schiuma 2007). Knowledge management has been co-opted in the data-information-knowledge-wisdom (or traditional) paradigm, where data are the most basic element and when aggregated can form information, some of which is distilled into knowledge. Computers are most effective at data processing and deriving useful (and nonuseful) information. At the highest level, knowledge is created and stored as wisdom in the minds of individuals and maybe computers.

Multiple perspectives exist on how knowledge is generated and shared, including (1) ideas are created in the minds of individuals, (2) knowledge comes from observing and analyzing human experiences (empiricists), and (3) linguistics is the building block of knowledge and learning. The empirical school of thought serves as the foundation for the development of computers as a technology for storing and processing large volumes of data (Geisler and Wickramasinghe 2009). The linguistics perspective emerged with the computer, which uses the logic of language as the basis for information and knowledge sharing (see Chapter 2). The value of computer technology increases according to its application, migrating from a backroom data-processing tool to a mechanism for retrieving and analyzing operations to an information system that performs complex computations to generate knowledge.

The traditional paradigm assumes that organizations have static structures with rapid-processing information systems made possible by sophisticated IT. Health informatics also supports the transformation of the structure of decision processes and the design of the organization itself. This focus emphasizes the importance of conceptualizing the nature of the problem being addressed in framing the need for information and data. Knowledge that comes from information and data contrasts with knowledge that defines the type and form of information and data needed to be gathered and analyzed. The latter perspective views the organization as being knowledge driven and not data driven. The reality is that knowledge is a two-way dialectic and thus a dynamic system.

Types of Knowledge

The science of clinical decision making relies on *explicit knowledge,* which is derived from research and science and is presented as measurements, relationships, and evidence for decision support. This knowledge can be generated from data files or the minds of individuals and can be expressed when needed. The art of clinical decision making, on the other hand, relies on other types of knowledge—*implicit, latent,* and *tacit*—stored in the memories and displayed by the creative capacity of individuals; this kind of knowledge has not been (and much of which cannot be) captured in text and data files (Nonaka and Takeuchi 1995). This natural knowledge includes practical knowledge, intuitive knowledge and wisdom, and expert reasoning (Lemieux-Charles and Champagne 2004, 1–17). Exhibit 8.1 defines each of the four types of knowledge that operate in healthcare organizations.

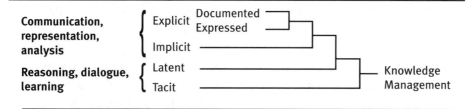

EXHIBIT 8.1
Types of Knowledge in Healthcare Organizations

Explicit ⌐Documented: Data, text, and other information stored in files, reports, etc.
       └Expressed: Information presented verbally or symbolically
Implicit: Not expressed but communicated and understood
Latent*: Present or existing, but in an underdeveloped form and not communicated
Tacit*: Hidden from the consciousness of the knower

Note: *Latent and tacit knowledge when discovered are converted to explicit knowledge.

Explicit knowledge is the focal area of clinical decision support system (CDSS). CDSS has the capacity to search, retrieve, and structure information, drawing on a vast reservoir of scientific evidence. Chapter 4 discusses the important consideration of the level of evidence and the science that supports CDSS. Certainly, much scientific evidence can be structured and presented within the clinical decision process, although not all of the existing evidence is captured. Only a portion of the explicit knowledge in most information systems is actually accessed, analyzed, and applied. Neither can the scientific understanding possessed by individual clinicians be totally encapsulated and entered into the CDSS or any form of IT. Information systems are primarily decision support and not decision making in nature. Clearly, the basic and clinical sciences bring new knowledge from the bench to the bedside at such a fast pace that CDSS can assist clinicians by incorporating the best available evidence in the decision-making process.

In the area of implicit knowledge, much information is communicated and understood within clinical teams but is never expressed. One needs only to observe a surgical procedure to understand the nonverbal communication that takes place among highly skilled clinical teams. Conceiving a method by which all of the available knowledge could be duplicated through data or information charts is difficult, although standard protocols such as checklists have reduced clinical errors by improving communications and by drawing on a broader knowledge base (Haynes et al. 2009). The restructuring of the clinical decision process in this instance might have implications on system efficiency, patient satisfaction, staffing quality, and surgical and other procedural outcomes.

Latent and tacit knowledge cannot be expressed, except through interaction with other humans who help frame issues, develop new mental models, generate new solution strategies, and engage in innovative thinking. Although considered as the art of decision making, these two types of knowledge draw on the science that supports each profession involved in the problem solving as well as on these professionals' collective experiential knowledge. There is great variability in the degree of involvement of multiple professions and the level of scientific evidence available, depending on the nature of the disease and whether the focus is on prevention or treatment. Clinical decision making that includes multiple professionals, each of whom brings his or her own scientific insight and understanding of the decision-making process, is complex. This acknowledges the human, social, and scientific aspects of knowledge within a clinical setting where communication becomes highly interactive (Thomas, Kellogg, and Erickson 2001). The nature of the problem being analyzed thus determines who is involved and the decision-making process.

For complex decisions, the greater the number of professions involved, the greater the understanding of the problem and the more scientific and experiential knowledge is brought into the decision-making process. This expands the total object field (which is perceived and considered) and the total evoked memory on which it draws (which in turn stimulates insight and innovation).

Knowledge Socialization

The concept of *knowledge socialization* recognizes human interaction as a means of conceptualizing new and innovative solution strategies. Nonaka and Takeuchi (1995, 65) define knowledge socialization as "a process of sharing experiences and thereby creating tacit knowledge such as shared mental models and technical skills." These problem-solving models transcend the mechanistic models assumed in applying scientific knowledge to clinical decision making (see Chapters 4 and 5).

Knowledge socialization supports the use of multidisciplinary teams, including the patient, in clinical settings. Knowledge of clinical condition and treatment approaches in team settings is elicited from each member on the basis of the relevant technical knowledge the team member can bring to the case. Relevance can be only assessed by the team—when it holds an open dialogue with its members about each person's professional expertise. Knowledge socialization seems to limit the degree to which clinical teams can function in different locations and at different times. However, the use of interactive communication software, such as IBM's Dialogue, enables team members to engage in dialogue over time and space (IBM 2006). Such interaction is based on the highly regarded Boem Dialogue, designed to extract tacit and implicit information through a rigorous, structured process (Thomas, Kellogg, and Erickson 2001). This technology enables highly skilled, expert professionals to form as a highly interactive team and function within a distributed community of practice whose culture thrives on teamwork and collaboration. The dialogue includes the patient and has the potential to improve decision making, problem solving, and patient compliance (which would evolve into the concept of "patient as co-producer").

The Community of Practice and Quality Improvement

The community of practice restructures the clinical process and provides considerable potential to improve quality and outcomes. Quality improvement techniques, such as Six Sigma, are frequently applied to departments or micro units, which are then bundled to form the clinical work process. However, system failure occurs in the process of bundling and the handoffs among clinicians and departments involved in the clinical process. Quality improvement techniques applied to the macro clinical process—not to individual practices, departments, or institutions—have been demonstrated to work, as they do in other service industries (Harris 2006; Margolis et al. 2009; Yang et al. 2012).

Clinical decision processes structured to involve all parties with scientific and experiential knowledge relevant to the treatment process are consistent with the principles of knowledge management. The mix of scientific and experiential evidence and the contributions of each profession in the process will be tested over time on the basis of optimal outcomes. Communities of practice can serve as the structural framework for federally mandated accountable care organizations and follow the principles of health maintenance, quality outcomes, patient satisfaction, and system efficiency. Linking organizations and clinicians within current structures of the clinical decision process will achieve suboptimal outcomes. A community of practice is a dynamic concept that is based on a collective or corporate work process but retains elements of professional autonomy. However, lack of training in IT and systems theory might limit the clinicians' ability to do so. They will need to work with organization leaders to create the vision and process for applying the best clinical and organization knowledge.

The Application of Knowledge Management

Knowledge management touches many facets of the healthcare organization. Decision support at the operations level has, historically, consisted of data-processing applications (Brown, Stone, and Patrick 2005). Thus, computer-supported decision making tends to be mechanistic in nature and applied historically at the operations level to repetitive decisions, primarily the business function. Meanwhile, clinical and complex enterprise and strategic management decisions relied on the information from databases and the knowledge (a combination of expert reasoning, intuition, and scientific analysis of research) of clinicians and organization leaders, respectively.

The application of IT as a communication science has increased attention to knowledge generation and management in general and the clinical domain in particular. Data on a patient's history, diagnostic tests, and treatment regimens can be integrated into the EMR and brought to the decision process as explicit knowledge. Information can be generated from the data and text files stored in an EMR and then transmitted as part of an information exchange to other parties by fax, e-mail, phone, or an integrated information system. The power of computers to record, store, retrieve, and report data is considerable once the issues of standardization, measurement, and relationships have been resolved (as discussed in Chapter 2).

Many operations/administrative-level staff members have viewed IT more as a data-processing rather than as a knowledge management mechanism. They do not recognize that the ability to access, integrate, and analyze data from disparate databases brings immense value to the decision-making process. This capability enables leaders and managers to generate a range of dashboard indicators as they measure, monitor, and manage performance (Nelson 2010). Much of this value, however, has not been realized because of social and technical impediments, including data mining and other analytical models applied to existing clinical and business databases. (These technical impediments are explored in Chapter 9.) Social impediments include silo thinking (where managers and clinicians view problems within the context of professional, functional, or operational silos and do not recognize the interdependencies between these silos) and concerns about privacy and security (which are discussed in Chapter 13).

Explicit knowledge contained in EMRs can be quickly and comprehensively gathered and reported to clinical decision makers. Clinical guidelines and protocols (traditionally stored in the memories of clinicians) also can be embedded in the EHR to provide additional scientific information. Capturing such knowledge without delay is crucial because much of it leaves the organization when the individual who possesses it moves on to other pursuits.

As mentioned, organizations are increasingly held accountable for clinical outcomes, such as the process measures mandated or recommended by The Joint Commission, the Centers for Medicare and Medicaid Services (see CMS 2011), and other regulatory bodies. These process measures are evidence based and thus can be justified and supported by public and organizational policy decisions. However, quality measured in terms of process indicators inherently view decision making from the micro perspective. When improvements in micro processes are considered collectively, they do not necessarily amount to macro-level optimization or offer a systems solution. As discussed in Chapter 4, we can optimize the performance of the emergency department in treating kids with asthma, but that does not address the question of why kids with asthma are being treated in the emergency department. Again, health informatics is a systems science and thus draws from all available and relevant knowledge, not just the knowledge of an individual, a department, or an organization.

Framework for Understanding Knowledge in the Context of Decision Making

Knowledge management does not provide a formula or prescription for clinical and organizational decision making. Rather, it presents a conceptual framework for understanding the dimensions of knowledge and how they can be used as the basis for evaluating different facets or concepts of what constitutes organizational performance. Knowledge-based decision support systems can be the basis for evaluating the structure of the clinical function, including who should be involved in the decision-making process based on what science each participant can bring to the process. Knowledge represents the accumulation of all that can be known about a patient's condition and effective treatment; it is not limited to individual institutional or professional contributions.

In this section, we explore the interrelationships among (1) knowledge, as the basis for assessing the potential contribution of (2) information technology (e.g., EMR, EHR), measured against (3) the structure of healthcare organizations and health professions and (4) system performance. Our premise assumes that all available knowledge should be used to achieve demonstrably optimum patient health outcomes and thus patient satisfaction. Exhibit 8.2 shows a model for conceptualizing the complex interrelationships among knowledge, IT, and systems structure. While information systems enable and support the transformation of clinical decision making, they do not cause the transformation. This requires changes in how the structure of decision making is conceptualized and changes in decision-making behavior. Information systems can thus be considered as a necessary but not sufficient condition. Similarly, the logic of information systems does not serve as the basis for the design of the clinical decision-making process; rather, it is adapted to that design. The design of the clinical decision process is based on the logic of process–outcome relationships, drawing on all of the data, information, and knowledge that can be accessed.

As clinical information systems become more sophisticated and widely used, the volume of clinical trials and other science-based reports, protocols, reminders and alerts, and other decision support tools will increase. This proliferation may mean that these decision support tools embedded in the IT could become more intrusive on the clinical decision-making process. To a degree, this intrusion can be justified, as evidence clearly indicates it ushers in an improvement in clinical outcomes and system performance (discussed in Chapter 4). The danger is that more sophisticated information systems might become inappropriately invasive of the clinical decision process if the logic of IT design is based on prescriptive rules of the traditional organization, where the tools are institutionalized and rigidly enforced (see Chapters 4 and 7).

Organizations have pursued many approaches to institutionalize guidelines and protocols, such as conducting training programs with a rational–empirical approach, which assumes that the more the users know how to use the tools the more they will accept and use those tools. These programs frequently fail because simply knowing how to use the tools does not make users more accepting and less resistant if they assume a change in the structure and behavior in the organization. What is needed is normative change, where users change their behavior according to demonstrated improvement in outcomes. Behavioral changes are frequently forced in traditional organizations, sought through coercive means, institutional mandates, financial incentives, and other controls. Such approaches cannot be justified as the means of changing decision-making behavior and will be and should be resisted by health professionals. Early approaches to implementing guidelines and protocols were not well informed and lacked a basic understanding of the relationship between the science of medicine and the practice of medicine that leads to superior clinical outcomes (Sonnad 1998). Knowledge management, in contrast, frames the issues of the art and the science of medicine, nursing, and other health professions and defines the proper role of organizations in creating a supportive clinical environment and an information system that enables that environment.

A plethora of information and knowledge exists on the business side of the enterprise, in areas of markets, workflow, productivity, utilization, staffing, budgeting, finance, and so on. These are structured to optimize the business function, primarily to boost financial performance and health outcomes (4 in Exhibit 8.2) but within a clinical function, based on the logic of the business function and professional role of physicians (2 in Exhibit 8.2, representing the existing structure of the system). As discussed, IT (3 in Exhibit 8.2) is based on the logic of the existing structure of the system but in part is based on its own technical logic. Information and knowledge about evidence-based clinical outcomes can, however, provide evidence-based management solutions for improving organization design. Thus far, the clinical data embedded in information systems have been a relatively untapped source of knowledge. Knowledge management should be considered from

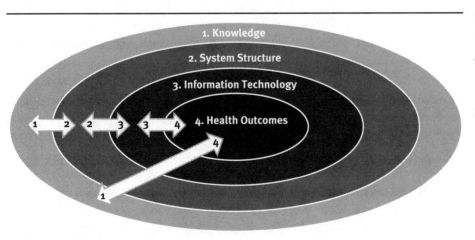

EXHIBIT 8.2
Interrelationship Among Knowledge, IT, and System Structure

the perspective of a dynamic system. Knowledge informs and enables changes in clinical decisions, decision processes, and the structure and culture of the organization.

A Systems Perspective of Knowledge Management

The first step in designing a strategy for knowledge-based decision making is to identify the level of knowledge needed to inform the decision process; the level of knowledge will define the needed IT and appropriate organization design. The existing design, IT, patterns of practice, and values of the organization frequently limit the level of knowledge incorporated into decision making. The justification for applying knowledge to clinical decisions is knowledge's ability to improve clinical outcomes, patient participation, and system performance. Many levels of knowledge can be used to inform decisions, all of which can positively affect system performance.

Selecting the level of knowledge depends on the aspiration of leaders, available resources, strategic orientation, market, and values of the organization. Resources include external forces, such as how services are reimbursed and regulatory mandates are applied. Clinicians and organizations cannot be expected to disregard their own individual performance in favor of optimizing system performance. However, their leaders may be asked to engage in the policy debate and participate in designing innovative knowledge-based IT that demonstrates how knowledge enhances clinical performance, patient satisfaction, and organizational efficiency.

Frontline clinical workers and visionary leaders are the greatest sources of real innovation. Some healthcare organizations have established centers of innovation to address and showcase how system transformation can be introduced into existing operations (see Kaiser Permanente 2012; CITIH 2012; Mayo Clinic 2012). Public policies and regulations can follow and support innovation, but they are not the most effective in leading it. Similarly, IT is essential in the change process when tailored to a knowledge strategy but on its own should not be expected to produce the change in knowledge-based decision making. The organization must view its IT not merely as a technical tool but also as a valued resource to support the transformation of decision processes and organization design. This orientation differentiates the concept of health informatics from that of information technology.

Four Types of Knowledge-based Decision Support

Knowledge-based clinical decision support is transformative in two ways. First, it can change clinical decision behavior and outcomes within the existing organizational structure ($1 \rightarrow 4$ effect in Exhibit 8.2). Second, it can change the basic structure of the organization and the clinical decision process ($1 \rightarrow 2$ effect). Knowledge-based IT systems might be conceptualized as consisting of four types of IT structure, each of which represents a layer of knowledge that informs and transforms the decision process. The first three types (EMR, HIE, and EHR) can change clinical decision making primarily within existing structures (they do not preclude changes in system structure and do not require it). The fourth (PHR) is transformational in nature.

All types function in an interrelated manner, but each imposes a different demand on the institution and its clinical decision support IT. The value contribution or marginal benefit of each type depends on the nature of the decision being made, the experience of the decision-making unit, and the aspiration of the organization. Each type may be considered as a stage or level in the decision support development, where leaders build and add information capacity to accommodate current (actual) and future (anticipated) needs.

Type 1: Electronic Medical Record

The most basic type of knowledge support is gathering, integrating, and reporting all patient-specific information. This explicit information may be obtained from clinical support areas throughout the organization, such as laboratory, radiology, and pharmacy, as well as from medical histories and existing databases (see Exhibit 8.3, EMR). Such data have been used by clinicians for decades—only they were recorded in paper medical charts.

Converting written records into digital format (the EMR) is a complex process (see Chapter 2). Once accomplished, however, digitized clinical data can be accessed, stored, integrated, analyzed, and reported by and to anyone who needs the information and can be tailored according to the user's

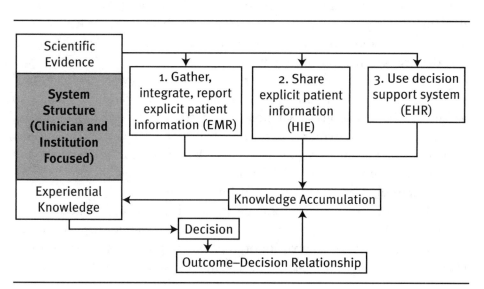

EXHIBIT 8.3
Traditional Structure of Knowledge-based Clinical Decision Process

preferred format. The EMR is a basic form of decision support, but it alone does not constitute a knowledge-based organization. Data on a patient's condition, treatment, and history that are complete, accurate, up-to-date, and compiled and presented in usable form contribute to change in clinical decision-making behavior and, in turn, improve clinical outcomes (Hillstad et al. 2005). In its most basic form, the EMR digitizes and automates the paper medical record. Digitization, in turn, increases access to information and allows the analysis and comparison of the patient's health trends and status. This capability converts data to information, giving caregivers additional explicit knowledge. In addition, the EMR can assist in coordinating care, increasing safety through technology such as bar coding and computerized physician-order entry, and being the foundation for other knowledge-based IT systems. When selecting and investing in an EMR, leaders must consider all the technology's value-added contributions to patient care, clinical work processes, and the health system (discussed in Chapter 14).

Doctors, nurses, and other health professionals draw explicit knowledge from the EMR to help them make clinical decisions. That explicit knowledge is supplemented by the knowledge accumulated by the individual clinician through formal training, reading literature, and clinical consultations as well as the clinician's experiential knowledge. There is a rigor to this decision-making process, although clinicians provided with the same information might reach different conclusions because of their training, how long ago they received that training, clinical experience, age, and other human factors. The decision-making process might be iterative, where the clinician's experiential knowledge may induce him to request more explicit information. The EMR alone typically does not include evidence-based decision guidelines or probabilistic relationships. It can provide trends and comparative statistics presented in meaningful graphics, derived from information contained in the EMR. This gives a clinician considerable flexibility to tailor her decision according to her experiential and other knowledge, her own clinical practice, and the needs of the individual patient.

The EMR as a knowledge source is the least invasive to the traditional structure of the clinical decision process and has the greatest probability of acceptance by physicians and nurses, when compared with other types of decision support. It requires change in behavior related to accessing and using information, and it might change the clinical decision and outcome but does not change the structure of the clinical process or how the clinical unit's membership and its interrelationships are structured. Such change might naturally occur, but it is not assumed by the decision support technology. Installing an EMR is a logical first step in developing an information strategy, given the considerable complexity of implementing it (see the discussion in Chapter 3). Clinical vocabularies, data standards, and the functional integration of clinical support areas in the hospital (such as laboratory, radiology, and pharmacy) change the logic of how information is structured from an individual department or clinician to an institutional focus. The fundamental change is on how information is represented and integrated in clinical decision making. Professional staff's acceptance of this change is an indicator of improvement, but improvement must also be measured by clinical outcomes. If clinicians do not realize or deny that they lack levels of knowledge essential to achieving optimal or even acceptable standards of practice, acceptance poses a particular problem.

Type 2: Health Information Exchange

A health information exchange (HIE) is the sharing of EMR data between institutions and clinicians involved in a patient's care (see Exhibit 8.3, HIE). HIE is a major development in health information technology in that it widens the reach of explicit information on a patient's history and condition. It has been touted as an effective strategy for developing a comprehensive national health information system and underlies much of the recent policy debate in the United States (Vest 2009).

HIE allows clinical information located in disparate EMRs to be accessed, integrated, and applied. This is not a trivial chore. It enables greater collaboration and integration of clinical decision making; as with EMR, however, it offers minimal change to the structure of the clinical decision process. HIE differs from EMR in one important way: It is integrated on a regional, national, and potentially global basis. The current policy expectation for HIE is to serve regional systems, but the properties of information are not regional by nature; they should be conceptualized as national and ultimately global.

Patient data (e.g., test results, diagnoses) shared through the HIE have differing levels of quality as exchange members do not all have the same level of accountability. The term *accountability* is used here to mean the measures and entities responsible for upholding the quality of individual tests and diagnoses in an organization, such as institutional accreditation, licensure and certification, and public reporting. Tests and diagnoses from one institution might be of acceptable quality but may not meet the quality standard of another institution that needs to use the information. This is an argument for increased quality standards and regionalization of institutions. (The interorganizational structure of regional decision support systems is discussed in Chapter 9.)

An HIE strategy has a major impact on EMR vendors, hospitals, and clinics (particularly small clinics) and brings additional information to the health professional but has a minimal effect on the structure of the clinical process itself. Having more complete and integrated EMRs allows an improvement in clinical decisions and patient outcomes. EMRs that are institutionally based become multi-institutional with HIE, enabling the information on patients who use more than one hospital or clinic to travel with the patient and inform all the health professionals involved in the care. This kind of access represents a change in perspective—from institution-centric to a systems orientation but still based on the medical record—but it also introduces increased concerns about the privacy and security of accessing and transmitting the data (which are addressed in Chapter 13). To address this problem as well as provide better access, the EMR information shared through the HIE is increasingly stored in data vaults or transferred though secure cloud computing.

Technology that supports the transfer of medical information is not a major technological advance, but it does reflect a significant change in how healthcare organizations view clinical information. One of the values of electronic information is that it can move easily across time and space, a fact belatedly accepted by many institutions. Data vaults and cloud computing have become the technological vehicle that enables the integration and transmission of information, which has traditionally resided in EMRs. The EMR of the future will be an integrated record, and future generations will look back and wonder why the EMR was ever institution based.

Type 3: Electronic Health Record
Scientific evidence derived from statistical analysis of large population studies can be brought to the point of decision making to inform and complement data in the medical record and knowledge derived from experience. Scientific inquiry through biological research and clinical trials is not a new phenomenon in the health sciences but has formed the basis of clinical science since the Flexner Report and served as the foundation of clinical education (Cooke et al. 2006).[1] What is new is that electronic systems (specifically the electronic health record or EHR) can present guidelines, reminders, alerts, and other decision support that are backed by evidence, ranging from closed clinical trials to expert opinion (Exhibit 8.3, EHR). The use of population-based decision support increases the level of empirical evidence in the EHR and differentiates it from the EMR. The fact that the support is population based, however, might not fit each individual patient and condition that requires individual clinician judgment. The challenge in introducing CDSS in EHR is not only technical- or information-related but both institutional and behavioral as well.

Institutional issues may include the following concerns about guidelines and other support presented in the CDSS and will affect acceptance by medical professionals:

- They are just "noise" and may interfere with or intrude on the decision process.
- They may slow down the decision process.
- The information may be perceived as offering no true value in terms of increasing quality.
- They are too prescriptive and mandated by hospitals, clinics, and financing and regulatory agencies.

Clinical decision making is a complex and dynamic process. It requires flexibility, a degree of professional autonomy and judgment, and full professional accountability. Traditional organizations, however, frequently do not acknowledge this dynamic, preferring instead to force the use of decision support by rules or mandates (see Chapters 4 and 7 for that discussion).

Behavioral issues need to be recognized, and the remedies must be based on sound theory and strategy. Physicians, nurses, and other clinicians are trained to respect and use scientific evidence to support clinical decisions, but in order to get them to use population-based evidence a substantial change in their decision-making behavior is necessary. Even guidelines based on the best evidence and presented in user-friendly format might be resisted. The reason for this is that such support alters the behavior and role of the clinicians, making them more dependent on the organization. However, when the application of clinical guidelines demonstrates improvement in clinical performance, health professionals and healthcare organizations have a shared moral obligation to use and contribute to them because of their quality and safety accountability to patients. The information age has demonstrated its contribution to increasing quality and safety. In doing so, it required the transformation of clinical decision making from one driven by independent clinicians to one driven by clinicians collaborating and being supported by complex IT while retaining a degree of independent decision authority. Special corporate models are required to support such collaboration and collective effort. A successful CDSS implementation might require changing clinicians' values, behavior, and attitudes. Part of this change process involves enlisting clinicians in the design of the CDSS. Training programs alone that merely teach clinicians how to use the IT are ill conceived and of limited value.

Keep in mind that while using population-based clinical guidelines and protocols changes the decision behavior of clinicians, these guidelines and protocols do not inherently change the basic structure of the clinical decision process—that is, how individual clinical decisions are made across different professionals often located in different clinics and over a span of time (see Chapter 4). Clinical guidelines remain very clinician- and institution-centric in their application (Exhibit 8.3, System Structure); that is, they are applied within a given structure (e.g., clinician, hospital) but do not inherently restructure the process. The HIE (Type 2) will likely leave out clinical guidelines and institutional knowledge and include only explicit data and information. As mentioned, HIEs simply inform the decision process. CDSS, meanwhile, changes decision-making behavior but only minimally disrupts the traditional clinician and institutional perspectives. In fact, clinical guidelines, protocols, alerts, reminders, and so on do reinforce the tenet that the clinician and organization are the locus of clinical activity. The justification for using decision support is that it transports clinicians and institutions into the information age by improving decision-making and thus clinical outcomes, although it does not fundamentally restructure the process (2 in Exhibit 8.2).

Type 4: Personal Health Record

Integrating patient health information into the clinical decision process brings additional knowledge and transforms the clinical decision process and those involved in it (3 in Exhibit 8.2). The patient not only is included in the process but also is the focus of the process, which has been called the "deification" of the customer (Fowler 2003). This results in the transformation of the EHR to the personal health record (PHR). Here, the clinical process is patient centered and thus must be integrated, with a view of the total medical and health needs of the patient. The PHR's sources of data and information include the EHR; the Internet; and health and wellness literature, much of which is based on sound evidence. Other information comes from the patient and family and includes their values; culture; and preferences, which might be derived from social networks (e.g., Facebook) and other online and offline activities.

The interactions between the patient and clinicians and between clinician team members both inform and transform the decision process. The clinical decision process does not simply conform to patients' desires but enlists them in the care process as co-producers. The decisions are based on evidence that the process will achieve improved outcomes and efficiency. Increased patient compliance is achieved when the structure of the process is patient-centric (Brown, Bopp, and Boren 2005). Decision making is designed to bring the most comprehensive, integrated, scientific information relevant to the case from a range of health professions, combined with experiential knowledge and patient preferences. The structure of the clinical process involves a multiprofessional team (also known as *knowledge workers*), whose members are selected by their specialty and its relevance to the patient's case. The team engages in dialogue to sift through the available collection of explicit knowledge to arrive at an evidence-based solution. The dialogue also gives the clinicians or team members a chance to draw from each other's experiential knowledge (Rothschild et al. 2004). The dialogue then should be of sufficient rigor to enable tacit and latent knowledge to be elicited from all participants. Depending on the case being considered, any given profession (e.g., nursing, medicine, psychiatry) might take the lead in coordinating the process. The common solution of having a separate and predetermined case manager only adds cost and formalizes what is essentially a team function (White and Wehlage 1995; Fjeldstad et al. 2012; Maccoby 2011; Kolfschoten et al. 2010; Faraj, Jarvenpaa, and Majchrzak 2011). Patient-centered clinical process requires a strong, team-oriented, dynamic environment with a culture of high commitment to quality. The current human resources management (HRM) function in most healthcare organizations has not created an environment that is supportive of knowledge workers (see Chapter 10 for a full discussion of HRM).

The multiprofessional team involved in a case need not be confined to a single location or organization. IT enables teams to form communities of practice, which come together to develop the best treatment plan and coordinate the delivery of services. Such an IT system does not require large monolithic institutions but loosely structured systems tailored to individual patients. These loosely structured systems form communities of practice that consist of professionals with high technical skills and are bound by a culture of cooperation, mutual respect, and integrity. If the common values of the community of practice are violated, the community may easily re-form. Exhibit 8.4 shows a transformed structure of clinical decision process—from one with a clinician and institution focus (Exhibit 8.3) to one that has a community-of-practice orientation. Opportunity exists for health system leaders to develop evidence-based, innovative, disruptive solutions for transforming the health system.

The basic question concerning the adoption of the PHR is the degree to which the PHR is valued and demanded by patients and the readiness of health professions, organizations, and insurance companies to develop

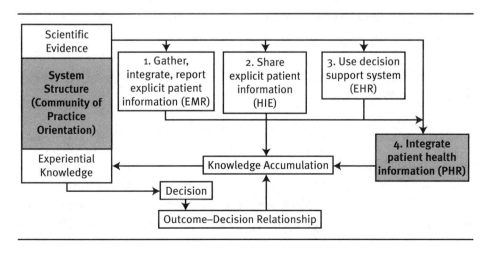

EXHIBIT 8.4
Transformed Structure of Knowledge-based Clinical Decision Process

and support it. Moving to a PHR requires the transformation of the clinical process and its support, which is a complex undertaking. However, the major obstacle is that everyone (except the patient vested in the process) has a self-interest in controlling access to information and will not press for PHR development. One determinant of acceptance and use by patients might be the degree to which they must assume responsibility for entering data and managing access, which would be a limiting or discouraging factor. The short life of Google Health reflects this reluctance by patients.

While not a significant IT breakthrough, PHR ushers in a profound change in terms of how information is structured and applied. A change in the structure of the clinical process represents a major shift in clinician, organization, information, and patient functions and values. Such a transformation is especially needed as the rate of chronic care cases rises in relation to the aging of the population. The current healthcare system is designed for acute episodic care. Patients, families, and public agencies are demanding greater accountability from healthcare organizations, including better integration and coordination of care data and information. This shift is associated with the changes in societal values, patterns of communications, and access-to-information expectations.

The transformation to a systems perspective necessitates a change in the traditional role of health professionals as independent or autonomous decision makers. It requires new values, behaviors, and skills designed to achieve superior outcomes. Such a system does not diminish but enhances, although it changes the role of health professionals. The institution may design a CDSS that contains specific population-based outcomes, such as the percentage of the population older than 65 years that has received pneumococcal vaccinations within the past 12 months (an existing metric for managed care organizations but not for hospitals). In addition, the organization may adapt its financing structure to the delivery process, not the other way around. Reimbursement may be based on valuation or the contribution to the care process, rather than on functional activities that inherently suboptimize the system.

Conclusion

This chapter is Part 1 of our discussion of knowledge-based clinical decision making; our discussion of knowledge management continues in Chapter 9. Understanding the basics of knowledge management and systems theory is important to understanding the sources of information for clinical decision making. EMR, HIE, and EHR are electronic systems that contribute considerably to accessing, integrating, and analyzing clinical information within and among institutions. Although such systems represent the profound advancements in health IT, they merely automate or digitize the existing information for clinical decision process. The PHR is more than just adding more information to the EHR. Instead, it makes assumptions about the redesign of both the clinical decision process (such as enlisting the patient as co-producer of her health outcomes) and the EHR that supports it. Chapter 9 delves deeper into how IT enables a higher order of analysis to guide the transformation or restructuring of the decision process to add knowledge and achieve improvements.

Chapter Discussion Questions

1. Name the four types of knowledge-based clinical decision support, and give examples of how knowledge is accessed in clinical settings.
2. What is the relationship between a knowledge-based organization and the human resources function?
3. Discuss why the clinical and business functions have not been well integrated. What is the potential value-added knowledge generated by integrating these functions?
4. In what ways can the existing design, IT, patterns of practice, and values of the organization serve to limit the level of knowledge incorporated into decision making?
5. Describe transformational research, and describe where within universities is the primary focus for research and development. Discuss the differences between translational and transformation research relative to the clinical process.

Note

1. Research-based clinical education has been termed *translational science*. Translational science or research refers to both bench-to-bedside clinical trials and translating basic research into practice. This discipline is worthy of exploration and is the subject of considerable national debate, discussion, and investment. The National Institutes of Health has invested in the development of the Clinical and Translational Science Institutes (CTSI), which focuses on levels of evidence to support clinical decisions. Such study is important to the development and acceptance of clinical decision support systems, but thus far the study has been limited to clinical decisions made within existing system structures and not the transformation of the systems themselves (Tufts CTSI 2012).

CASE STUDY	Knowledge Management in Accountable Care Organizations

Gordon D. Brown

The Setting

A large psychiatric specialty group practice in a metropolitan area provides a range of psychiatric services. The practice has grown rapidly and has thrived since its formation in the 1980s, as a result of the development of managed care plans, including the state Medicaid program that follows a carve-out model for behavioral health services. The psychiatrists carry out extensive translational research and use evidence-based protocols in their practice. They also develop these science-based protocols and embed them into their individual practices.

Several psychiatrists are concerned about the impact of the new federal mandate to develop accountable care organizations (ACOs). The mandate identifies 65 performance measures that the standard ACO must meet under the Shared Savings Program. These measures span five quality domains: patient experience of care, care coordination, patient safety, preventive health, and at-risk population/frail elderly health. The only behavioral health measure mandated is in the preventive health domain, a measure for depression screening.

Some leaders of the group feel that mental and behavioral health, as a specialty area, and the clinical volume would not significantly change. They do not think they should develop an ACO strategy and have resolved to take a wait-and-see approach. Another set of leaders, including the CEO, believes that ACOs do present some threats but at the same time provide an opportunity for the group to transform itself into an information-driven practice.

Evidence-based Strategy

The practice forms a multidisciplinary team to explore an ACO strategy. The team comprises two psychiatrists, one psychiatric nurse, the practice CEO, and one healthcare management intern. The team agrees that it will entertain all ideas and proposals as well as research the literature to bring in the best explicit information and experiential knowledge available. The relevant literature topics include ACO basics, knowledge management, and managed care organizations' limited acceptance and success since the 1980s.

The management intern, Marjorie, is interested in the medical-offset effect and its potential as a strategic asset. She presents to the team 30 years' worth of research on the concept, including closed clinical trials. Studies on medical offset measure the impact of providing effective behavioral health services on the utilization of medical care, including physician consults and visits to the emergency department. Marjorie is impressed by the extensive studies that include a wide range of populations and conditions, including Medicaid patients and chronic care diagnoses. The findings consistently demonstrate a savings of 10 to 20 percent from reductions in medical care utilization. The psychiatrists met these studies with skepticism, however. Although they think the science behind the research is valid, they reason that the practice has a specialty in mental health and not prevention or behavioral health, so the studies are not relevant to what they do.

In a brainstorming session, the team explores alternative scenarios on how the practice might add value to the ACOs that are developing within its area. The first scenario is to embed specialty psychiatric knowledge into the ACO's decision support system. The second scenario is to develop formal affiliations with as many ACOs as possible to capture their referrals for specialty care. The third scenario is to extend the practice's decision support protocols to address prevention, early detection, and aggressive management of behavioral health issues. This last idea is suggested by the psychiatric nurse, who points out to the team that the nursing staff and social workers have considerable (but untapped) expertise in behavioral health. The psychiatrists worry that developing behavioral health decision support protocols would result in a loss of status for the psychiatrists and thus would be strongly opposed. They are also concerned that the strategy would result in loss of prestige and reputation for the practice as a whole.

After considerable discussion and debate, the team agrees to respect the existing culture but to pursue the collective (corporate) interest of the practice rather than one group (psychiatrists). They begin to develop a proposal for the third strategy.

(continued)

Case Study Discussion Questions

1. Create a strategy to leverage the knowledge base of the practice against the value of knowledge within the developing ACOs. Consider the following guidelines and questions for this exercise:

    - What change will be made on who accesses knowledge generated by the practice and how would it be used?
    - Address each of the five quality domains specified by the ACO mandate, and justify their inclusion or exclusion. What are the implications of each on the structure of the clinical process and on the information system that supports the process?
    - What new properties of the decision support system must be included within the proposed strategy? How might tacit knowledge within the practice be leveraged by primary care physicians, other specialists, and patients?
    - What form of organizational structure would be formed with the ACO? What are the implications of collaborating with more than one ACO? Should the psychiatric group serve as the focal organization for developing an ACO?
    - What value is brought to the ACOs, and how would it be assessed? How would the practice be paid for its value-added services?

2. Comment on the environment of the practice and its readiness for strategic change. Who might you want to add to the team that is exploring an ACO strategy?
3. In the face of strong evidence, why do you think that managed behavioral health has been slow to develop and has developed as a niche industry by carving out behavioral health and managing it separately? What are the reasons for this, and what alternative strategies might be considered?

PREDICTIVE ANALYTICS IN KNOWLEDGE MANAGEMENT

9

Gordon D. Brown, Kalyan S. Pasupathy, and Mihail Popescu

Learning Objectives

After reading this chapter, students should be able to

- Critically assess data mining applications in healthcare organizations
- Classify data mining applications based on method and structure of databases
- Critique applications of modeling to alternative problem scenarios
- Develop a conceptual model of a community of practice
- Discuss the contribution of the EMR, EHR, HIE, and PHR to a knowledge-based system

---

KEY CONCEPTS

- Knowledge-based systems
- Data mining
- Organizational (business) intelligence
- Analytical models
- Discrete, agent-based, and systems dynamics modeling
- Learning or knowledge organizations

Introduction

This chapter builds on the concepts from Chapter 8. Specifically, it explores how data and information are accessed and analyzed and how knowledge is generated within the health system. The development of information technology (IT) applications to support clinical decision making has been significant and rapid, overcoming complex issues in establishing vocabularies and integrating systems. However, only a limited amount of real innovation and systems transformation, which are frequently enabled by advanced IT, has occurred. In this chapter, we explore the concepts of data mining and analytical modeling and their potential to generate sources of knowledge that can be used to improve health outcomes and increase system efficiency.

Electronic medical record (EMR), health information exchange (HIE), and electronic health record (EHR) generate large and valuable databases, which have spawned decision support tools, dashboard indicators, and other metrics—all claiming success in improving decision making and performance. However, organizations and clinicians have been reluctant or unable to apply higher-order analytics to these databases to add knowledge of complex relationships to guide clinical decision making. Scholars conclude that with the information age, most organizations have "increasing amounts of data but don't analyze the information to inform their decision making" (Davenport, Harris, and Morrison 2010, 9). In this chapter, we explore the concept of data mining as a higher-order analytical tool and its potential to generate sources of knowledge from clinical and management databases.

The personal health record (PHR) makes inherent assumptions about the transformation of the structure of clinical processes, aided by changes in organization structure, financing, and other support systems. Developing and testing the transformation of these interrelated and complex systems require a higher order of analysis. We examine the practicality and utility of analytical models as tools. The PHR can be used as the basis for conceptualizing innovative and transformational models for healthcare delivery, such as the development of accountable care organizations, but in itself will not transform healthcare delivery. The level of complexity is too great, and the health system is prone to apply new labels to old delivery models. We explore modeling as a technology that supports innovation.

Data Mining and Analytics

The EMR is a warehouse of accumulated information that includes relationships and patterns about a given patient or group of patients. IT applications, such as bar coding, have facilitated the use of technology for information integration, process improvement, and safety. In this respect, the EMR is still rather inert and characteristic of many electronic databases within hospitals and clinics. Health informatics enables the collection, integration, and presentation of patient-specific information from the EMR at a more rapid rate, allowing the presentation of more trend data than was possible with paper charts. However, limited data mining and modeling have been done with the patient-specific information drawn from the EMR, making such information systems function as did the paper charts. Embedding clinical decision support systems (CDSS), such as clinical guidelines and protocols, into an EHR does substantially change decisions and clinical outcomes. These guidelines, however, are made up of general, population-based information and not based on specific patients.

Large databases are a natural outgrowth of electronic information and represent considerable potential value to enterprises. Known as **Big Data**, these large databases in healthcare contain considerable information on behaviors; individuals; or small population sectors, such as a physician's panel of patients or a subpanel made up of a specific meaningful pattern of individuals. Here, the meaningful pattern is unknown going in, but using analytics can identify and describe this pattern. Big Data can define the pattern as the accumulated information for a single patient, for patients with similar diagnoses seen by a single clinician, or for patients with similar diagnoses seen by a community of practice.

Business intelligence and analytics, including information on customers, have become valuable assets to organizations and have been identified by corporate leaders as priorities for business development (Davenport, Harris, and Morrison 2010; IBM 2011). Service and product industries consider business intelligence and analytics to be the competitive differentiator in many future markets. It is difficult to see how the health system will not be impacted directly and indirectly by these new technologies that capture, analyze, and guide operational and strategic decisions.

Data Mining

In Chapter 8, we discuss the four types of knowledge-based IT systems—namely, the EMR, HIE, EHR, and PHR—that inform the transformation of clinical decision making. Each of these databases supports a Level 1 analysis, including measurement, trends, comparisons, and tests of statistical significance. In this chapter, we explore data mining as a higher order, or Level 2, analysis.

Data mining of electronic health records, financial, utilization, and other organizational and clinical files uses mathematical algorithms to convert the accumulated experiential knowledge embedded in data files into explicit knowledge. **Data mining** (Type 5) is the use of sophisticated search capabilities and analytical techniques on large databases to discover patterns, correlations, and trends that can be leveraged to produce knowledge. What constitutes a large database is relative and depends on the application and the types of analytics that are to be deployed. The size of the database is defined by the statistical tool and level of analysis being performed. For example, typically, a database is "small" if it stores less than a few hundred thousand records, and a database is "very large" when it has more than 1 billion records. This technique is commonly used to identify relationships within an existing decision-making structure, but it can be used as the basis for transformational change (see Exhibit 9.1). Data mining extracts accumulated knowledge embedded within an EMR (and through HIE) of individual patients and/or populations of like patients of an individual clinician or a group of affiliated physicians. Such accumulated knowledge forms a level of empirical evidence that complements the memory and recall (tacit knowledge) of clinicians. A clinician could choose to mine patient-specific information from an EMR to examine relationships that might confirm, refine, or refute population-based clinical guidelines contained in an EHR. The findings of the analysis of relationships within a patient's electronic record allow a clinician to balance the continually accumulated empirical evidence with experiential knowledge. These data are not high-level scientific evidence based on clinical relationships that can be generalized to an entire population, but they can complement decisions because they represent the experiences of a patient or groups of patients. In addition, they might be used to support clinical decisions that deviated from population-based guidelines. Patient preferences on appointments, referrals, and other matters; patterns of compliance with medications; wellness behaviors; and other information can be generated as well to tailor services to individual patients. As patients become more informed consumers, such information might be of considerable value as a basis for selecting and retaining a clinician. (Privacy concerns related to data mining are addressed in Chapter 13.)

Exploring the value-added potential of data mining requires a level of understanding of the context in which it is applied and the analytics that drive it. The degree to which clinical data can be accessed has practical limits, some of which are institutional restrictions and some are technical challenges. The EMR and HIE serve as the initial, primary data source because they are viewed as the property of the institution and because the knowledge they generate may add value to the organization and its clinicians. The EMR

EXHIBIT 9.1
Knowledge
Generation
Using Data
Mining

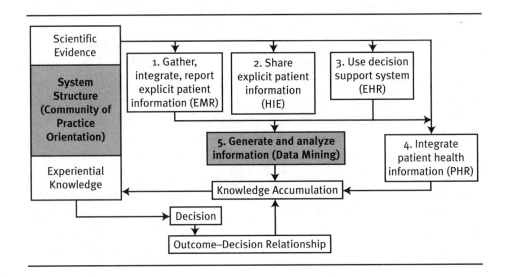

limits data mining because data are frequently structured in a manner that makes data mining difficult. Extracting information from medical records in other institutions through a health information exchange (Type 2) might be technically possible if the disparate data share a common vocabulary and architecture, which would create a larger database. However, that too is limited because issues of organization politics, legal restrictions, and privacy and security are involved. Some institutions are also not willing to allow valuable patient and clinical information (a market asset) to be extracted from their EMRs because such data may be used by competitors to gain a competitive advantage. This illustrates that the problems of data mining through HIE are not associated only with IT or clinical capability but with market and competition.

As discussed in earlier chapters, the interrelationship among the technical, clinical, and institutional (business) perspectives are inherent in health informatics. Data mining and analytics enable looking into this interrelationship and guiding the strategy for innovation and system transformation. Extracting value from knowledge gained from such analysis likely fosters changes in system structure and creates new systems-based forms that integrate the technical, clinical, and business functions that previously competed with each other and functioned in isolation.

Healthcare leaders must understand the potential value and technical challenges of data mining. Data mining has two main components: stored data and mathematical algorithms. *Stored data* are the various databases available, and the relationships of many of these databases have never been analyzed. *Mathematical algorithms* are the set of precise rules followed by the computer in calculating relationships in a database used for knowledge extraction. The underlying data storage technology has a great impact on the nature of the data mining methods used.

Database Types and Their Impact on Data Mining

The four main types of databases are pre-relational, relational, object oriented, and resource descriptive format (RDF):

- *Pre-relational database* stores data in tree-like hierarchies. Some EMRs are pre-relational formatted, such as the EMR of the US Department of Veterans Affairs; the EMR of Epic Corporation in Verona, Wisconsin; and MUMPS, the healthcare database originally developed for the Massachusetts General Hospital in the 1960s.
- *Relational database* is currently the most widespread database format. It is used in some EMRs, such as those produced by the Cerner Corporation in Kansas City, Missouri. It keeps the data in tables that represent real objects and the relations between these tables (hence the

name "relational"). For example, the "patient" table has columns such as "patient last name" and "patient age," while another table called "visit" represents the relation between patients and physicians. This structure is powerful and adaptable as a CDSS, but it is somewhat inflexible. This is a problem with information architecture designed for a given purpose and is not well adapted for any other function. If the problem context changes, modifying the tables to reflect the new situation is not easy. For example, two different EMR databases may have different data dictionaries (e.g., the column "patient last name" may be called "last name"), which will result in great difficulties in data exchange.

Another, more subtle drawback is that relational databases are not conducive to data mining. First, the relational format minimizes data redundancy and is suitable for multiple input-output operations. For example, in the "visit" table, the information about each patient (e.g., last name, age) at each visit is not repeated. Instead, only an identifier that can be found in the "patient" table can be used. As a result of this structure, searching many tables (maybe tens of tables in a typical EMR) is necessary in order to retrieve the desired data. For this reason, it is not generally a good idea to conduct data mining experiments on an EMR relational database. To alleviate this problem, a variation of the relational framework—a data warehouse—might be created, either within a given institution or in a common warehouse among institutions that serves the HIE. A *data warehouse* is a relational database with a special format that is more conducive to analysis than to transaction processing. For example, if one wanted to relate finance and clinical information, a data warehouse would facilitate extracting and transforming different data formats into a common analytical framework. The data warehouse is highly optimized for output (fast data retrieval) but not for input. Second, the table format of the typical EMR does not allow the discovery of relationships among data that are not already known when the database was built. For example, in an EMR that contains data from four generations of the same family, finding a link between great grandparents and their great grandsons is hard technically because the EMR designers did not anticipate that generational relationships were clinically relevant. In the era of genomic medicine, generational relationships will be.

- *Object-oriented database* is more flexible than a relational database in several respects. First, it can deal easily with a variety of objects, such as image sequences that are abundant in medical practice. Second, it integrates data with code under the object-oriented paradigm, resulting in a more structured representation of the problem domain.

Third, it introduces the concept of class hierarchies, which allows for an incremental refinement of the domain model. However, from the knowledge-discovery point of view, an object-oriented database is not fundamentally different from a relational database. Most of the current EMRs are either in relational or object-oriented format. This online analytical processing (OLAP) architecture is highly optimized for fast data input/output or for satisfying the demands of the medical personnel during the care delivery process. However, this data representation does not lend itself to more complex questions that usually arise in mining a clinical database to determine relationships and patterns emerging from EMRs. For example, a search for patterns related to a given clinical diagnosis usually involves relationships among numerous tests and diagnostic areas. For this reason, any complex data mining question might take weeks to produce an answer in a regular EMR. Instead, an OLAP architecture, such as a data warehouse, should be used for a fast answer to such problems.

- *Resource descriptive format* (RDF) addresses most of the problems inherent in the other database types. In an RDF database, data are stored in just one table that has three columns: subject, predicate, and object. All information is stored as triples. For example, "patient id 11100" (subject) "has-LastName" (predicate) of "Brown"

IMPACT OF THE INTERNET

The Internet has significantly affected the traditional data mining process along multiple dimensions. The first and most notable is the removal of the middle operative from the mining process. Traditionally, the process involved three entities: database, analyst, and decision maker (clinician or manager). The main drawback of this setup is the delay between the situation reflected by the data and the decision time (which is analogous to dressing today based on weather conditions one month ago). The new data mining process provides just-in-time knowledge for the decision process. For example, when you go to Amazon.com to buy a camera, you instantaneously know what other customers who bought this camera also viewed; this way, you do not need any other report about cameras and their features. In this case, the middleman has been replaced by sophisticated ("intelligent") computer program, reducing the decision lag. In the clinical setting, the clinician would know at the time of each consult the complex interrelationships among clinical conditions and among conditions and treatment patterns.

The second impact of the Internet is the interconnected architecture of the underlying database and its intelligent algorithms. Extraction of Type 1 (EMR) clinical knowledge requires a statistically significant amount of data that can be acquired only from multiple institutions. As mentioned in Type 2 (HIE), the EMR interconnection provides the architecture necessary for this endeavor. At present, the required data are acquired by mandatory reporting of individual institutions and deposited in registries (e.g., cancer registry) or national data sets (e.g., Healthcare Utilization Dataset or HCUP [Healthcare Cost and Utilization Project]). EMR interconnectivity eliminates the need for reporting and reduces the decision lag. As a consequence, the data can be mined and reports generated by the decision makers in real time. Obviously, this powerful capability has its own security challenges.

(continued)

However, both the banking industry and online commerce proved that society can find a balance between utility and security. The third change in the traditional data mining process inspired by the Internet is represented by the semantic orientation. As explained in Chapter 2, controlled vocabularies and ontologies are required for extracting knowledge from diverse and complex data.

Currently, several data mining frameworks coexist:

1. Framework 1: Data are extracted from the EMR or business database of a single organization and then processed by the analyst who makes a report for the decision maker (manager or clinician). This approach is typically employed for institutional management and quality assurance.

2. Framework 2: Knowledge is automatically generated just in time for the clinician and manager. In this case, the analyst is involved in method development but not in knowledge creation per se. If the decision process is knowledge intensive, a data warehouse might be necessary.

3. Framework 3: Data from multiple institutions are obtained by reporting, analyzed, and then published. This approach is appropriate for Type 3 guideline production (EHR) and for strategic healthcare management (see "System Structure" in Exhibit 9.1).

4. Framework 4: Knowledge is extracted from the entire healthcare organization, just in time for the decision process. Unlike the third framework that can generate general clinical guidelines, this fourth framework is able to account for local experiential knowledge. For example, it might be interesting to find out what clinical methodology is employed by some highly experienced physicians who consistently achieve above-average outcomes but who systematically draw on experiential knowledge and do not strictly follow published clinical guidelines.

(object or value). This format is extensible and thus easy to interconnect and conducive to mining. RDF databases, however, still require (as do relational databases) a way to "chunk" the information into triples—through natural language processing, for example. In fact, natural language processing (NLP) is increasingly employed in contemporary EMRs to enable searching of unstructured text fields, such as physician notes or discharge summaries. In a sense, NLP is contributing to the transition from Type 3 (EHR) to Type 5 (data mining/analytics) knowledge management systems.

These four types of databases follow the historical evolution of information systems: file based (single desktop computer) to relational and object oriented (desktop computer and local network) to RDF (desktop computer and Internet).

Data Mining Methods

From a research perspective, data mining methods are distinguished from the hypothesis-driven data analysis (Wickramasinghe et al. 2008) in the sense that data mining generates hypotheses rather than verifies them. While there is some truth in this statement, we believe that the distinction is rather artificial. According to the data-information-knowledge-wisdom paradigm, knowledge and data have a feedback relationship, and we need to know something about problems before starting data mining. In our point of view, data mining includes statistical analysis.

We consider the term *data mining* restrictive because it connotes that the analysis part is performed after a large quantity of data has been accumulated. While this approach is part of data mining, it does not account for just-in-time knowledge generation (see frameworks 2 and 4 in the sidebar). Moreover, in some instances, knowledge-discovery methods use current data that are acquired online while the application is running. Imagine, for example, an intelligent mammography system that assists the physician during the screening process. While the image is acquired, an automated system suggests to the clinician a possible area of concern. The area will be further investigated by the acquisition of further images. To include this kind of decision support system, the term "pattern recognition" is probably more suitable to describe all knowledge-discovery methods. However, for the sake of consistency, we use "data mining" throughout this chapter. A detailed discussion of data mining methods is beyond the scope of this text but should be included within clinical, managerial, and informatics curricula. Students are encouraged to draw on any general reference for gaining more knowledge about this important area of analysis (Witten and Frank 2005). Here, we provide some context for thinking about data mining in healthcare organizations.

Three main types of data mining methods exist: classification, clustering, and association rule mining:

1. *Classification* is an algorithm that attempts to assign an unknown object to one of the available classes of known objects. For example, when a patient is chronically late for clinical appointments, we might want to know as soon as possible if he will or will not show up for a visit. In this situation, we have two classes: "show" and "no show." The classification algorithms can be data driven or knowledge driven. In the data-driven algorithms, previously stored data are used together with the known class labels to develop classification models, such as neural networks, support vector machines, or simple Bayes ones (Theodoridis and Koutroumbas 2009). In the "no show" case, a data set is needed that includes examples of patients described by several relevant characteristics (e.g., age, complaint, insurance, distance from the clinic) and the related show/no show labels. After we trained the classifier, we can use the data online (just in time) to find the status of a scheduled patient. In some applications, however, either we do not have classification data available or the problem domain can be easily described by simple rules. In this case, we use rule-based classifiers, such as fuzzy rule (FR) systems, first-order logic (FOL) rules, or description logic (DL) rules (Brahman and Levesque 2004). For example, we want to design an automatic system for detecting heart attacks on the basis of a set of body sensors. Sensors

can be designed for this purpose, but it is hard to collect sufficient data to construct the algorithms needed to provide the alert. This problem is related to the power calculation in clinical trials, and in the case of an innovative medical system, the analysis is not afforded that luxury. Instead, we can set clinical rules (implemented as FR, FOL, or DL) provided by clinicians. When the class labels are not known, such as "show" or "no show," we need to group the available objects to discover possible similarities or relationships.

2. *Clustering* is the quintessential data mining problem, where the number of groups and the relationships between the objects are typically not known. Using the same "no show" example, before implementing the classifier, we can ask ourselves, How many types of patients does the clinic have? and What is the profile of the patient from each group? A large variety of clustering algorithms is available, such as k-means, hierarchical clustering, and self-organizing feature maps (Theodoridis and Koutroumbas 2009), each of which has its own advantages and disadvantages. Note that no perfect data mining algorithm exists, but a range of techniques (each designed to fit a problem at hand) is available. The key is to select the algorithm that fits the problem.

3. *Association rule mining* is another typical data mining algorithm that tries to find corelationships among characteristics of objects stored in a database. The discovery is based on the frequency of association; that is, if two characteristics associate often, then their relation might be relevant to the problem being analyzed. In the "no show" example, we might be able to discover a relation between distance from home to the clinic and "no show" status. We can then use the correlation in a rule-based classifier.

There are no prescriptive rules for employing various data mining algorithms. Rather, the set of data mining methods should be seen as a rich tool chest available to the knowledge engineer for addressing a large range of information needs.

Dynamic Systems Modeling

Knowledge management is described in Chapter 8 as a concept "that promotes an integrated approach to identifying, managing, and sharing all of an enterprise's information needs" (Lee 2000). Here, "enterprise" refers to the system, which includes all units that bring knowledge to the services being delivered. It extends beyond individual clinicians, the organization, and the healthcare system into other sectors, such as education and social services.

The structure of the enterprise is defined by the nature of the problem being addressed and the collective knowledge needed to serve the consumer(s). Through this process and interactions among all participants in the system, knowledge is gathered and integrated. In the healthcare system, part of the enterprise is the community of practice. An accountable care organization (ACO) may be defined as a community of practice, but it is not necessarily so. The ongoing political debate in the United States raises caution against assigning a label to ACOs that could imply more traditional structures. Chapter 8 discusses community of practice from a systems perspective, which necessitates change in the traditional roles of health professionals (values, behaviors, and skills); new delivery, financing, and legal and regulatory structures; and new relationships with suppliers and other sectors (e.g., education and social services). The complexity inherent in such analysis cannot be understood through statistical analysis and data mining alone and by using traditional decision models, but it requires a dynamic systems perspective.

Applying knowledge management includes considering how the clinical and business enterprise might be structured to bring maximum knowledge to bear on a problem being considered. In a dynamic enterprise system, one can test the impact of alternative designs, such as the change in the structural orientation from a static system that focuses on clinicians and the organization to a patient-centered system with a community of practice that focuses on the patient. The latter is characterized by considerable variability and complexity and thus lends itself to modeling, our Type 6. Modeling starts with building conceptual models that challenge current assumptions and introduce futuristic thinking. Analytical models can then be developed and applied to test assumptions, refine the conceptual model, and present alternative futures. PHR (discussed fully in Chapter 8) stimulates the need to redesign elements of the healthcare system, and modeling is the process through which change in complex systems is framed and analyzed. The analytical process is too complex to be carried out using traditional data and information-driven models.

Organizational leaders who are engaged in the process of IT design bring with them, to some degree, traditional ways of thinking, professional and institutional perspectives, and desire for stability. All of these can impose demands that conflict with innovative IT models and change. In order for organization leaders to effectively develop new models, they need tools that frame the issues and test alternative assumptions. These tools draw from several theories, including knowledge management, organizational learning, and complex systems. Building conceptual mental models is a process of finding a common framework. It draws on the perspectives of each participant but also challenges and extends these perspectives. An outside facilitator might be helpful in this exercise if the leadership team is new or if the institution is transitioning from a defender (relying on existing strategies) or reactor (reacting to others) to a prospector (innovator) (Miles and Snow 1978). The pursuit of coming together as a team to build knowledge-based IT has increased the amount of research on complexity leadership (Lichtenstein and Plowman 2009). Complexity leadership is characterized by leadership teams that interact within and across organization domains and emphasize both informal and positional leaders (Hanson and Ford 2010).

Exhibit 9.2 adds modeling (Type 6) as a means of increasing knowledge for both clinicians and organization leaders. As mentioned, data mining brings together disparate databases and identifies relationships that raise important questions about service delivery and that serve as a framework for new delivery models. Modeling differs in concept from various data mining techniques that provide information and knowledge extracted from various databases (Pasupathy 2010). Data mining increases knowledge of clinical and operational decisions and is useful for framing larger systems questions. However, to increase systems knowledge and to engage in transformational decision making, IT should progress from an operational perspective to a strategic and systems perspective. Because today's healthcare organizations are highly complex, an individual's mental models or data mining alone cannot provide the necessary analytics and evidence to support learning and decision making. Individuals' mental models are restricted by personal assumptions, which they have learned or observed from their life experiences.

Modeling is a method of studying, understanding, and then replicating the complexities of the real world in order to design, change, and

EXHIBIT 9.2
Knowledge
Generation
Using Modeling

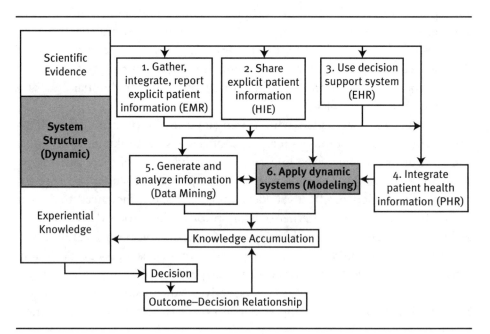

improve information systems. This process, in turn, introduces and increases learning. The system structure thus becomes dynamic (see Exhibit 9.2). Modeling also helps to validate information generated by data mining models. A simple modeling process is shown in Exhibit 9.3. Here, information from the real world provides some understanding that forms the paradigm or mental model of the decision makers. The modeler uses this paradigm to act (i.e., build a model). The simulated model, along with additional information from the real world (through data mining, for example), brings about a paradigm shift. This process is repeated until the model represents the real world sufficiently, and along the way, the decision maker gains knowledge or learns. The model built can then be used to predict future states of the system and to evaluate what-if scenarios. Finally, the decision maker uses this information and knowledge to act in the real world. Models can be statistics based, optimization based, or simulation based. These models can be used to study static and dynamic systems. Because healthcare organizations have a high degree of variability and are dynamic, our discussion focuses on simulation-based models.

Models do not come without limitations. Models are all "wrong" from an idealistic standpoint, as they cannot represent each and every aspect of reality. However, they can replicate the essential elements of a system and in doing so frame key questions and propose solution approaches (Sterman 2002). The validity of models is important to ensure that they succinctly and sufficiently capture the real-world system. Models are built by human beings and are restricted by the assumptions built into the paradigms (Silvert 2001). However, the modeling process in itself helps to challenge and break down mental models (or silo thinking) and prompts paradigm shifts. In short, models can evaluate existing systems and what-if scenarios and predict future states.

Modeling has three basic types, which should be considered when testing different assumptions and interrelationships: discrete event, agent based, and system dynamics.

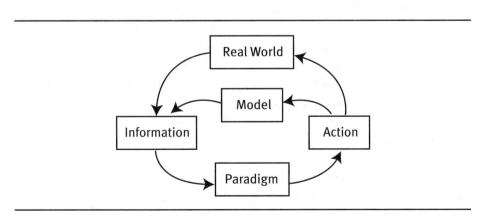

EXHIBIT 9.3
The Modeling Process

Discrete Event Modeling

Discrete event (DE) modeling is used to study processes, streamline them, and reduce bottlenecks through better resource allocation, capacity utilization or standardization, and mechanization of routine processes (Law and Kelton 1991). This type of modeling has been used in healthcare settings over the years (see Murray and Berwick 2003; Brandeau 2004; Schaefer et al. 2004). Most of these applications have been to improving processes in (not the restructuring of) healthcare organizations and systems, which is consistent with the typical use of DE modeling—the operations in a system, termed "decomposed systems," where the process has the greatest potential value. Examples of such applications include centralizing the information center in physician clinics in order to manage all nonmedical operations (Swisher et al. 2001) and studying the flow of medication orders in inpatient pharmacy settings (Shimshak, Gropp Damico, and Burden 1981; Ghandforoush 1993; Dean et al. 1999; Buchanan 2003; Zhang and Pasupathy 2009). The medical informatics and bioinformatics literature also reflects the use of complex systems models to understand the clinical progression of specific diseases, which is a context similar to data mining (Cross et al. 2008).

The application of DE models typically focuses on operations (including processes that transcend professional and institutional boundaries) within a fixed, stated, or assumed strategy (Fowler 2003). Application of DE modeling to knowledge systems, however, should focus on operations but is considered within the dynamics of alternative strategies. Fowler (2003) is correct in stating that it is,

> erroneous to delegate operations to the status of an after thought. Rather it should, as the custodian of the value adding process, be promoted into a much more central role as a potentially rich source of understanding and creativity within the dynamic systemic paradigm of strategic thinking.

Knowledge-based systems require insights into the dynamic working of the total system and the total value-adding potential of work processes and their interrelationships. Such an approach focuses on information systems to support operations within alternative strategies and not on operations within a given structure. With such a model, information itself can, and frequently does, become a strategic asset (Davenport and Glaser 2002).

Because DE modeling concerns the flow of entities (e.g., patients, medication orders), understanding queuing theory is necessary. The skills required to perform DE modeling include flowchart or process mapping, data collection, fitting arrival and service distributions, model building in simulation software, and quantitative analysis for staffing/capacity planning. Some of the software available to perform DE modeling include Arena (www.arenasolutions.com), ProModel (www.promodel.com), and Simio (www.simio.com).

Agent-based Modeling

Agent-based (AB) modeling is used to study the behavior of systems on the basis of the interactions between agents or entities. Such an approach uses the behavior of individual agents under given circumstances to model the overall changes in the system over time. Departments or divisions, people, projects, products, and services have served as agents to be modeled in traditional applications in healthcare systems. This approach is also related to DE modeling or bottom-up approach, where the agent is typically an individual or a functional area of an organization. Even applications that seem to be systems-based are driven by individuals (agents) and their behavior. For example, AB models are applied in public health informatics to study patterns of individual behavior and its relationships, such as the link between exercise and health status and the impact of food prices on dietary disparity as a result of low income (Maglio and Mabry 2011). Such analysis derives information from the PHR to inform the consumer (patient) and the clinical process, but it does not address the issues that alter the structure of the clinical process. Specifically, it provides the basis for examining the relationships among sectors, such as health, social services, and education, that have traditionally been structured and that function in relative isolation. This examination can lead to system transformation, broadening the concept of community of practice.

The strength of AB modeling is its interdisciplinary nature; that is, it can synthesize knowledge from different disciplines. The disciplines relevant to the discussion depend on the level of analysis within the system. Health informatics addresses the complexity of sectors and systems to enable leaders to develop the most complete understanding of the interactions among disparate systems. Here, the question is not the relevance of the models applied to the problem but the problem that these models address.

Some of the theories underlying AB modeling are game theory, artificial intelligence, and complexity science. The skills required to perform this approach include developing state charts, modeling interactions, data collection, model building in simulation software, and scenario analysis. For instance, AB modeling can be used to study smoking patterns (where smokers can influence their friends to take up smoking), sexual behavior (where teenagers without proper sex education are likely to engage in unprotected sex), and other behavioral issues. Some of the software available for AB modeling include AnyLogic (www.xjtek.com/) and NetLogo (http://ccl .northwestern.edu/netlogo/).

System Dynamics Modeling

System dynamics (SD) modeling is used to model complex nonlinear relationships between components and to study the dynamics of the system over time. This framework operates under the premise that structure predicts behavior over time.

The underlying principle behind SD modeling is complexity theory. Complexity theory views the organization as a learning system (Senge 1990) that uses knowledge to drive the organization's strategies and structures. In addition, complexity theory challenges the school of thought that promotes prescriptive structures, plans, and strategies (Fowler 2003). Leadership in such learning organizations is team based, includes informal leaders, and guides a process within which strategies and vision emerge as a co-involving supra system (larger unit that encompasses subsystems and components). The skills most relevant for SD modeling include systems thinking, cause-and-effect formulation, data collection, stock-and-flow modeling, differential and integral calculus, building the model in the simulation software, and analysis for decision making and policymaking. Several SD models have been developed over the years and are discussed in the literature; see Sterman (2000), Lattimer and colleagues (2004), and Taylor and Dangerfield (2005). The software used for this approach include Vensim (www.vensim.com/) and iThink and STELLA (www.iseesystems.com/).

In the healthcare field, SD modeling has been applied primarily to free-standing institutions and population groups, but it has equal (if not greater) potential when applied to higher-order systems (Hirsch 1979). This traditional application is not due to the limitation of this modeling type but because of the lack of vision of the leaders who use it. The value given to higher-order systems applications has been low because of the highly regulated and subsidized nature of the healthcare industry, the power held by health professionals, and healthcare leaders' traditional orientation toward the business function. Current health policy that looks to regulating the healthcare system to become a high performance and integrated system is a fallacy. Government initiatives and regulations can cause disruption that might lead to the healthcare system transforming itself. The challenge to enterprise leaders has always been developing systems that are innovative and that address the issues of costs, quality, safety, continuity of services, wellness, and patient-centeredness. These are not new issues, but they will require new solutions.

Comparison of the Three Modeling Approaches

The three modeling approaches differ in their level of abstraction and the amount of details required for modeling. While DE modeling is at the middle-to-low level of abstraction, it requires medium-to-high amount of details for modeling purposes. SD modeling is at the high abstraction level and is used for strategic decision making and policy analysis. AB modeling spans a wider range of abstraction, including high, middle, and low levels of abstraction. DE and AB modeling are predominantly discrete, while SD modeling is continuous; this comparison is shown in Exhibit 9.4.

Because healthcare systems are highly complex, one modeling approach does not suffice to capture all aspects (strategic, tactical, and operational) of a real-world system. A combination of modeling approaches may be used. For example, DE and SD modeling can be used together to study the nuances of operations and to learn the impact of strategic decisions. Regardless of the type applied, modeling helps in better understanding systems and in increasing the knowledge and learning among workers (see Chapter 10).

Conclusion

In the decision-making literature, the first step in the process is to identify the correct problem. This chapter focuses on defining the problem, using complex health systems as the frame of reference. This is the correct perspective for designing a knowledge-based information system. It is true that almost any analysis or use of evidence will add knowledge to a process, but it does not necessarily maximize the performance of the process. Such an approach might undervalue IT as a knowledge asset. An information system is optimized when it contains the collective knowledge of all agents, who engage in dialogue to define the problem and to develop an optimal solution strategy.

The EMR, HIE, and EHR are all valuable sources of data and knowledge. Application of the best evidence derived from CDSS has improved clinical outcomes and safety. However, such decision support systems draw on only a fraction of the clinical data available within these electronic records, and some of the data could be used to tailor solutions to individual clinical problems. Data mining represents a range of analytical techniques for accessing and

EXHIBIT 9.4
Three Modeling Approaches

Modeling Approach	Level of Abstraction	Time Basis for Simulation	Amount of Details Needed	Uses
Discrete event	Middle to low	Discrete	Medium to high	Tactical, process
Agent based	Wide range (high, medium, and low)	Discrete	Varies depending on the model	Multiple
System dynamics	High	Mostly continuous	Less detail	Strategic decision, policy analysis

analyzing such data and, in so doing, increases the volume of information and knowledge and the level of evidence that can be brought to bear in a given clinical decision. Data mining has been applied in the healthcare system, but the application has been limited to large databases such as those containing insurance company enrollees (we mine where the data are not the sources of the most usable knowledge). Linking these databases with CDSSs is difficult.

CDSS exists within given structural contexts and in itself does not provide the basis for analyzing and improving the performance of the overall system to optimize performance, including clinical outcomes. PHR provides an information system that inherently changes assumptions about the optimum structure of the clinical process, systems, and supporting IT. PHR could provide the framework for analyzing system performance on tailoring treatment protocols that emphasize wellness and efficiency. The danger is that PHR may be used as an expanded EMR or EHR, evaluating outcomes within existing structures but not transforming those structures.

Systems change is complex and examines the structure of clinical processes and organizations; the role of the professions; financing; laws and regulations; and the potential contribution to healthcare of other sectors, such as education and social services. Innovation is needed in the healthcare system and is supported by analytical models, which test complex interrelationships of alternative assumptions. Such models are carried out by visionary leaders and innovation centers that build and test conceptual and physical models. A system that is truly knowledge based not just improves operations but also innovates and transforms. This is the contribution of the science of health informatics.

Chapter Discussion Questions

1. Identify technical and clinical factors that limit the application of data mining tools within the EMR and EHR.
2. What information will you include in an analytical model focused on identifying individuals within a given diagnostic category who have the highest repeat visits and resource consumption? Where will you go to access this information?
3. What impediments do healthcare leaders face in applying modeling as an approach to guide the transformation of the healthcare system?
4. What types of evidence for improving clinical outcomes are introduced by analytical modeling and are not included in clinical guidelines because they present much evidence derived from clinical trials?
5. Differentiate the three types of modeling and give examples of how they might be applied to the healthcare system.

CASE STUDY	Analytics for Disease Management and Wellness

Gordon D. Brown, Kalyan S. Pasupathy, and Mihail Popescu

Central Medical is a multispecialty group practice that has embraced the community-of-practice concept of an ACO. The practice forms a multi-professional committee to identify services to improve clinical outcomes, maintain health in the population, and increase efficiency. Central maintains around 60 physicians and 4 clinics spread in different locations. Two are primary care clinics that focus on family medicine, internal medicine, and obstetrics/gynecology. One is a specialty clinic with a multidisciplinary staff devoted to metabolic disorders, and the remaining clinic is the largest and offers a range of clinical specialties. All four clinics are centrally managed with an EMR, which has the capacity to present clinical information in meaningful and actionable ways, including trend lines for patients, evidence-based clinical guidelines, and integrated treatment protocols.

Central has multispecialty teams whose composition is tailored according to the needs of the illness, including primary care physicians, chronic care nurses, therapists, nutritionists, and health educators. After the start-up period, these teams have developed a level of comfort and respect that enables members to bring the best discipline-based evidence to support diagnosis and treatment, healthy patient lifestyles, and the total-person concept of patient care. Because of Central's emphasis on improving the patients' knowledge and behavior about healthy lifestyles, the decision is made to invite patients with a specific disease to join the multispecialty team focused on that illness. Two patients and their respective family caregivers are added to the committee organized to identify and treat high-risk, chronic-care patients.

Central's committee identifies the investment in institutional capacity for processing information as a key resource, one whose knowledge on wellness and health maintenance can be embedded in treatment protocols. The committee agrees that the planned strategy's focus should be on quality, safety, and efficiency, with later emphasis on reimbursement strategies. This approach is consistent with the philosophy and values set forth by the ACO—address the overall health of patients, not just treat their illness.

The patient population of Central is demographically diverse and covered by a range of insurance companies, each with different eligibility criteria and benefit packages. Among the insurance providers is Health First, a large capitation-based plan with more than 1 million members,

(continued)

including 20,000 of Central's patients. Health First is generally accepted as an insurance carrier, primarily because it enrolls a significant number of patients, but the carrier's mission conflicts with that of the medical practice. Central is concerned with quality, while Health First is focused on finance and profit. As a strategy, Central entered negotiations with Health First by overstating costs and taking a rigid stance in reaching acceptable capitation and utilization rates. Both organizations accept their adversarial relationship, which they consider to be inherent between the health delivery and health insurance industries.

Central's committee moves forward with developing a strategy for carrying out its mission to achieve greater quality and efficiency using evidence-based medicine. The group focuses on disease management of complex chronic illnesses, such as Type 2 diabetes, learning from available research that intensive interventions such as life coaches demonstrate a 20 percent reduction in glycosylated hemoglobin (HbA1c) within 6 months for some patients. However, the committee cannot justify the cost of additional staff needed for intensive health maintenance for the Type-2 diabetes patient population. This particular population is inherently high risk, although some patients (critical cases) use resources at a much higher rate than others with the same condition. By systematically identifying diabetes patients who are at highest risk, the committee could better focus its intensive maintenance strategy, improve health, and increase efficiency. When the committee determines the criteria that define patients at high risk, many judgments must be made, such as patient age, comorbidities, and length of time (number of years) with the disease. These considerations, however, are not based on any evidence. The question becomes how high-risk patients within the patient panel of a given physician can be identified with any confidence.

The committee's review of the literature reveals that predictive models have been deployed by managed care plans to identify high-risk patients on the basis of their resource utilization (Axelrod and Vogel 2003; Zhao et al. 2003). By analyzing population-based enrollment data, managed care plans can predict the 1 or 2 percent of all diabetes patients who account for up to 30 percent of the total cost for this diagnostic group. Variables used in the predictive models include total annual prescriptions, unique (disease specific) annual prescriptions, physician visits, hospital utilization (including emergency services), comorbidities, age, gender, occupation, family composition, benefit coverage, treatment history, and attending physician.

Central's committee concludes that by deploying predictive models, a focused strategy could help the team select patients who require interventions, such as life coaches and other intensive treatments, the most. The evidence derived from the literature brought out several questions for the committee:

1. How many of the variables used in the predictive studies are available in the EHR?
2. What information can be accessed from the EHR, and can it be mined? What data needed to analyze an individual physician's patient population are not included or discoverable in the EHR?
3. Is the population size for individual physicians sufficient to support predictive modeling?
4. What are issues to consider in using the patient population for the entire clinic to support the statistical analysis? Can these considerations generalize from the clinic population to individual clinicians?
5. Can the clinic use the patient population covered by Health First to generalize to patients of individual physicians?
6. What are the advantages of the Health First database? What are some concerns related to the reliability and predictive validity of the Health First data set?

Case Study Discussion Questions

1. Present arguments for including patients and families in the initial team discussions.
2. What does "confidence" in this case mean? Is it based on intuition, collective judgment (experience), or statistical analysis?
3. How can information on high-risk patients be brought to the point of clinical decision making to guide physicians?
4. Is there sufficient data in Central's EHR and in a form to be mined to build predictive models for identifying high-risk patients for all physicians? Individual physicians? What questions regarding the structure of data in the EHR would you ask?
5. What might Central's committee propose given the potential conflict between the mission of the ACO to improve the health of the patients and the fee-for-service plans of Health First to reimburse based on utilization?

(continued)

6. How can the knowledge derived from population data sets inform clinical decision making by individual physicians? How can these data be accessed by clinics or physicians at the point of care?
7. What are the different perspectives on outcomes as defined by Central and Health First? Does predicting areas of decreased resource consumption equate with potential areas of quality improvement?
8. Are insurance claims data valid measures of clinical diagnosis and treatment?
9. Can the predictive model generalize to patients in other diagnostic categories?

THE CRUCIAL ROLE OF PEOPLE AND INFORMATION IN HEALTHCARE ORGANIZATIONS

10

Naresh Khatri, Kalyan S. Pasupathy, and Lanis L. Hicks

Learning Objectives

After reading this chapter,[1] students should be able to

- Understand the implications of knowledge intensiveness and service orientation in healthcare organizations
- Appreciate the fundamental role that human resources management (HRM) and health information technology (HIT) functions and capabilities can play in healthcare organizations
- Develop an understanding of the complementarities between HRM and HIT functions and capabilities

---

KEY CONCEPTS

- HRM capabilities
- HIT capabilities
- Complementarities between HRM and HIT capabilities

Introduction

Healthcare organizations are facing the dual challenge of providing high-quality patient care at an affordable price. In this chapter, we argue that the role of people (human resource management [HRM]) and information (health information technology [HIT]) is crucial in surmounting this dual challenge. Specifically, we contend that HRM and HIT are fundamental resources (not merely support functions), and healthcare organizations need to build internal capabilities in both HRM and HIT to manage these resources effectively. The HRM department or function in a healthcare organization is the overseer of all workforce issues, such as recruitment, training, compensation, and performance management. The HIT department or function in a healthcare organization, on the other hand, manages information technologies—both hardware and software.

A few exceptional healthcare organizations have built both HRM and HIT capabilities and have derived significant complementarities between HRM and HIT that, in turn, have allowed them to be leaders in value-based healthcare delivery. Several healthcare organizations have developed capabilities in either HRM or HIT but not in both, and still many others have developed capabilities in neither function. Outsourcing of HRM and HIT is likely to hamper the integration and embedding of these functions in organizational operations. HIT has attracted significant attention from policymakers and healthcare organizations alike, but that is not the case with HRM. Most large-scale HIT initiatives that proceed without strong HRM capabilities are likely to result in disappointing outcomes. This occurs because the organization change and development embodied in major HIT initiatives often cannot be sustained without strong HRM capabilities.

We expound on these arguments in this chapter. Specifically, we note that healthcare organizations are not factories or fast-food restaurants; rather, they are highly service-oriented and knowledge-based entities. Then, we define HRM and HIT capabilities and highlight their critical role in the healthcare delivery process. This is followed by a discussion of the significant complementarities between HRM and HIT in delivering high-quality healthcare.

Two Major Features of Healthcare Organizations: Service Orientation and Knowledge Intensiveness

Service Orientation

Service organizations like those in healthcare are different from manufacturing corporations in important ways (see Exhibit 10.1). Unlike in manufacturing, in the service industry customers interact with the production process. In doing so, customers inject a high degree of variability and customization into the production process. To meet this challenge of variability, service organizations need employees who are empowered and are proficient at diagnosing problems, thinking creatively, and developing novel solutions (Herzenberg, Alic, and Wial 1998; Korczynski 2002; von Nortdenflycht 2010).

Understanding the customer is fundamental to service work (Korczynski 2002). To be responsive to customer needs, service workers need to be given more discretion. Consequently, the service organizations need to manage the worker–customer dyad instead of the management–worker dyad, which typifies the traditional industrial model. Here, the more flexible "interpretive model" of decision making is more appropriate than the fixed and structured "engineering model" (Herzenberg, Alic, and Wial 1998). The

Healthcare Organization	Manufacturing Organization
Services and processes are variable and thus less amenable to standardization	Processes are mechanistic and not flexible
Constant contact occurs between employees and customers (e.g., patients, family)	Little to no contact occurs between workers and customers
Employees must have greater discretion in overcoming or solving issues related to service/process variability and customer complaints	Workers rely on chain of command and protocols to resolve issues
Customer satisfaction is mediated by employee satisfaction	Customer satisfaction has no bearing on worker satisfaction
Employee–customer dyad is the key to managing services effectively	Manager–worker dyad is the key to managing manufacturing processes

EXHIBIT 10.1
Basic Differences Between Manufacturing and Healthcare

human element takes on a central role in effective service operations because people produce the service product and because the interactions of frontline employees with customers form key attributes of the service product itself.

Using the industrial model to manage service-based organizations makes as little sense as using farm models to run factories (Davis 1983). Research evidence suggests that service firms often have difficulty improving performance by using organizational practices devised for manufacturing firms (Drucker 1999; Gera and Gu 2004; Grimshaw and Miozzo 2009; Karreman and Alvesson 2004). Healthcare organizations built on the industrial model have become trapped within bureaucratic structures that do little to meet customer needs, and too often they are structured to meet outdated ideas of internal efficiency (Herzenberg, Alic, and Wial 1998). To be effective, healthcare organizations need to adopt the logic of service production and delivery rather than the logic of manufacturing goods (Schneider and White 2004; Khatri et al. 2010).

Knowledge Intensiveness

Knowledge management is a relatively new management tool that organizations are trying to incorporate into their management systems. The capacity to learn is considered critical to organizational adaptation and long-term survival. According to Pearlson (2001, 193), "ultimately an organization's only sustainable competitive advantage lies in what its employees know and how they apply that knowledge to business problems." Despite the increasing realization that knowledge management and organizational learning are sources of sustainable competitive advantage, current knowledge management practices in most healthcare organizations are elementary. The work on the productivity of the knowledge worker has barely begun, and in terms of actual work on knowledge-worker productivity, organizations are roughly in the same phase that they were in 1900s in terms of the productivity of the manual worker (Drucker 1999; Khatri et al. 2010). Balas and Boren (2000) in their review of the medical literature conclude that healthcare organizations take about 17 years to adopt a mere 14 percent of existing medical knowledge and that physicians adopt unproven methods in treating patients, which results in a greater number of medical errors and a significantly higher cost of care.

About 42 percent of organizational knowledge is housed exclusively in the minds of the employees (Hansen and Thompson 2002). Healthcare organizations can exploit this knowledge by designing learning-oriented HRM systems that (1) promote positive learning attitudes and (2) nurture a self-renewal organizational climate (Jaw and Liu 2003). Doing so, however, requires human resource professionals to play a pivotal role in designing, shaping, and reinventing the work context—that is, implementing organizational change and development strategies. Similarly, HIT is essential in managing information and knowledge in healthcare organizations by providing the underlying infrastructure for organizational change and renewal.

Crucial Role of HRM and HIT Capabilities in Healthcare Organizations

Healthcare organizations are service oriented and knowledge based, and research seems to suggests that HRM (people) and HIT (information) are fundamental rather than support functions for the effective management of such organizations (Gera and Gu 2004; Pollak 2012; Robertson and Hammersley 2000; Schneider and White 2004). While healthcare organizations have generally overlooked the critical role that HR can play in furthering their performance (Buchan 2004; Khatri 2006a), their investments in IT have not produced the desired results either (Fernandopulle and Patel 2010). This is the result, at least partly, of healthcare organizations not developing internal HRM and HIT capabilities that are essential to conceiving and implementing effective HRM and HIT initiatives.

HRM Capabilities

The importance of HRM in healthcare is evident from the simple fact that salary and wages constitute about 65 to 80 percent of the total operating budget in a typical healthcare organization, making people the single largest input in the healthcare delivery process (Dussault and Dubois 2003; Khatri 2006a; Leggat et al. 2010). It is only logical that healthcare organizations use their HR maximally if they want to improve their clinical and financial performance. However, many HRM systems and practices in healthcare are built on a traditional manufacturing model of management and thus are highly inadequate for managing knowledge-based and service-intensive healthcare entities (Drucker 1999; Khatri et al. 2006; Schneider and White 2004; Tataw 2012). Healthcare organizations that use such practices are not able to make the leap from traditional HRM practices to innovative HRM systems because they lack the necessary capabilities to do so (Khatri 2006a; Lawler and Mohrman 2003).

HRM capabilities can be defined as an organization's capacity to acquire, develop, and deploy HR resources for achieving organizational goals. Healthcare organizations are finding themselves in the midst of a revolution in organizing and managing people as a consequence of competition, globalization, and continuous change in markets and technology. A flatter, less bureaucratic, less hierarchical, faster, and more responsive organization is emerging as the model for the future (Beer 1993; Bonias et al. 2010; Hempel 2004). Although HRM can contribute significantly to such a transformation, HRM in most organizations lacks the capability and credibility to help with the needed transformation (Beer 1993; Lawler and Mohrman 2003; Tataw 2012). Two major obstacles hold back HRM in this respect (Beer 1993):

1. *The capability of most human resources (HR) professionals.* In many companies, the traditional HR role and the rewards that typically go with that role make attracting professionals with the required talent difficult. The new role of the HR specialist demands a deep understanding of the business and expertise in organizational design, organizational change, and intervention methods (Buchan 2004; Tataw 2012).

2. *The attitudes and assumptions of the top management team.* Chief executive officers and other healthcare leaders say they want a more strategic HR function but often do not understand what this entails. Many still judge HRM by its effectiveness in delivering administrative services and keeping the company out of trouble with regulatory agencies. Many top managers and HR professionals limit the scope of HRM by pursuing a legal-centric approach rather than an organizationally sensible approach (Roehling and Wright 2006).

Without HRM capabilities, healthcare organizations fall short of the challenge of creating the next-generation work environment—highly collaborative and capable of not just fostering but also encouraging the instant and seamless movement of ideas and expertise (Ruona and Gibson 2004). Conventional notions of organizational structure rest heavily on such concepts as division of labor, unity of command, and grouping of similar tasks. In contrast, the view of the firm as an integrator of knowledge provides a different perspective on the functions of organization structure (Grant 1996; von Nortdenflycht 2010).

To learn in a cooperative manner, healthcare workers need to be given autonomy so that they can decide how to work, how to schedule work, and how to assign resources to their work (Janz and Prasarnphanich 2003). Further, team orientation is a key characteristic of the organizational learning process. Team-oriented work environments provide opportunities for employees to learn from colleagues with expertise who are supportive and willing to help one another through working together and sharing information (Bonias et al. 2010; Cabrera and Cabrera 2005; Tataw 2012). Instituting these new practices and processes requires a sophisticated HR department.

Healthcare organizations have high levels of communication between customers and employees, intimacy of communication, and richness of information exchanged during contact (Goldstein 2003). Healthcare work involves extensive employee knowledge and skills and is unpredictable, requiring employees to make continuous and multiple nonprogrammed decisions. Thus, employees must have the ability and authority to achieve results for the customer (Heskett, Sasser, and Schlesinger 1997; Khatri et al. 2010). Many healthcare organizations spend substantial resources on factors, such as better rooms, that directly attempt to improve patient experience. However, Goldstein (2003) has found that such initiatives are not successful and thus recommends that healthcare organizations focus instead on their employees, who are ultimately responsible for delivering care, to improve customer satisfaction. An employee-focused approach includes developing work systems, training programs, and services for employees. Service organizations, such as Southwest Airlines, have found that this approach produces exceptional customer satisfaction.

HIT Capabilities

A disproportionate amount of healthcare literature on the realized benefits of HIT comes from a small set of early adopter institutions that implemented internally developed information systems (Buntin et al. 2011; Chaudhry et al. 2006). These institutions had considerable expertise in HIT and implemented the systems over long periods in a gradual, iterative fashion. Moreover, many of the HIT initiatives in these institutions were funded by research-granting agencies and foundations. Thus, the cost of HIT initiatives was not an overriding concern. Of course, if we allocate more money, effort, and expertise into something, we can often do it better and derive more benefits.

In most healthcare settings, studies have reported a huge gap between HIT's purported benefits and accrued benefits. For example, Grossman and colleagues (2007) examined physicians' experiences with commercial e-prescribing systems in 21 physician practices, the majority of which had fewer than 100 physicians. E-prescribing, even in these less complex settings, was found to fall well short of the advocated benefits. The physicians reported barriers in all major aspects, including maintaining complete patient medication lists, using clinical decision support, obtaining formulary data, and transmitting prescriptions to pharmacies electronically. In addition to product limitations and use of specific product features, implementation challenges posed as major hurdles in e-prescribing. Similarly, O'Malley and colleagues (2009) studied commercial ambulatory care electronic medical records (EMRs) in 26 physician practices. The EMRs in these practices were in place for at least two years. O'Malley and colleagues reported limited benefits from the EMRs, such as they facilitated within-office coordination and improved billing and documentation. However, the EMRs failed to support coordination between clinicians and settings, did not adequately capture the medical decision-making process, and resulted in information overflow for clinicians. From the perspective of ambulatory care clinicians, the EMRs did not reflect the natural flow of patient care and dynamic coordination process within and across practices that are absolutely necessary.

Multiple studies in other industries show that IT investments produce operational improvements and sustainable competitive advantage *only* when they are accompanied by the development of effective IT capabilities (Bharadwaj 2000; Khatri et al. 2010; Powell and Dent-Micallef 1997; Ray, Barney, and Muhanna 2004; Yeh, Lee, and Pai 2012). Ross, Beath, and Goodhue (1996) argue that a firm is successful not because of any particular leading-edge IT applications but because it has developed a capability for applying IT to ever-changing business opportunities. Hence, we define the HIT capabilities of a healthcare organization as its ability to acquire, deploy, and adapt HIT-based resources to enhance firm performance (Bharadwaj 2000; Khatri 2006b). In the absence of internal HIT capabilities, healthcare organizations tend to return to paper records or to use partial information recorded in both electronic and paper-based systems (Curry and Knowles 2005; Fernandopulle and Patel 2010; Metzger et al. 2010). Under either approach, information is lost, work time is increased to retrieve data, and decision support systems are undermined and underutilized.

Healthcare organizations have made significant investments in HIT, with wishful thinking that because they have written a big check in acquiring IT, the efficiencies should spring up magically (Pare 2002). Unfortunately, too many healthcare organizations have spent huge amounts of money and have frustrated countless people on wasted IT implementation efforts (Curry and Knowles 2005; DesRoches et al. 2010; Feld and Stoddard 2004; McDermott 1999). Most of these organizations pursued the early computer-era practice of buying the latest technology, without knowing how it might effectively be employed in achieving organizational goals. If an organization just invests in HIT rather than in HIT capabilities, it is likely to be merely acquiring HIT components (i.e., hardware, software, and vendor-provided services) that it may not really understand and may not be capable of fully applying to achieve enterprise objectives (King 2002; Smith, Buller, and Piland 2000; Yeh, Lee, and Pai 2012).

For example, Smith, Buller, and Piland (2000, 22) studied more than 300 multispecialty and 600 single-specialty groups and arrived at this conclusion: "Simply throwing resources at staffing or at major equipment support, such as computer hardware and software, probably does not necessarily lead to financial success.... More is not always better. Thus, procuring the right IT design with appropriate capabilities for tasks and goals could produce high returns rather than simply ensuring that IT is in place."

From studying IT implementations in various industries, Feld and Stoddard (2004) found that companies had created and populated dozens of information systems. The IT architecture in these companies was made up of a series of silos. Various divisions of each company used different applications and disconnected databases, leading to redundancy, increased costs, and overall organizational dysfunction.

Similarly, healthcare organizations have relied heavily on the fragmented HIT vendor market in which vendors do not offer an open architecture and have been unwilling to offer electronic interfaces that would make their "closed" systems compatible with those of other vendors (Fernandopulle and Patel 2010; Metzger et al. 2010; Weiner et al. 2004). As a result, healthcare organizations are hamstrung because they have implemented so many different technologies and databases that information stays in silos.

In addition, simply moving from paper-based to electronic information systems does not address the fundamental problem of silos prevalent in healthcare organizations. The barriers to information sharing posed by the healthcare cultures and management systems embodied in paper-based information systems typically remain intact; they impede and fragment electronic information to the same extent as they did in the paper-based systems. However, by building HIT capabilities, healthcare organizations are more likely to implement HIT effectively and bring about necessary changes in healthcare cultures and systems.

HRM and HIT Complementarities

Information and communication technologies affect both how employees work and how they relate to customers when their interactions are mediated, replaced, or constrained by technology (Blount, Castleman, and Swatman 2005). Thus, during HIT assimilation, changes in behavioral systems, as well as technical systems, are to be expected. As a result, the effective integration of HIT and HRM perspectives is likely to offer significant benefit (DeVore and Figlioli 2010; Martinsons and Chong 1999; Pollak 2012). Healthcare organizations are investing billions of dollars in technologies that generate huge volumes of transaction data. However, these investments do not live up to their potential, unless healthcare organizations are able to build broad capabilities—both technical and human—to convert data into knowledge and then into business results (Buntin et al. 2011; Davenport et al. 2002; DeVore and Figlioli 2010).

For example, several studies using nationwide, cross-industry business surveys find higher performance among businesses that adopt both innovative work practices and information technologies (Brynjolfsson and Hitt 2000; Gera and Gu 2004; Khatri et al. 2010; Ichniowski and Shaw 2003). Although IT may be applied to improve performance with few organizational changes, the successful application of IT is often accompanied by significant organizational changes to policies and rules, structure, workplace practices, and culture, among other areas (Melville, Kraemer, and Gurbaxani 2004). However, to make substantial changes in organizational structure, culture, and workplace practice is an arduous task that is beyond the reach of HIT capabilities alone. A strong partnership of HIT with HRM can go a long way in ensuring successful transformations in organizational structures and cultures when implementing new information technologies.

Elaborating on this insight, McAfee and Brynjolfsson (2008), two leading IT scholars, studied all publicly traded U.S. companies in all industries from the 1960s through 2005. They observe that, since the mid-1990s, a new competitive dynamic has emerged: Bigger gaps exist between the leaders and laggards in an industry, markets have become more concentrated, and there is greater churn among industry rivals. This accelerated competition coincides with a sharp increase in the quality and quantity of IT investments. McAfee and Brynjolfsson note that businesses entered into a new era of increased competitiveness in the mid-1990s, not because they had so many IT innovations to choose from but because of how some of these technologies enabled improvements to companies' operating models and then replicated those improvements more widely. Thus, the deployment of IT is a key success factor for competitive advantage and remains a critical management challenge. Importantly, McAfee and Brynjolfsson found that companies that successfully use IT are more proactive in their HRM strategies. They argue that embedding IT in organizational processes is hard to achieve without the support of reconfigured HR practices. This presents a clear lesson for healthcare organizations: Either they set their house in order by building internal capabilities in HIT and HRM, or they lose their place to competitors.

Knowledge management is important in healthcare organizations. The current approach to knowledge management is problematic, however. Robertson and Hammersley (2000) and Zarraga and Bonache (2005) point out that, when academics and practitioners refer to knowledge management, they often mean IT. As Medina-Borja and Pasupathy (2007) suggest, organizations that allocate most of their IT resources to data collection are data rich but information poor. The dominance of technological initiatives comes as no surprise, if we bear in mind that most knowledge management systems are run by information-processing departments. This reflects the assumption that knowledge exchange is essentially technical in nature. Indeed, developing high levels of organizational capital is difficult without creating or providing an underlying **IT infrastructure** that supports knowledge management and codification (Yeh, Lee, and Pai 2012; Youndt and Snell 2004). However, overemphasis on technical aspects of knowledge management and marginalization of the vital people-management aspects results in "expensive and useless information junkyards" (McDermott 1999, 104). This is because knowledge involves thinking with information. If all we do is increase the circulation of information, we have only addressed one of the components of knowledge. To leverage knowledge, we need to enhance both thinking and information, which involves a unique combination of human and information systems.

The shortage of workers is seen as one major problem facing healthcare organizations. HIT can be a useful tool in overcoming this major challenge. For example, by leveraging IT investments during the 1990s, banks saw a 25 percent reduction in branches and a 20 percent reduction in full-time employees (Blount, Castleman, and Swatman 2005). However, the benefits of HIT investments have not been realized fully in healthcare; this partial realization of benefits occurs because HIT interventions are not coupled with essential organizational changes. Effecting changes in organizational cultures and management systems using HIT requires an IT department that possesses technical HIT expertise and insights into organizational cultures and management systems. In other words, healthcare organizations need IT departments that have both technical and change management capabilities.

Most research on the HRM and IT link centers on the role of IT in HRM rather than on what role HRM can play in IT initiatives. Maguire and Redman (2007) examined this aspect using a case study of a large, U.K. public-sector organization employing more than 200,000 people. They concluded that IT failure is often associated with a lack of attention to "softer" management practices, such as cultural change, and HRM was the key success factor that was neglected in failed IT initiatives. Moreover, they argue that IT should be organized around business processes rather than the other way around.

A few exceptional healthcare organizations have built internal capabilities in both HRM and HIT. Two examples of such organizations are Arkansas Children's Hospital and the Mayo Clinic. Arkansas Children's Hospital, with a total of 4,500 employees, has 45 professionally trained HR employees and about 100 full-time IT professionals. The hospital has an internally developed HIT system and has been frequently ranked on the list of "Best Places to Work in America." Both HRM and HIT work together; for example, HRM proactively sought the help of HIT in designing an online recruitment and selection system six years ago. Further, HRM is currently working with HIT in developing an electronic performance-management system. Similarly, HRM is involved in helping HIT establish a new automated scheduling system for nurses. HRM is also supporting HIT in redesigning the hospital's website. Similarly, the Mayo Clinic has built a strategic HR function along with an internally developed and well-integrated HIT system. HRM and HIT enable each other to enhance their support of healthcare delivery.

Some healthcare organizations, such as community hospitals, do a relatively good job in developing HRM capabilities but lack HIT capabilities. On the other hand, the US Department of Veterans Affairs has developed a powerful enterprisewide HIT system, but its HR practices and systems are outdated. Unfortunately, a sufficiently large number of healthcare organizations have low capabilities in both HRM and HIT and will face great difficulties in providing high-quality care while containing costs.

Because of the Institute of Medicine's (IOM 2001) report *Crossing the Quality Chasm*, marketing by HIT companies, and new funding for HIT contained in the HITECH (Health Information Technology for Economic and Clinical Health) Act of 2009, the American media and public-policy focus on how HIT can improve healthcare has increased. Ironically, there has been a dearth of news and policy initiatives on HRM and its strategic role in transforming healthcare organizations. In view of the complexity of healthcare organizations and the critical role of culture in transforming healthcare organizations, we argue that HRM capabilities must be improved first before HIT initiatives can be successful. Unless we get HR practices and systems right, many of the HIT initiatives and investments will achieve disappointing results, in part because of either the lack of use by health professionals or the workflow inefficiencies introduced or aggravated by the new HIT.

Unfortunately, many HIT initiatives focus solely on achieving technical deployment, and in the process ignoring the vital HRM success factors that enable or inhibit the strategic use of HIT within the healthcare organization. Arguably, this unintended consequence happens because a typical healthcare organization lacks sufficient HIT and HRM capabilities and, as a result, approaches IT projects naively. In terms of HRM and HIT capabilities, a healthcare organization may be classified into one of the following four categories:

1. High capabilities in both HRM and HIT
2. High capabilities in HRM and low capabilities in HIT
3. Low capabilities in HRM and high capabilities in HIT
4. Low capabilities in both HRM and HIT

As illustrated in Exhibit 10.2, we propose that as these capabilities diminish, the probability of a successful HIT initiative decreases. Moreover, the types of successes that can be achieved will vary depending on whether HRM or HIT capabilities are strong or weak. On one hand, healthcare organizations with high levels of HIT capability but low levels of HRM capability are likely to be successful in achieving widespread technical deployment of a HIT initiative, such as an electronic health record (EHR). Where this initiative likely will falter is in the strategic and widespread use of the EHR by health professionals. On the other hand, healthcare organizations with low levels of HIT capability but high levels of HRM capability are likely to be successful in achieving the use of EHRs by health professionals, but they will likely falter in its widespread technical deployment. For healthcare organizations with low levels of HRM and HIT capabilities, we believe they should invest in building internal HRM capabilities before investing in HIT (see arrows in Exhibit 10.2).

EXHIBIT 10.2
Relationship
Between
HRM and HIT
Capabilities and
Probability of
HIT Success

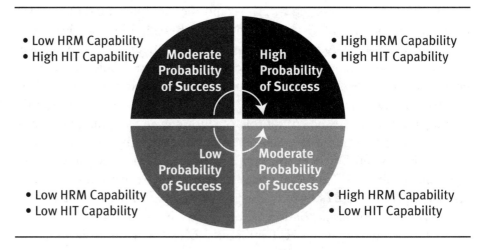

Conclusion

While HRM and HIT are crucial in achieving high-quality patient care, they are not particularly well managed in healthcare organizations. This shortcoming occurs because healthcare organizations have failed to build both their HRM and HIT capabilities. Nonetheless, development of HIT capabilities in healthcare organizations is gaining attention. Unfortunately, despite the centrality of people in the care delivery process, HRM continues to receive inadequate attention and strategic focus from many healthcare executives.

Just as individual departments cannot improve healthcare delivery and quality in isolation, HRM or HIT alone cannot do so either. Together, however, they have the power to bring service orientation and knowledge management, which can go far to transform the organization. The inadequacy of HRM and HIT capabilities is both a challenge and an opportunity (with a call for improvement) rather than a drawback. Healthcare organizations should focus on the personnel growth and technological innovation that go beyond supporting day-to-day procedural operations with a short-term focus and enable the entire organization to sustain gains and reap long-term benefits. Such a transformation cannot be done in isolation within any of the functional areas—be it clinical, HR, IT, or operations.

HRM and HIT personnel should acquire an in-depth understanding of the clinical and managerial aspects of the organization. For instance, HRM should be involved in organizational change efforts to foster and grow clinical and interprofessional collaboration and teamwork. Using HRM capabilities in this way can enable health professionals to break down process barriers and silos and thus see the broader picture of the process—the entire breadth of the service encounter between the patient and various clinicians. This initiates the creation of organizational learning and the collection of knowledge, knowledge that relies on HIT capabilities to help manage and disseminate throughout the enterprise.

Chapter Discussion Questions

1. What key features of service organizations differentiate them from manufacturing firms? What are the implications of such a differentiation in managing healthcare organizations?
2. What are the underlying reasons for the failure of HIT initiatives?
3. In its prescription to reduce medical errors and improve quality of care, the IOM report put a lot of emphasis on HIT but not on HRM. Do you see any flaw in such an approach?

4. If you were the chief executive officer of a hospital, what immediate steps would you take to improve the healthcare delivery in your organization?

Note

1. This chapter has been adapted from Khatri, N., K. Pasupathy, and L. L. Hicks. 2010. "The Crucial Role of People and Information in Health Care Organizations." In *Advances in Health Care Management*, Volume 9, edited by M. D. Fottler, N. Khatri, and G. T. Savage, 195–211. Adapted with permission from Emerald Group Publishing Limited.

CASE STUDY   University Hospital

Naresh Khatri

University Hospital is a 300-bed acute care facility that serves the residents of one of the Midwestern states in the Unites States. It is part of a large university health system that employs more than 8,000 faculty and staff and that has an annual operating budget close to $1 billion. In addition to the University Hospital, the health system consists of a medical school, a nursing school, a children's hospital, a regional hospital, and a cancer center. University Hospital operates the region's only Level 1 trauma center, only burn and wound intensive care unit, and only kidney transplant program. It receives more than 50,000 visits to its emergency department annually.

Human Resource Management

Because University Hospital is part of a health system, recruitment and selection of physicians are done at the level of the medical school, and the allocation of their research and clinical time is governed by the medical school in concert with the hospital's administration. While the hospital deals with most of the human resource management (HRM) aspects of nurses and other employees, its HR policies and programs are affected by the university's HR policies. All of this makes HRM issues at the hospital complex, because three different entities (university, medical school, and hospital) need to work together to manage the HR function of the hospital. The hospital's HRM department is headed by Luz Salvador, the vice president who was hired about four years ago to transform the HR function. Luz has more than 20 years of experience in healthcare management, although she does not have specific professional education or training in HRM.

On average, the hospital has one HRM employee per 200 FTEs (full-time equivalents), as compared with one HRM employee per 100 FTEs in companies of similar size in other industries. This ratio shows that the hospital's HRM department is grossly understaffed, which is reflected in a lot of the clinical staff's complaints about the slow filling of vacant positions. Recruiting employees take several months, and many times the hospital loses the qualified applicants to other healthcare organizations in the region. Employee turnover at the hospital during normal economic conditions is about 22 percent, which is above the industry average. Employee morale at the hospital is low, and most employees feel a sense of helplessness and frustration.

Luz is expected to solve these problems, but most of the promises she made upon her hiring have not been fulfilled. However, she thinks she has done an excellent job thus far in reforming the HRM department's practices. While she thinks HRM plays an important role in the hospital, most other department heads and managers are not aware of this role or any of HRM's contributions and purported changes. These leaders think that the department is as slow in responding to their needs as it was before. Some of them prefer that HRM assume a policing role rather than a strategic, supportive role. Clinicians in the hospital dominate the decision making. While they expect a lot of support from HRM, they do not consider it important, do not provide it with sufficient resources, and do not give it enough authority to manage its own function and implement changes. As a result, HRM remains weak, poorly led, and highly understaffed and fulfills only the traditional personnel management tasks.

Health Information Technologies

Ten years ago, with a view to taking the lead in implementing health information technology (HIT) (e.g., electronic medical records, physician order-entry system, billing system), University Hospital outsourced its IT to a private company that specializes in health information management systems. For several years, the hospital maintained its own workforce of 100 IT workers and received supplemental services from the vendor. Maintaining a large IT workforce and paying an annual contractual amount

(continued)

to a vendor were expensive. Two years ago, the vendor agreed to absorb the hospital's IT workers.

The individuals who headed the hospital's IT initiatives were physicians who did not use technologies much and did not understand or care to know about existing and emerging IT systems. The former chief information officer (CIO) at University Hospital has a PhD in genetics but zero knowledge of computers and information technologies. Meanwhile, the point person at the vendor company is adept at marketing and selling its services, making it easy for the company to mislead the CIO and other hospital leaders by promising IT enhancements that the company had no capability of delivering. However, the hospital's enthusiasm faded quickly as users found that the installed system was dysfunctional and woefully inadequate to handle the complexities of healthcare delivery. Most physicians complained about the serious problems, but the CIO and senior management persisted with using the system and the vendor.

Two years ago, the hospital appointed a new CIO—a senior nurse manager, who also has no IT background but a firm belief that clinical knowledge is all that is needed to oversee the planning, design, and implementation of the HIT. Today, the HIT at University Hospital remains in disarray and is holding back the hospital from delivering efficient, affordable, and high-quality patient care.

Case Study Discussion Questions

1. Do you think the scenario in this case is unique to University Hospital, or do other academic medical centers approach HRM and HIT in a similar piecemeal, ad hoc fashion?
2. What suggestions would you provide to the senior management at University Hospital to improve its HRM and HIT functions?

E-HEALTH AND CONSUMER HEALTH INFORMATICS

11

George Demiris and Blaine Reeder

Learning Objectives

After reading this chapter, students should be able to

- Identify and differentiate the different platforms that support e-health applications
- Describe consumer health informatics concepts and their role in the design of e-health systems
- Construct the essential elements of a health social network
- Critically assess implications and barriers of health social networks
- Examine the relationship between e-health and methods of reimbursement

---

KEY CONCEPTS

- E-health
- Consumer health informatics
- Personal health record
- Social media
- Health social network site
- Telehomecare, telemedicine, and telehealth
- Patient empowerment

Introduction

E-health encompasses the use of telecommunication platforms, mobile and ubiquitous hardware and software, and advanced information systems to support and facilitate healthcare delivery and education. Therefore, e-health triggers a fundamental redesign of healthcare processes, integrating electronic communication at all levels and affecting all stakeholders. This also supports patient empowerment—namely, the transition from a passive role where the patient is the recipient of care services to an active role where the patient is informed and involved in or even leads the decision-making process. Feste and Anderson (1995) emphasize that the patient empowerment model introduces "self-awareness, personal responsibility, informed choices and quality of life."

E-health bridges both the clinical and nonclinical sectors and includes both individual and population health–oriented tools. It encompasses different platforms, such as

- telehealth applications (e.g., videoconferencing) that bridge geographic distance,
- web portals,
- personal health records,
- online services for patient and family support groups,
- consumer information services,
- social media, and
- portable or even wearable monitoring tools that capture physiological parameters.

In addition, e-health delivers healthcare information, diagnosis, treatment, and care in a nonlinear manner, where traditional hierarchies are obsolete and patients enter the system at an infinite number of points and with their own terms of usage frequency and pattern. Healthcare lawyers are challenged "to determine whether they are dealing with the sale of a product or the supply of a service [and] whether to apply strict products liability or professional negligence" (Terry 2000).

Advances in telecommunication technologies have introduced innovative ways to enhance communication between health professionals and patients. The implication is a shift of focus for informatics researchers and system designers who had primarily focused on designing information technology (IT) applications that met the needs of healthcare providers and institutions by using data models that included episodic patient encounters as one group of healthcare-related transactions. The emerging model aims to evolve around the life course of the individual patient and to ensure continuity of care. New technologies and informatics approaches call for the development of informatics tools that support patients as active consumers in the healthcare delivery system. This shift from institution-centric to patient-centric information systems calls for new design and evaluation approaches that examine and maximize the systems' effectiveness.

Consumer health informatics is the area of health informatics that focuses on the implementation and evaluation of system design to ensure that it interacts directly with the consumer, with or without the involvement of healthcare providers. Such a system can include community informatics resources available to the general public (e.g., community online networks, support groups, general health–related web portals) and clinical resources for specific populations. As Eysenbach (2000) argues, consumer health informatics is concerned with the analysis and modeling of consumer preferences and information needs, the design of applications that support consumers in obtaining high-quality information, and the development of a methodology that allows for the integration of consumer needs in clinical information management systems (Eysenbach 2000). Furthermore, consumer health informatics studies ways to increase the effectiveness of health information and the effect of informatics tools on public health. Consumer health informatics has emerged from and is focusing on the shift from traditional institution-centric to patient-centric information systems. The applications and systems described in this chapter are all within the domain of consumer health informatics, as they focus on the individual patient's needs and preferences and aim to support consumers and their families in the context of healthcare.

Review of Patient-Centric Systems

Consumer informatics applications reach out to patients in their homes or in clinical settings, facilitating their access to personal health documentation or supporting their management of health information; linking them to friends, peers, and others; actively engaging them in health decision making; and providing them with tools to manage a disease or maintain wellness. In this section, we review home-based e-health applications and social networks and discuss the challenges, barriers, and facilitators to the successful adoption of such patient-centric systems.

Home-based E-Health Applications

E-health applications offer a platform to support disease management for home care patients diagnosed with chronic conditions and their families. Such applications address numerous diseases or conditions. An example of Internet utilization for asthma management is the home asthma telemonitoring (HAT) system (Demiris, Speedie, and Finkelstein 2001a). The HAT system provides patients with continuous, individualized help with the daily routine of asthma self-care and coping, and it alerts healthcare providers if specific conditions or patterns emerge. It is operated by the patient and/ or an informal caregiver and involves a spirometer that assesses the patient's lung capacity. Data sets from these assessments and web questionnaires are transmitted regularly to healthcare providers.

Similarly, e-health applications have been implemented for diabetes management, including the following:

- The Center for Health Services Research developed the web-based Diabetes Care Management Support System (DCMSS) in Michigan to support the routine care provided to patients with diabetes (Baker et al. 2001). A nonrandomized, longitudinal study demonstrated that web-based systems that used clinical practice guidelines, patient registries, and performance feedback had the potential to improve the rate of routine testing among patients with diabetes (McKay et al. 1998). The study explored the feasibility of a web-based tool for diabetes self-management that emphasized personalized goal setting, feedback, and social support. Patients who participated in that study appreciated the social support and the availability of information.

- The Telematic Management of Insulin-Dependent Diabetes Mellitus (T-IDDM) project implemented a distributed system for managing insulin-dependent diabetes. The goal of the project was to support patients and clinicians with a range of automated services, from data collection and transmission to data analysis and decision support (Riva, Bellazzi, and Stefanelli 1997). T-IDDM included a module that enabled patients to capture and transmit readings of a blood-glucose monitoring device to a hospital information system. It gave clinicians a set of tools for data visualization, data analysis, and decision support (Bellazzi et al. 2002).

Web-based e-health systems are also available for chronic conditions that are common in home care, such as congestive heart failure and chronic obstructive pulmonary disease as well as wound care requirements. The TeleHomeCare Project at the University of Minnesota, for example, relied on low-cost, commercially available monitoring devices and an Internet application designed for patients diagnosed with congestive heart failure and chronic obstructive pulmonary disease as well as those who needed wound care. The system included interfaces that were customized to address the information needs of individual patients. The daily questionnaire asked about symptoms, vital signs, overall well-being, and compliance with dietary guidelines (Demiris, Speedie, and Finkelstein 2001a).

Cancer treatment also benefits from e-health tools. In a study by Basch and colleagues (2005), 80 patients who had gynecologic malignancies and were about to begin standard chemotherapy regimens were enrolled in the web-based system and encouraged to log in to report their symptoms at each follow-up visit; alternatively, they were asked to access the system from home. Patients reported the symptoms they experienced during chemotherapy, and their communication using the web platform often led to clinical interventions and changes in the care plan. This indicated that such web-based asynchronous regular communication can be effective for the treatment and monitoring of cancer patients at home (Basch et al. 2005).

Finally, post-transplant care is an appropriate domain for e-health, because it requires an ongoing and regular monitoring of health status. Consistent spirometry monitoring of lung-transplant recipients is critical to early detection of acute infection and rejection of the allograft. A prospective study investigated the impact of a telemonitoring system that directly transmitted home spirometry to the hospital. The study found that "home monitoring of pulmonary function in lung-transplant recipients via the Internet is feasible and provides very reproducible data" (Morlion et al. 2002).

Most of the earlier studies of e-health applications in the home were either pilot, exploratory projects or feasibility studies with limited sample sizes. One of the earliest clinical trials in the area of telehealth in home care was a study by Johnston and colleagues (Johnston et al. 2000). This was a quasi-experimental study where newly referred patients diagnosed as having congestive heart failure, chronic obstructive pulmonary disease, cerebral vascular accident, cancer, diabetes, and anxiety as well as those who needed wound care were randomly assigned to either standard home care or an e-health intervention, which included a remote video system with peripheral monitoring devices that enabled nurses and patients to interact in real time. The study had a total sample of 212 subjects; 102 subjects were enrolled in the experimental (e-health) group and 110 in the control group (standard care). Findings demonstrated no differences in the quality indicators (i.e., medication compliance, knowledge of disease, and ability for self-care) or patient satisfaction.

A recent randomized clinical trial of home-based e-health was the Informatics for Diabetes Education and Telemedicine (IDEATel). This project compared e-health case management with standard care among older, medically underserved Medicare beneficiaries with diabetes who resided in medically underserved areas of New York State (Shea et al. 2009). The sample size included 1,665 Medicare recipients with diabetes, aged 55 years or older. Findings demonstrated that e-health case management resulted in net improvements in HbA1c, LDL-cholesterol, and blood pressure levels over the span of five years (Shea et al. 2009).

Personal Health Records

E-health applications support not only the transmission of data from one's home to a clinical setting but also the design of tools that allow patients to store and manage their own health information as a personal health record (PHR). The National Alliance for Health Information Technology (2008) defines a PHR as "an individual's electronic record of health-related information that conforms to nationally recognized interoperability standards and that can be drawn from multiple sources while being managed, shared and controlled by the individual." Thus, a PHR is a tool to use in "sharing health information, increasing health understanding and helping transform patients into better-educated consumers of health care" (Kahn, Aulakh, and Bosworth 2009).

In recent years, several initiatives have emerged to explore the design and implementation of such PHR tools. The Veterans Health Administration launched a PHR system called MyHealtheVet (US Department of Veterans Affairs 2012). MyHealtheVet documents and manages appointments and medication requests. It also assists veterans with selecting and obtaining a variety of healthcare services. Epic, the electronic medical record (EMR) software vendor, has also introduced a PHR application that is currently used by Kaiser Permanente, the Cambridge Health Alliance, and other healthcare organizations. These systems are widely used by consumers because they offer important functionality that could lead to improved health (Mechanic 2008).

PHRs enable the sharing of information, such as health finances (e.g., billing, insurance paperwork), diagnoses or conditions, allergies, immunizations, and medications, to assist patients with managing their own health (Hassol et al. 2004). In such systems, the patient (not any healthcare facility or provider) owns and controls/manages her data. The PHR developed by Microsoft (HealthVault) aims to give consumers access to their health information online without having to sign an organizational agreement or use special hardware. Traditional EMRs, in contrast, are owned by healthcare organizations and maintained by clinicians and other staff.

The integration of EMR and PHR systems is a synergistic model, where PHR data can augment EMR data and allow a collaborative continuum of care. Several challenges have served as barriers to realizing this synergistic vision, including legal, regulatory, and sociotechnical issues (e.g., clinicians' lack of trust in the data owned and generated by patients, acceptance of the patient's active role, changes in clinical workflow).

Social Media and Consumer Health Informatics

Social media and social networking have seen widespread adoption in the past decade. The sharing of personal details, including health information, has increased since the advent of social media and social network sites. Networking has been the subject of social science research since the 1950s (Ackerson and Viswanath 2009; Berkman 1984; Berkman et al. 2000; Bott 1957; Burt and Schøtt 1985; Fowler and Christakis 2010; Heckathorn 1979; Israel 1982; Milardo 2000). Our discussion focuses on networking brought on by the Internet and social media technologies that connect consumers to health information.

What Is Social Media?

Social media allows new forms of communication of information (health and personal) between individuals and groups—in contrast to the old, one-way channels of communication from care providers to patients—by using Web 2.0 technology and user-generated content (UGC). Consumer health informatics focuses on the analysis of an individual's health information needs and preferences and the creation and implementation of technology based on models that make health information accessible to consumers (Eysenbach 2000). One of the challenges of discussing social media is the lack of universally accepted definitions for social media or Web 2.0, which creates confusion (Adams 2010; Doherty 2008). In addition, many different types of social media exist.

Doherty (2008) notes that Web 2.0 "is essentially a set of technologies and the range of affordances made possible by those technologies." Kaplan and Haenlein (2010), meanwhile, define Web 2.0 as "a platform whereby content and applications are no longer created and published by individuals, but instead are continuously modified by all users in a participatory and collaborative fashion." They define UGC as content that is publicly available on a website, shows creative effort, and is created outside of professional practices.

Social media uses Web 2.0 applications and UGC that allow multi-way communication, collaboration, and democratic content management (Orsini 2010). This technology also facilitates communication by breaking down language barriers through natural-language processing and machine translations (McNab 2009). Social media exchanges are instantaneous; conversations rather than directives; active not passive; connective, linking people with similar conditions and concerns; and representative of how lessons from experiences can be shared. This capability gave rise to Health 2.0 (Doherty 2008), Medicine 2.0 (Eysenbach 2008), and Public Health 2.0 (Wilson and Keelan 2009), which are concepts that leverage social media in the healthcare context. Health 2.0 is defined as "the affordances of Web 2.0 technologies for the healthcare community whilst recognising that these affordances are manifest in a variety of ways" (Doherty 2008).

As a means of sharing personal health information, social media is a substantial tool. More than 32 percent of the world's population were Internet users in 2011, and that number continues to grow (Internetworldstats .com 2012). The question now about using social media for healthcare purposes is how control of personal health information will shift from government and healthcare organizations to individual patients supported by private service providers (Kidd 2008). A related question is what impact such a shift might have on patient–provider relationships, quality of care, and efforts to equalize health disparities (Bacigalupe 2011).

What Types of Social Media Exist?

Kaplan and Haenlein (2010) classify social media into six broad categories:

1. Blogs
2. Collaborative projects
3. Content communities
4. Virtual game worlds
5. Virtual social worlds
6. Social network sites

Each of these categories can be used to exchange personal health information. Collaborative projects, content communities, and virtual game worlds are not structured for personal information sharing and thus have lower levels of self-disclosure than are possible with blogs, social networks, and virtual social worlds (Kaplan and Haenlein 2010). Higher levels of self-disclosure, however, increase the risks of privacy abuses by people and organizations outside of the social media community. Each of these categories is discussed below, but social network sites are explored in a separate section later in this chapter.

Blogs

The blog (a contraction of *web* and *log*) is the earliest form of social media. It amounts to an online diary or a personal website written, designed, and managed by a single blogger but typically open to comments from readers who wished to interact with the blogger. One popular blog site is Blogger (www.blogger.com), which offers templates and other services to those who want to maintain a blog. Over the years, blogs have grown in type, scope, and function, covering news, business, marketing, and other nonpersonal interests. For example, www.thehealthcareblog.com is a robust blog run by a community of healthcare insiders and experts and publishes news, opinions, and features about different health settings and sectors. Twitter is another type of blog—a microblogging variety—that allows frequent posts of messages (as well as responses and reposts) that are limited to 140 characters. As such, it has the potential to improve health communications among its users (Hawn 2009; Scanfeld, Scanfeld, and Larson 2010). Specifically, "Twitter and similar services may provide a venue to identify potential misuse or misunderstanding of antibiotics, to promote positive behavior change, and to disseminate valid information...behavior change interventions delivered by mobile telephone short-message service can be used as a model for such Twitter-based reminders" (Scanfeld, Scanfeld, and Larson 2010). In addition, Twitter has been used to raise awareness for a global surgery campaign, to track H1N1 cases, and to share information about clinical trials and disease (Jatem, Casey, and Kushner 2011).

Collaborative Projects

A collaborative project invites many people to participate and enables them to create or contribute to a social product with the use of web-based applications. It relies on crowd sourcing—that is, engaging volunteer labor (Kaplan and Haenlein 2010; McFedries 2006). A popular example of a global collaborative project is Wikipedia (www.wikipedia.com), a crowd-sourced web encyclopedia. Wikipedia includes articles on health-related topics and is a prominent health information site as a result of its high search rankings (Laurent and Vickers 2009), although its mental health entries have been shown to contain inaccurate information (Mercer 2007). Meanwhile, there is also the health community wiki, a "collaborative website authored by a group of patients or by medical professionals" (Doherty 2008). WikiSurgery (http://wikisurgery.com) is an example of a health community wiki.

Content Communities

Also known as an information community, a content community is "form[ed] around people's needs to get and use information in ways that they perceive as helpful" (Fisher, Durrance, and Unruh 2003). YouTube (a video-sharing site) and Flickr (a digital photo-sharing site) are two well-known content communities. Analyzing archived messages from three online cancer communities, Civan and Pratt (2007) identify three types of support that have been exchanged in traditional support groups and waiting rooms:

1. "Informational support (e.g., exchange of advice, explanations, opinions, and experiences) helps patients understand and learn to cope with their illness."
2. "Emotional support can bolster interpersonal connectedness and self-esteem as well as reduce distress through the expression of feelings, such as anxiety, concern, empathy, or reassurance."
3. "Instrumental support involves the exchange of practical assistance and material goods (e.g., financial support, transportation, or help with household chores)."

In another health-related implementation, one municipal health department used an information community as a new channel to disseminate information about the use of public funds via the Internet (Fisher, Durrance, and Unruh 2003).

Virtual Game Worlds

Virtual game worlds "are platforms that replicate a three-dimensional environment in which users can appear in the form of personalized avatars and interact with each other as they would in real life" (Kaplan and Haenlein 2010). World of Warcraft (http://us.battle.net/wow/en/) is an online role-playing game that is representative of a virtual game world. Virtual game applications have the potential to engage consumers in activities that can promote health literacy or cognitive function.

Virtual Social Worlds

Similar to virtual game worlds, virtual social worlds place users in real-life scenarios (Kaplan and Haenlein 2010). Second Life (http://secondlife.com) is one example. Pilot studies on relaxation have been conducted by clinicians within the Second Life environment, while the Centers for Disease Control and Prevention (CDC) maintains podcasts, holds virtual health fairs, and has conducted private interviews with online participants about HIV/AIDS (Bruck 2008).

What Is a Social Network Site?

According to boyd and Ellison (2007), a social network site consists of "web-based services that allow individuals to (1) construct a public or semi-public profile within a bounded system, (2) articulate a list of other users with whom they share a connection, and (3) view and traverse their list of connections and those made by others within the system." Other authors also contribute their definitions and characteristics of a social network site, including the following:

- "An online location where a user can create a profile and build a personal network that connects him or her to other users" (Lenhart 2007)
- "Involves the explicit modeling of connections between people, forming a complex network of relations, which in turn enables and facilitates collaboration and collaborative filtering processes" (Eysenbach 2008)
- Enables "users to connect by creating personal information profiles, inviting friends and colleagues to have access to those profiles, and sending e-mails and instant messages between each other. These personal profiles can include any type of information, including photos, video, audio files, and blogs" (Kaplan and Haenlein 2010)
- Makes "it possible for users to branch into different conversations and create special relationships" (Landro 2006)

Health Social Network Sites

Health social network sites emerged from social networking and its breadth and capacities. As technologies that support the accessibility and exchange of health information for consumers, they are considered consumer health informatics resources. With a health and wellness focus, a health social network site is powered by Health 2.0 applications. Swan (2009) provides this definition: "a website where consumers may be able to find health resources at a number of different levels." The types of interactions or communications that a health social network site supports are patient to patient, patient to provider, and provider to provider (Doherty 2008). Patient-to-patient and patient-to-provider communications are most relevant to a discussion of consumer health informatics.

Understanding what the health implications of social network sites are entails learning who uses these sites. Lenhart (2009) has found that "one third (35%) of American adult internet users have a profile on an online social network site, four times as many as three years ago, but still much lower than the 65% of online American teens who use social networks." In addition, a background paper from the Canadian Library of Parliament reports that younger Canadians have social network site profiles to a greater degree than do older Canadians (86 percent for ages 18 to 34 versus 44 percent for ages 55 or older) (Dewing 2010). A survey of 2,251 American adults who use social network sites states that 51 percent have multiple profiles on different sites for professional and personal uses, while 43 percent had but a single profile (Lenhart 2009). An analysis of data from the 2007 Health Information National Trends Study in the United States also indicates that among web users, social networking sites (23 percent) are more popular than blogging (7 percent) and online support-group participation (5 percent) (Chou et al. 2009).

The wants and needs of patients and other customers must be central to the design and features of a health social network site. Civan and colleagues (2006) determine the three goals, through a group study of participants interested in managing their personal health information, that a health social network site should deliver: "monitoring and assessing health, making health-related decisions and planning preventive or treatment actions." Meanwhile, Weiss and Lorenzi (2007) offer four considerations when designing and rolling out a pilot health social network site for patients with cancer: Sites (1) should have a mechanism that informs patients whether information is actively sent or passively posted, (2) should have clearly delineated spaces to avoid unintentional personal disclosures, (3) should offer a spell-check feature, and (4) should ensure that patients' family members do not think site invitations are spam. In a study of breast cancer patients, Skeels and colleagues (2010) argue that the site's features should support dissemination of caregiving information and management of help requests and offers, and these features should be implemented using the Facebook Connect platform.

According to Eysenbach (2007), people get health information through three ways: (1) intermediation, where the person receives information from a health expert or information gatekeeper; (2) disintermediation, where the person eliminates the information gatekeeper; and (3) apomediation, where the person receives guidance from network intermediaries. Use of a web portal with content vetted by health experts (e.g., www.webmd .com) is an example of intermediation, use of a patient-initiated web search is an example of disintermediation, and use of a health social network site is an example of apomediation (Eysenbach 2008).

The value of health social network sites lies in their capability to connect a person with others with similar health conditions and with whom he can share information (Swan 2009). As Ancker and colleagues (2009) note, people can obtain or give "advice, interpretation of medical language or events, and personal experience. Such patient-generated information is likely to be written in common terms, rather than in medical jargon, and it may be easier to understand by those with lower health literacy or numeracy." A *folksonomy* (a combination of *folk* and *taxonomy*) is generated when people tag digital information with their own keywords and classifications for later retrieval or use; these tags are then found by other searchers (Dye 2006). On health social network sites, folksonomies are a source of insight about how patients use clinical terminology and understand their conditions; for example, some patients discuss Type 1 diabetes as a symptom and not a disease (Smith and Wicks 2008).

Swan (2009) notes that 20 health social network sites have launched in the past few years and can be grouped into three categories: "patient-focused general multi-condition websites, patient-focused cause-specific websites and physician-focused social networks." Examples of health social network sites are OrganizedWisdom, DailyStrength, PatientsLikeMe, Everyday Health (formerly Revolution Health), HealthSpace, Group Loop, and HealthVault. These sites use folksonomy tagging and offer information sharing and emotional support and some "may emphasize one area more, such as information and research citations (example: OrganizedWisdom) or social connection and support (example: DailyStrength)" (Swan 2009).

- PatientsLikeMe (www.patientslikeme.com) enables patients diagnosed with Amyotrophic Lateral Sclerosis, Multiple Sclerosis, or Parkinson's Disease to share information and experiences (Smith and Wicks 2008). These shared information and experiences help patients understand what outcomes can be expected or are possible and what plans can be created to reach those outcomes (Wicks et al. 2010).

- Everyday Health (www.everydayhealth.com) provides vetted content and hosts user communities interested in "risk assessments, healthcare ratings, a symptoms checklist, portfolios for organizing health records, and free newsletters" (Brynko 2007).
- HealthSpace (www.healthspace.nhs.uk) operates out of the United Kingdom and "allows patients to record selected data in their own Internet based health record, with control over how they share this record with healthcare providers" (Kidd 2008).
- Group Loop (www.grouploop.org) connects teens with cancer in the United States and nine other countries by leveraging collective experiences with Facebook and Myspace (Landro 2006).
- With a focus on exchange of information, "Personal Health Application platforms such as HealthVault...have APIs for other applications to connect to" (Eysenbach 2008).
- With regard to provider-patient communication, Kaiser Permanente offers physician home pages with profiles that are similar to those seen on social network sites like Facebook (Orsini 2010). However, it remains to be seen whether patients want this type of interaction with their clinicians, given that in a survey of 450 upper-extremity patients "only 31% of patients surveyed were interested in using social networks to communicate with their physicians" (Rozental, George, and Chacko 2010).

A survey about online behavior and HIV/STI risk factors among 201 homeless youth served by a drop-in agency in Los Angeles reveals these mixed findings: Online interactions increase the likelihood of meeting a sex partner, but online discussions about love and sex add to knowledge about HIV and sexually transmitted infections (STIs), and mere membership in a health social network site increases the likelihood of getting tested for STIs (Young and Rice 2011). In addition, networked communication used during the treatment of youth with mental health problems reduces symptoms and improves quality of patient–provider encounters, but whether this type of communications can be integrated into other types of consultations is unclear (Martin et al. 2011).

Reliability Concerns

The information on health social networks sites is crowd-sourced and thus may be unreliable or inaccurate. One study report on the "very low quality user-contributed health information on three different sites. Half of all postings containing medical information were incomplete or contained errors. Of these, over 80% were potentially clinically significant...[and thus may] compromise patient safety as a distribution platform for persuasive, personally tailored, but harmful misinformation" (Tsai et al. 2007). The issue with Web 2.0 technology as a health information communication channel is that it provides an online environment for consumers with alternative health beliefs to engage in group discussions with other consumers who can share and validate viewpoints that may or may not be true (Wilson and Keelan 2009). With regard to HealthSpace, the majority of consumers prefer a summary care record and control over entities that are granted access to such resources but are not interested in entering their own information (Kidd 2008). Some organizations, like the American Cancer Society, recommend that content on health-related web resources be validated by health experts (Landro 2006); however, doing that could create a credibility risk for site operators if the content on their site is filled with errors (Kidd 2008).

Barriers and Opportunities

In 2006, Landro observed that "it is still too early to tell whether health social-networking sites will flourish, since they will depend on how vigilant members are about keeping them going." Six years later, that observation remains applicable. In 2007, boyd and Ellison (2007) recognized the limited understanding of who does and does not use social network sites, their reasons, and the implications of using these sites. Four years later, Bacigalupe (2011) points out that given "the accelerated adoption of these technologies in the last decade, the collaborative health world seems to be developing without paying enough attention to the phenomenon."

McDaniel, Schutte and Keller (2008) identify these barriers to integrating PHRs with health social network sites: "low health literacy; inaccessibility due to lack of knowledge, skills, or technology; legal concerns of providers; and economic sustainability (i.e., who should pay for the development and maintenance of personal health record systems)." In addition, Rozental, George, and Chacko (2010) observe that "[e]xpanding use of social networking in health care will thus benefit only patients who are already online, and efforts should continue to target patients without computer and Internet access with traditional printed media." Health social network sites also must be designed for usability. HealthSpace has experienced slow adoption because of user frustration with using the system (Kidd 2008).

Many opportunities are available for health in social media. Because more people use social network sites more than they do blogs and online support groups, health social networks are prime for health communications (Chou et al. 2009). Swan (2009) observes "emerging patient-driven technology-enabled health care models have focal points at every node of the wellness cycle, particularly at earlier stages, targeting prevention rather than therapy." This may enable small health communities to interact with each other and larger groups to negotiate contracts with insurance providers (Swan 2009).

Future health consumers and patients likely will come to expect the use of social networking as part of the services offered by their healthcare providers (Bacigalupe 2011). These sites "may someday replace other traditional forms of patient–physician or researcher subject communication, such as the telephone, or even newer forms of communication, such as e-mail" (Moreno et al. 2009). If and when that happens, providers must be prepared to engage in real patient dialogues enabled by Health 2.0 rather than continue to deliver the monologues supported by the traditional provider–patient contact.

Challenges in E-Health Applications

Factors that are critical for the success and diffusion of e-health applications include privacy and confidentiality, reimbursement, and accessibility.

Privacy and Confidentiality

An important and continuing issue in e-health and consumer health informatics is the privacy and confidentiality of personal health information. Privacy is a person's right to be free from and refuse interference, attention, observation, and other types of invasion. In the context of healthcare, privacy is assurance that one's health information is collected, accessed, used, retained, and shared only when necessary and only to the extent necessary and that the information is protected throughout its life cycle using fair privacy practices consistent with applicable laws, and regulations and the preferences of the individual. Confidentiality is the obligation of every HIPAA-covered entity to enact and enforce policies that protect the patient's privacy. (Privacy and security are further discussed in Chapter 13.)

HIPAA (Health Insurance Portability and Accountability Act of 1996) introduced the need for comprehensive, national safeguards from privacy and confidentiality threats, mandating the implementation of standards to keep individual health information safe, secure, and private (HHS 2000). Compliance with these standards greatly affected the design and functions of e-health applications. Multimedia transactions (e.g., video and audio recording, transmission of still images) not only must be able to conceal identifiable data but also must be performed through the most-secure infrastructure or platform (e.g., phone, satellite, Internet). The widespread usage of the Internet and Web 2.0 has widened HIPAA compliance issues. For example, web-based applications for disease management drive organizations to assess issues of data ownership and access, such as who owns the information stored on a vendor's or a third-party's server and who has the authority to use those data and information. Similarly, personal health applications that empower patients to collect, store, and maintain their own information must also be examined, and their ownership, access and monitoring rights, and potential confidentiality violations must be defined.

Privacy and Social Media

High levels of personal health information disclosed or posted on health social networks create risks for privacy abuses. Using Facebook as a framework, Grimmelmann (2009) conducts an in-depth analysis of the social and psychological factors behind people's use of social network sites and their privacy expectations. Grimmelmann asks, "What motivates Facebook users? Why do they underestimate the privacy risks? When their privacy is violated, what went wrong?" He argues that failure of site operators to ask similar questions of their users will result in privacy policies that do not work.

Some of the privacy issues related to health social network sites include the following:

- Some people may not know the potential risks of giving up their anonymity (thus undermining their privacy) when they participate in social networking (Adams 2010).
- Personal information disclosed on social network sites may "reinforce existing stereotypes, making them more intractable" (Ellison, Lampe, and Steinfield 2009).
- "Personal information may be misused by marketing agents or used for nefarious purposes such as stalking, bullying, and identity theft" (Ellison, Lampe, and Steinfield 2009).
- Personal information requests are more likely to be granted to "friends" via a phishing scheme on a social network site (Jagatic et al. 2007).
- Social network users must find a balance between the ease and convenience of widely publicizing their information to a network of people and the need to protect their identity and associated information by customizing their privacy settings, which limits the risk of privacy invasion (Pratt et al. 2006).

In a survey of 205 college students about privacy concerns and risk-taking attitudes "almost 10% of the participants provided their phone number on their social network profile" (Fogel and Nehmad 2009). However, boyd and Hargittai (2010) find that the majority of young consumers on Facebook are engaged to some degree with management of their privacy settings. Regardless, Moreno and colleagues (2009) recommend that providers and parents understand social network sites to help mitigate the potential risks and benefits for teenagers who use these sites, while Fogel and Nehmad (2009) recommend that allied health professionals, consumer groups, and communication professionals promote policies that would display warnings about privacy risks before young consumers are permitted to create social network profiles. Favoring the positive, Swan (2009) points out that "patients are the only ones who can avoid HIPAA privacy regulations and open source their own data to the benefit of the greater community, patients can skirt the social taboos that other health care ecosystem members may encounter regarding economic issues...[and] providers would be forced to develop consumer-presentable health service offerings and pricing."

Reimbursement

A recent policy statement issued by a diverse group of healthcare providers called for recognition of telemedicine in healthcare reform and the need to reimburse telemedicine on par with in-person visits. In 2011, the Centers for Medicare and Medicaid Services (CMS) announced a revised rule that makes it easier for hospitals to credential physicians for reimbursement of telemedicine visits (HHS and CMS 2011). The revised law took effect on July 5, 2011. The new CMS rule should increase the use of telemedicine, as most physicians receive reimbursement through state Medicaid programs. In the past, only 19 states offered Medicaid reimbursement to physicians for telemedicine services (Naditz 2008). Private payers also lagged in adopting reimbursement policies for telemedicine, but progress (albeit slow) is being made toward changing that (Pamela and Lorraine 2007).

Many insurance companies reimburse healthcare organizations for specific types of telemedicine services. In many instances, providers can use their patient charts to indicate to certain service providers or reimbursement companies (such as Kaiser Permanente or Blue Cross) that the patient visit took place via a telecommunication network. For home-based applications such as telehomecare (broadly defined as the use of telehealth in the home setting), the issue of reimbursement becomes more challenging. The Health Care Financing Administration (now CMS) initially denied Medicare reimbursement of telehomecare because the service was not yet proven to be cost effective. Evidence emerged, however, that demonstrated the cost effectiveness of traditional disease management. For example, a retrospective analysis of 7,000 patients found a $50 per member, per month savings in diabetes treatment costs over 12 months and an 18 percent decrease in admissions (Rubin, Dietrich, and Hawk 1998). The results of a telemedicine cost-effectiveness study in an intensive care unit were mixed, but they indicated that telemedicine is cost effective for the sickest patients (Franzini et al. 2011). In addition, a study of a collaborative-care telemedicine intervention in rural settings found the intervention to be effective but expensive. These results suggest that additional evidence is necessary to determine the models that might be cost effective or allow long-term cost reduction through utilization of the Internet and advanced telecommunications in disease management and home care.

The Balanced Budget Act (BBA) of 1997 allowed for telemedicine reimbursement in specific cases—especially for providers in rural locations, which the BBA defined as healthcare professional shortage areas. In these cases, reimbursement is provided for Medicare patients who stay at home and receive healthcare services via telemedicine. In 2000, a new means of paying for home care—the prospective payment system (PPS)—went into effect. PPS apportions payment per episode of care (using 60-day periods), instead of payment for each visit, allowing home care agencies to integrate virtual visits within the care plan as they see fit.

Cost analysis and/or cost effectiveness studies will contribute to discussions about possible reimbursement issues of web-based monitoring or telemedicine services, including who will bear the costs of implementing and maintaining these services. One of the reasons that reimbursement of telemedicine has not garnered attention (or that progress in this area has been slow) is the lack of a federal e-health authority. In the last few years, state and federal health agencies have focused on increasing the number of high-quality online health resources. Several healthcare institutions and agencies of the US Department of Health and Human Services have been sponsoring e-health-related initiatives. The two major federal agencies with regulatory authority over e-health matters are the Federal Trade Commission and the Food and Drug Administration.

Accessibility

A significant segment of consumers who require home care services or who manage multiple chronic conditions comprises older adults who have functional limitations. Such limitations are related to a decrease in cognitive, motor, or sensory abilities as a result of temporary or permanent injury, illness, or aging. E-health systems enable members of this population to manage their own health and inform their healthcare decision making. With this consumer informatics application, however, those oldest, with severe limitations, or without computer experience or proficiency are at a disadvantage because hardware and software designers often fail to consider their needs. Addressing cognitive, functional, or sensory limitations and recognizing the diversity of user skills and abilities are essential to designing consumer informatics systems. Doing so increases the system's accessibility and practicality as well as the number and diversity of users. Designers need to develop functional system features and subject them to rigorous tests by a wide range of consumer groups with differing capabilities, interests, and motivations. Existing resources—such as design recommendations developed for web systems for older adults (Demiris, Finkelstein, and Speedie 2001) and considerations in implementing telehealth systems to accommodate functional, cognitive, and other consumer needs (Stronge, Rogers, and Fisk 2007)—can guide designers who aim to maximize the accessibility of their products.

Another dimension of accessibility is the availability of the appropriate technological infrastructure that supports the e-health system. Broadband Internet, for example, may be required to operate a system but may not be available in a residence or geographic region. Likewise, web-based applications may require a peripheral device for synchronous communication, such as a camera or a microphone, but the consumer may not have such equipment. Before software is designed, implemented, or widely distributed, infrastructure and hardware needs must be determined and evaluated to ensure that current and potential users can gain access and those in rural communities and in institutions with limited resources are not excluded. Inaccessibility greatly contributes to the digital divide.

Success Factors for E-Health

Factors determining the success and sustainability of e-health applications include outcomes, processes, cost, patients' and family members' acceptance, and providers' acceptance.

Outcomes

If e-health applications are to be adopted as part of the standard care, their outcomes should be at least the same as (or better than) that achieved by traditional care. The impact of e-health on clinical outcomes has been investigated to some extent, but large randomized clinical trials are needed that would clearly demonstrate such an impact (Johnston et al. 2000). For example, when telehomecare's effect on medication compliance and ability for self-care was examined in a quasi-experimental study with a control group (receiving traditional care) and an intervention group (receiving traditional care and access to a remote videoconference system), the effect was found to be no different from that of traditional care (Jerant, Azari, and Nesbitt 2001). However, when conducted in a one-year randomized trial, which involved congestive heart failure patients equipped with a two-way video-conferencing device with an integrated electronic stethoscope, telehomecare showed its ability to reduce hospital readmissions and emergency visits for this patient population.

The assumption about most technology applications used in telemedicine is that they enable more intensive and frequent physiological monitoring, which then leads to early detection and intervention. In addition, they can monitor medication and treatment compliance and promote patient education. The time has come to test this hypothesis by measuring the technology in large clinical trials rather than small-scale feasibility studies.

Processes

During a face-to-face visit, addressing technical issues (e.g., focusing the camera, adjusting the audio) is not part of the patient–provider communication. But these issues can be common in, or even dominate, a virtual visit. Thus, studying care delivery processes that use telemedicine is of great importance. It is not fully understood whether video-mediated or web-based communication affects or significantly alters the relationship between clinicians and patients and how these virtual encounters may be a barrier to the relationship and the care processes. Use of technology during the clinical encounter may intimidate patients and result in their limited participation in their care or reduced communication with their providers, as face-to-face interactions are considered "more spontaneous, and free-flowing" than technology-enabled contact (O'Conaill and Whittaker 1997). This diminished willingness or ability to participate and engage because of the technology is a serious threat to caregiving, as patients greatly value the opportunity to ask questions and voice concerns when interacting with their clinicians (Ende et al. 1989; Street 1992). Active patient participation contributes to greater satisfaction with care, treatment adherence, and improved health outcomes (Lerman et al. 1990; Kaplan, Greenfield, and Ware 1989).

One study reviewed 122 virtual visits and performed content analysis to determine the themes of interaction that emerge from these visits (Demiris, Speedie, and Finkelstein 2001b). The research showed that visit time is spent on these categories of communication: assessing the patient's medical status, promoting medication and treatment compliance, addressing psychosocial issues, exchanging informal banter, educating the patient on health issues, discussing administrative and technical issues, evaluating patient satisfaction, and ensuring continued accessibility to the provider. Clearly, some of these topics should not be covered during a virtual visit, but overall the discussions indicate e-health has the potential to enrich the care process. Further studies and direct comparisons between actual and virtual visits will provide insights into the process of virtual patient–clinician encounters—for example, whether e-health enhances or inhibits a patient's communication to the provider of her physical discomfort, medical symptoms, and emotional state and, conversely, whether it encourages or prevents a clinician's communication to the patient of treatment instructions or expression of empathy (Oliver and Demiris 2010; Bashshur 1995).

Cost

A comprehensive evaluation of e-health applications must include a cost analysis to compare the inputs and outputs associated with e-health with those of traditional healthcare. Telemedicine evaluation methods have improved in recent years but more work needs to be done (Bergmo 2010) to ensure that the benefits and outcomes are balanced with the cost and other inputs. Here, the inputs include medical expertise, facilities, technology, service personnel, and client characteristics. During a cost analysis, the effects of known quantities of traditional healthcare (e.g., episodes of care, hospital stays) should be assessed. Cost savings from the use of e-health can be realized if the following outcomes can be demonstrated:

- Reduction of unnecessary visits to the emergency department
- Reduction of unnecessary/unscheduled visits to the physician's office
- Early detection and intervention
- Patient education that leads to improvement of lifestyle choices and medication adherence
- Prevention of repeat hospitalizations, or overall decrease of rehospitalization rates
- Reduction of indirect costs and burn-out by easing the burden on caregivers

The number of face-to-face consultations could, in some cases, be reduced if the visits are substituted with virtual or web-based consultations, which in turn eliminate travel time and travel costs. Using portable devices and e-health technologies, vital signs data can be collected and interpreted several times during the course of a day rather than only at scheduled visits. This allows for early detection and intervention, which is especially important if signs of deterioration or problems are missed or misidentified. In addition, telemedicine technologies enable family members or other caregivers to participate in a collaborative care process, adding to the patient's support network.

Patients' and Family Members' Acceptance

One of the unique aspects of e-health is that the required technology is installed in the patient's home and operated by the patient and/or her surrogate. The success of this form of healthcare delivery hinges on the patient's and family's acceptance of its use. What influences this acceptance (and diffusion) is the understanding of the concept of e-health. Considering the patient's possible functional limitations and inexperience with the e-health technology, this initial acceptance is essential.

Not many instruments that have been tested for reliability and validity can measure patients' perception of or satisfaction with e-health applications. One such instrument is the TMPQ (Telemedicine Perception Questionnaire) (Demiris, Speedie, and Finkelstein 2000), which was developed by the University of Minnesota to assess patients' perceptions of the advantages and disadvantages of e-health. TMPQ was tested extensively and was found to show high levels of internal consistency and test-retest reliability. Its domains include the following (Demiris, Speedie, and Finkelstein 2000):

• Perceived quality of and access to healthcare
• Time and money (e.g., time savings for the patient and nurse, reduced costs for the patient and the healthcare agency)
• Components of the virtual visit (e.g., ease of equipment use, equal acceptability of virtual and real visits, protection of privacy and confidentiality, lack of physical contact, reduced sense of intimacy, patient's ability to explain her medical problems in a virtual environment)
• General impression of telehomecare and its role in the future

Providers' Acceptance

The success of e-health applications that involve healthcare providers (e.g., through videoconferencing) does not depend only on patients' acceptance but also on the acceptance of care providers themselves. Many e-health applications alter providers' practice patterns and affect their workflow. Thus, they have to accept this alternate mode of care delivery and to be comfortable using the required equipment to interact with their patients.

As is the case with all technological innovations, organizational commitment is essential to optimum telemedicine utilization. This dependency can be a challenge as many complex, institution-centric information systems do not support (at least not currently) the e-health infrastructure or endorse a strategic agenda for e-health applications. Adoption of e-health implies a restructuring of the institution and redefinition of its services.

Conclusion

E-health and consumer health informatics have seen significant advancement in recent years. New technologies and pilot implementations in a variety of settings have emerged, showcasing a potential shift to patient-centered care. The landscape of modern healthcare has undergone a transformation as a result of new laws and policies, particularly in the United States. The viable models and long-term effects of e-health and telemedicine interventions have yet to be determined, but people, aided by technology and acting as collaborators of care providers, are destined to play a large role in their own health and wellness. To determine the most cost-effective cause-and-effect models of e-health, studies in many different areas must be conducted.

On the consumer side, researchers can determine who is using new technologies, in what ways, for what purposes, and how that use allows people to be empowered and to manage their own health and related information. On the clinical side, studies should explore how technologies, such as social media, can be integrated into the information systems in clinical settings. In addition, researchers must find ways to improve the reliability of the information that new technologies make available to healthcare providers, as these technologies can change the roles of everyone who has a stake in the health and wellness of an individual. Healthcare leaders and administrators, for their part, must engage and include providers in planning, selecting, designing, or implementing new technologies that change the dynamic of the patient–provider relationships. From an administrative perspective, all stakeholders must help determine how an integrated healthcare system can keep pace with new technologies and can adjust reimbursement models to make them sustainable.

Privacy and confidentiality are paramount in e-health and consumer health informatics. The questions of who owns personal health information, who can access and use it, and for what purposes it may be used must all be answered, and better means of protecting such information must be developed. In addition, the benefits and risks of emergent technologies to populations and communities must be weighed, particularly in the context of improving community and population health and engaging traditionally marginalized or disenfranchised populations. Equally important is understanding how new technologies can be used to address and minimize healthcare gaps and disparities and how they widen the digital divide between people who have access to the Internet and technology and people who do not.

Chapter Discussion Questions

1. What are the different platforms that support e-health? Give examples of each.
2. Define consumer health informatics, and differentiate it from traditional clinical informatics approaches.
3. Discuss the types of social media, and give examples of how social media can be applied to e-health.
4. How would you design a reimbursement system that recognizes the value of e-health applications?
5. Identify the success factors in e-health.

6. How can inadequate or lack of access to communication technology (the digital divide) lead to care inequality in the emerging e-health model? Identify the social and ethical issues associated with modern health IT.

7. What are some of the cultural challenges in shifting from a centralized health IT controlled by the organization to a decentralized health IT controlled by the patient?

CASE STUDY   **Blue River Home Care**

George Demiris and Blaine Reeder

Blue River Home Care is a for-profit home care agency affiliated with the Blue River Hospital, a private 60-bed hospital. The agency is an early adopter of telehomecare services that are now integrated into the care plans of patients suffering from chronic diseases. The telehomecare technology integrates data from portable monitoring devices, including spirometers, blood pressure cuffs, digital weight scales, and videophones. After eight years, the agency is beginning to reap the benefits of investing in the telehomecare infrastructure, which enhances the quality of delivered services and reduces costs. Specifically, regular patient monitoring enabled by technology has reduced the staff's travel costs and time, made scheduling home care visits more efficient, and (in many cases) intervened proactively to prevent adverse events. Thus far, it is too early to tell if rehospitalization rates for home care patients with chronic conditions will be reduced, given that the technology enables early detection of symptoms and signs, but anecdotal evidence of such reductions is positive.

Currently, Blue River's administration is looking for ways to keep pace with emerging technologies, which would give the agency a competitive advantage. The leaders are examining the integration of a PHR and a health social network site into the existing telehomecare infrastructure. Proposed features of this social network include the ability for patients to access and manage their personal health information, for patients to find and connect with others with similar conditions for support and sharing, and for family members and caregivers to participate in virtual support groups. Blue River has held informal meetings with its healthcare providers regarding this plan. While some clinicians are supportive of the communication and information opportunities that the plan will afford patients and their caregivers, other clinicians have some worries, including the following:

- The health social network site might propagate unreliable or wrong information.
- PHR integration could pose privacy (and thus liability) risks.
- Patients may not use the site.
- Physician compensation could be affected (and how so) by the online patient–clinician interaction.
- Patients, especially older adults and those without experience with technology, may find using the PHR and the site to enter, manage, and find health information (especially to improve health literacy) difficult.

These reactions are indicative of the diverse views and attitudes of healthcare providers, administrators, patients, and family members toward consumer health applications.

Solutions and Considerations

Following are factors Blue River (and other healthcare organizations) should consider and discuss when proposing and implementing an integrated PHR and health social network site:

- Communication between patients and their formal and informal caregivers will greatly improve. This, in turn, may lead to better health outcomes because such a system would
  1. form or strengthen the social support for patients,
  2. serve as an early detection tool of new health or medical events,
  3. ease care coordination across various caregivers and care networks, and
  4. increase the patient's feeling of independence.
- The viewpoint of each stakeholder group should be solicited and taken into account.
- The potential benefits of an integrated PHR and health social network site may be offset by problems introduced by the new technology.
- More information may be available to patients but they may not know how to interpret it for decision-making purposes. Most patients lack medical knowledge, so health research findings, notes, discussion, and other information could confuse or be misunderstood by the patients. The same holds true for family members who have access to their loved one's PHR and social network profile.

(continued)

- Different approaches to integrating PHRs and health social networks should be tried. For example, patients may be left to own, manage, and control their own data, but first the organization should develop a web portal that enables patients to access, annotate, or share their own information. This may address the patients' desire and willingness to play a more active role in their own healthcare.

- The technology will introduce new privacy and information reliability issues. Specifically, family members' access to their loved one's information and the ability of other members of the social network to view each other's profile or pages could breach a person's privacy and confidentiality. In addition, with the patient in charge of his PHR, concerns about the reliability of the available information will emerge and will affect the provider's clinical decision making.

- The organization must assess the usability and compatibility of system interfaces, regardless of whether the system or software was purchased from a vendor or created for the institution's use. It cannot be difficult to operate or navigate, especially for frail or elderly people (as is the case for Blue River) or those with little or no experience with technology or computers. User friendliness must be maximized to enable and encourage access to the system. Initial and ongoing training and customer support must be offered whenever feasible.

- Because the proposed integrated PHR and health social network site is touted to facilitate frequent communication among members of the network and allow patients to get involved in the decision-making process, the organization should build an IT infrastructure that supports these functions.

- To gain institutional support, leadership must demonstrate that the new system will yield concrete benefits for the organization and its staff (such as increased marketability and competitiveness, improved quality of care, and reduced inefficiencies) without placing undue burden or additional tasks on the staff. Furthermore, leadership must show evidence that the proposed system has proven effective in other clinical settings or similar organizations.

Case Study Discussion Questions

1. Name some of the challenges in ensuring continuity of care for patients with chronic conditions. How can emerging technologies solve or at least ease these challenges?

2. List some of the benefits of integrating a PHR with a health social network site for patients with chronic illness, their caregivers, and the organization.

3. Name the specific impacts of adopting e-health and social media applications on the structure and strategies of a healthcare organization.

4. How might the adoption of an integrated PHR and health social network site change the interaction and relationship between patients and health professionals?

GENOMIC MEDICINE: INFORMATICS IMPLICATIONS AND OPPORTUNITIES

12

Mark A. Hoffman

Learning Objectives

After reading this chapter, students will be able to

- Articulate the basic principles of genetics and genomics
- Understand the roles of genetic and genomic information in clinical practice and health management
- Understand trends that will lead to greater precision in determining a care plan for a patient
- Recognize clinical decision support opportunities related to genomics
- Discuss the opportunities and challenges related to consumer genomic testing
- Understand the current state of standardization related to clinical genomics and the solutions to the standardization problem

---

KEY CONCEPTS

- Genomic health
- Consumer genetics
- Clinical genetics
- Molecular pathology
- Bioinformatics
- Pharmacogenomics
- Molecular diagnostics
- Decision support
- Personalized medicine
- Standardization

Introduction

The goal of this chapter is to survey the informatics issues and opportunities related to genetic and genomic information in the context of medicine and healthcare management. After a brief overview of genetics and genomics, we discuss the use of DNA-based information in current clinical practice. Next, we address pharmacogenomics to illustrate the emerging opportunities related to genomic health. Information technology (IT) initiatives that enhance the ability of the care provider to better use genomic information in the delivery of healthcare are then described. The chapter concludes with a discussion of genetic and genomic information as it relates to wellness, including disease prevention and risk management.

Why Genomic Medicine and Health?

Advances in surgical techniques, imaging modalities, point-of-care testing, and other innovations have all contributed to the continual improvement in healthcare. However, few advances in biology have generated more hope for substantial change than our rapidly growing understanding of the human genome. Because the genome stores the instructions for building and maintaining the human body, is largely static throughout a human life (with exceptions that are discussed later), and is inherited, the widespread expectation is that deeper understanding of the genome will correlate with radical advances in how we approach medicine (the treatment of disease) and, increasingly, health (the avoidance of disease or injury). As these expected advances materialize, they bring novel information management challenges and opportunities.

The expected benefits of the increasing use of genome-based information to improve medicine and health include the following:

- Improved ability to predict disease risk and take preventive action
- More sophisticated diagnostic tests
- New classes of therapeutic agents
- New approaches to managing clinical conditions
- Improved ability to prevent adverse reactions

Raw genomic data are complex, accepted interpretations of genomic information are continually changing, and the mathematical algorithms involved in using genomic information to support predictive medicine are sophisticated. The computational capacity to process large volumes of genomic information has given rise to the field of bioinformatics (see Chapter 1). Many of the informatics opportunities relate to managing the dynamic and complex nature of genomic information and ensuring appropriate patient and clinical context. Some of the challenges relate to ensuring that privacy issues are adequately addressed (see Chapter 13), presenting the information and interpretations in an appropriate context, and enabling integrity and granularity of information across venues.

Current State of Genetic Medicine

The current state of the art is most accurately described as **genetic medicine,** the practice in which clinical decisions are made on the basis of information about a single gene. Genetic medicine is a mature discipline, unlike genomics. *Genomics* is a systems approach to the complex interplay between the full set of genes found in an organism—in this case, a human being. Thus far, genomics is not widely practiced, but it is an area of major research investment. Currently, the genomic approach to health is focused on the consumer, generating summary reports of individual risk for various diseases and conditions as well as information about nonclinical traits and ancestry. Meanwhile, genetic medicine is demonstrated in two areas: clinical genetics and molecular pathology. Before we cite examples from these two areas, we provide a general introduction to genetics.

Overview of Genetics

All genetic conditions have as their basis a change in a molecule called *deoxyribonucleic acid* (DNA). In humans and all other higher organisms, DNA is packed into cellular structures called *chromosomes*. Normally, a human inherits 23 unique chromosomes from each parent, for a total of 46. The full complement of DNA included in these chromosomes is a genome. The information stored in the DNA molecule is referred to as a *genotype*, and an observable state influenced by a genotype is called a *phenotype*. For example, sickle cell anemia is a phenotype caused by a change in the genotype of the hemoglobin gene.

DNA is a long threadlike molecule made of four types of building blocks (nucleotides) represented by the letters A, C, G, and T. The precise sequence of these letters in DNA—for example, "ATGCTATTAGGC"— provides the instructions that determine how proteins (another category of biological molecules) are assembled. Proteins perform the majority of the activities in the body—whether generating energy, providing structural support, or protecting the body from pathogens.

Variations from the "normal" sequence of a gene (generally the instructions for a single protein) can often have severe physiological consequences. For example, a change in a single nucleotide in a gene called *CFTR* can lead to cystic fibrosis. When a change in DNA causes a functional change in the protein encoded by the gene, it is called a *mutation*. Other DNA changes that cause functionally neutral variations are called *polymorphisms*. Polymorphisms are important clinically because many commonly tested characteristics, including blood type, are based on functionally neutral variations. Macro-level variations in chromosomal structure can lead to the exchange of entire regions of chromosomes or even the complete duplication (or deletion) of a chromosome. For example, Down's syndrome is associated with a duplication of chromosome 21. Accurately and rapidly detecting these genetic variations is the basis for most of the diagnostic capabilities used to deliver the current "genetic medicine."

Clinical Genetics

Many diseases are hereditary. Well-known examples include cystic fibrosis, Huntington's disease, sickle cell anemia, and Tay Sach's disease. Furthermore, susceptibility to some chronic diseases, including diabetes and hypertension, is influenced by complex interactions between genetics and environmental factors. Clinical genetics involves integrating the knowledge of a patient's family history with diagnostic testing to allow the clinical geneticist or genetic counselor to make an informed diagnosis and then make recommendations for a patient.

The catalogue of diagnostic tests available for use in the clinical genetics workflow is rapidly growing. In early 2011, there were 2,109 tests listed in GeneTests. While some serological and biochemical tests continue to be used to support the diagnosis of genetic conditions, most currently performed tests fall into one of two categories—molecular diagnostics or cytogenetics. The boundary between these two fields (or methodologies) is fading, as molecular techniques are increasingly applied in cytogenetics, especially comparative genomic hybridization arrays (Edelmann and Hirschhorn 2009).

Molecular diagnostics is the collective term for methods that provide precise findings about DNA. For example, a method called *polymerase chain reaction* (PCR) can provide results that confirm whether a patient has a disease-causing mutation in a gene. PCR has reduced the cost of genetic testing and is one of the driving forces behind the increased availability of many new genetic tests. Some laboratories perform diagnostic DNA sequencing, in which the entire DNA sequence of a gene or the clinically significant region of a gene is determined. While more expensive and labor intensive than PCR, DNA sequencing yields more comprehensive results than PCR does. Advances in DNA sequencing technologies are reducing the cost for both single-gene and even genomic sequencing through initiatives connected to the $1,000 genome concept (discussed later in the chapter).

Cytogenetics involves making a diagnosis based on chromosome-level observations. For example, the diagnosis of Turner's syndrome is based on the presence of only a single X chromosome (and the absence of a Y chromosome). Cytogenetics involves the use of molecular techniques. One method that is widely used is fluorescent *in situ* hybridization (FISH), which applies segments of DNA labeled with a colored dye to determine whether unusual chromosomal rearrangements or deletions have occurred. Sophisticated image-analysis applications are now a mainstay of the clinical cytogenetics laboratory. These applications introduce significant data-management issues, as a high-quality FISH image can require multiple megabytes of storage capacity. The seamless integration of cytogenetics images into the electronic medical record (EMR) is currently under development and will serve as a useful resource in the future.

Molecular Pathology

The key difference between molecular pathology and clinical genetics is that molecular pathology deals with detecting and classifying DNA changes that have occurred after one is born (somatic mutations), while clinical genetics is primarily concerned with hereditary or congenital conditions. Most somatic mutations are benign, but some can result in uncontrolled cell growth, which leads to cancer. In molecular pathology, many of the methods discussed so far (i.e., PCR, DNA sequencing, FISH) are applied to the detection or classification of malignancies. For example, most patients with chronic myelogenous leukemia have a detectable chromosomal rearrangement between the 9th and the 22nd chromosomes. By detecting this rearrangement, the clinician is able to make a definitive diagnosis. Quantitative methods can then be used to track the prevalence of malignant cells compared with cells that lack the rearrangement and thus track how well or poorly a patient is responding to therapy.

Some analyses relate to both clinical genetics and molecular pathology. For example, susceptibility to breast cancer is influenced by mutations in two genes—BRCA1 and BRCA2. Risks of developing other malignant conditions, including some forms of colorectal cancer, are also mediated by genes. Evaluating and communicating patient risk, rather than an actual diagnosis, are clearly challenging tasks for the clinician. These risk-conferring traits have significant implications for family members as well. Designing and implementing a clinical genetics system that appropriately manages the privacy and security of these results that have potentially life-altering consequences are major factors in building a system to support genomic medicine.

Current Informatics Approaches

The current state of the art in information systems used by the cytogenetics or molecular diagnostics laboratory indicates some of the informatics challenges ahead. Many bioinformatics platforms are designed for the research setting, which leads to a common misperception that these research applications can be extended easily into the clinical diagnostics laboratory. Here are some of the information requirements that differentiate the clinical genetics laboratory from others:

- Ability to document and respond to orders from clinicians for genetic tests
- Ability to capture discrete results
- Ability to generate reports that comply with regulatory guidelines, including the Health Insurance Portability and Accountability Act (HIPAA), the Clinical Laboratory Improvement Amendments, 21 CFR part 11 (electronic signatures), and other requirements of self-governing organizations such as the College of American Pathologists
- Support for systemwide compliance with HIPAA, including the persistence of an audit trail
- Ability to integrate with applications that are capable of generating appropriate billing documents

Interviews with multiple molecular diagnostics laboratories reveal the three common approaches to meeting these requirements:

1. *Use of a niche application for documenting genetics observations or laboratory workflow.* Generally designed for the smallest of laboratories, these applications are often low-cost and were built with limited or no capability to integrate into a larger clinical system. Importantly, many such systems were built using architectural components that were not designed to be fully compliant with HIPAA. For example, HIPAA requires that transactions be logged to trace user inquiries against specific elements of the database.
2. *Custom implementation of an off-the-shelf database application.* Many laboratories have engaged consultants to design customized systems for their laboratory. These implementations often share the HIPAA concerns cited in number 1 and frequently are inadequately supported. As customized development projects, they are typically not structured to be easily extended.
3. *Use of commercial anatomic pathology systems.* These systems were designed to support the textual reporting of pathology information and are generally able to integrate with other clinical information system features, whether through architectural integration or HL7 messaging. These systems lack the ability to manage the discrete results generated by the molecular laboratory and are not designed to accommodate the unique workflow of the genetics laboratory.

To address the limitations of these three approaches, in 2005 Cerner Corporation released Millennium Helix, a laboratory solution designed specifically for the workflow and results-management needs of the molecular diagnostics laboratory. Millennium Helix combines the discrete results and textual reporting capabilities needed in the molecular diagnostics laboratory with workflow capabilities designed specifically for that lab.

Several informatics challenges emerge as a result of the wider adoption of molecular diagnostic technologies. One is the accurate presentation of the precision of various methods. Variations of PCR remain the most commonly used methods for generating molecular diagnostic results. A typical PCR test is designed to ask the question, "Is this specific mutation present or absent?" or "Has this region of DNA been duplicated?" Information generated by this method should be presented in this context because the patient could have a rare or as-yet undiscovered mutation other than the target of the testing. These potentially clinically significant findings would not be detected by PCR-based screening but would be by a well-designed DNA sequencing test. Accurately and consistently specifying the method used to generate a result is thus an important capability for the molecular diagnostics lab.

Another challenge is the use of information systems to support the protection and privacy of highly sensitive genomic findings. The opportunity is provided by the unique capability of healthcare information systems to log transactions and manage access to information. The challenge is implementing appropriate policies that ensure that the appropriate care providers have access to necessary results while personnel without the "need-to-know" are restricted from accessing sensitive information.

The current utilization of genetic technology for patient care is stronger

THE GENOME

In the late 1990s and the beginning of the 2000s, an international consortium of public organizations, including the National Institutes of Health (NIH) in the United States and the Burroughs Welcome Foundation of the United Kingdom, raced against a private company, Celera, to determine the full DNA sequence of the human genome. These projects applied the latest in robotics, computing, and biology to accomplish this aggressive goal by 2001 along with the coordinated publication of the findings generated by both Celera and the international consortium (Lander et al. 2001; Venter et al. 2001). Subsequently, a complete draft was published in 2004 (see Collins et al. 2004).

These efforts yielded the DNA sequence of each of the 25,000 human genes, providing a wealth of information for researchers and technology companies to use in seeking a better understanding of human biology. Of equal importance to the solution of the genome sequence was the development of the first databases that describe human variability at a population level (Sherry et al. 2001). This work identified the positions in genes at which variations are most likely to occur, allowing researchers to focus their efforts more precisely. Subsequent work has included the development of a database of identified genomic variations (dbSNP) (see www.ncbi.nlm.nih.gov/projects/SNP/) and an analysis of the genomic variabilities shared by human populations (the HapMap) (Manolio and Collins 2009).

The determination of the complete DNA sequence of the human genome in 2001 was widely expected to usher in a new era in healthcare. Promises of new medications, new diagnostic tests, personalized medicine, and gene therapy generated significant public enthusiasm. Yet, with the exception of a few new diagnostic tests, few tangible benefits from the human genome project

(continued)

have emerged for most patients. Multiple reasons can explain this lag:

- The development cycle for new drugs averages 7 to 11 years.
- Gene therapy has had limited successes and major failures. Establishing a long-term, viable ethics framework for testing gene therapies will be a long-term effort.
- Single-gene disorders were well understood before the completion of the genome sequence. Deciphering the genetic influences involved in complex disorders such as diabetes will be a lengthy undertaking.
- Identifying a genetic variant and preliminary evidence of its biological role is vastly different from having a solid understanding of the clinical impact of the variant and modifying the standard of care to reflect those new insights.

Training clinicians to use existing genetic knowledge, much less how to adopt the still expanding body of new knowledge, has proven difficult. The transition from a deep understanding of single-gene disorders to adopting a systems approach to learning about complex conditions has benefited from a particular technology—the microarray analysis.

A microarray is typically a glass or plastic surface with thousands or millions of spots, each of which includes a unique DNA probe. Microarray tests can be used to measure levels of gene expression, with the goal of determining which genes are either over- or underexpressed in various malignancies or diseases. Work with this technology has demonstrated that gene expression patterns can be used to predict the outcome for otherwise similar breast cancer cases. This technology has also been applied to forms of leukemia and other malignancies. Armed with this new prognostic tool, the clinician will be able to use these results as a factor in determining whether a mild treatment or a highly aggressive (but risky) one is needed. The eventual need to incorporate microarray results into clinical information systems is a daunting prospect, as each assay can yield thousands

(continued)

than many would acknowledge. The application of genetic information is increasingly used to improve the delivery of patient care.

Standardization

As discussed in Chapter 2, standardizing clinical information delivers a number of benefits. The use of controlled vocabularies, such as SNOMED-CT and LOINC, enable organizations to exchange clinical orders, results, and other information through HL7 or other messaging systems. However, these vocabularies lack the sufficient concepts required to describe the detailed findings of the molecular diagnostics or cytogenetics laboratory. Bioinformatics resources, including those provided by the National Center for Biotechnology Information (NCBI), were developed to meet the needs of the researchers (Pruitt and Maglott 2001; Maglott et al. 2000; Sherry et al. 2001) and are generally not appropriate for the clinical setting because of the variability that results from the lack of quality-control processes required to support clinical practice.

One resource developed to address the gap between the clinical vocabularies and bioinformatics resources is the clinical bioinformatics ontology (CBO) (Sherry et al. 2001; Cerner 2012). The CBO is a curated resource that structures observations, generated by current clinical practice, in a semantic network (Noy, Rubin, and Musen 2004; Hoffman, Arnoldi, and Chuang 2005). It allows the association of complex reference data. For example, the CBO maintains information on the chromosomal band(s) in which a gene is located—the intron or exon in which a mutation is found or the mode of inheritance for a given gene. The CBO information is structured in formats that are machine readable, such as comma space value (CSV) and rich data format (RDF). These formats allow developers of clinical information systems to integrate this genomic reference information into their applications and support the exchange of clinically significant results using a standardized format.

Standardization of genomic test results allows one to accomplish multiple clinical and research goals, including the following:

- *Facilitate the communication of clinical orders and results between organizations.* For example, standardization enables reference laboratories to improve the way they send results to the clinicians who ordered tests. Multi-institutional integrated delivery networks, such as Kaiser-Permanente and Tenet Healthcare, also benefit from the standardization of genomic results exchanged between facilities. Information exchange networks, made up of disparate institutions, can also share clinical orders for given patients.

- *Enable the design and delivery of prepackaged clinical decision support rules.* The use of standards reduces the need to perform customization during a clinical system implementation.

- *Optimize the data for inclusion in a data warehouse or research repository.* By standardizing results at the point of capture, the need to perform data mapping in the data warehouse organization is reduced.

These are the general benefits attributed to any data standardization effort. In genomic medicine, however, the absence of a clear standard for documenting molecular findings could create a barrier to the recognition and realization of many of this field's anticipated benefits.

---

of data points. The volume of data, combined with the currently high level of variability among individual assays, will require progress in data normalization and compression, both areas of active research in the bioinformatics community. Operational decisions regarding the retention of every data point or only those of known significance will need to be made, again raising questions about whether to sacrifice findings that can be reinterpreted in the future. An appealing middle ground is to use genomewide expression scans to identify those genes for which up or down regulation is diagnostically significant and then make those genes (a more manageable subset of the genome) the basis for diagnostic testing.

Clearly, the genomic approach to medicine will alter diagnostic practices and provide many opportunities to improve patient care. The detection of a single mutation for a patient does not create a "genomic" record but rather a "genetic" record, as it is based on a single gene. The systems approach to genomic medicine will require EMR systems capable of seamlessly integrating genetic and clinical information and accurately representing the complex relationships between these sources of information.

Emerging Trends

So far our discussion has focused on the ability of genomic medicine to support advanced diagnostic practices and the development of new therapies. Of equal or greater significance are emerging trends that will alter physician behavior and decisions based on these diagnostic findings. Increased patient access to genetic tests is also an emerging trend of significant importance to the designer of healthcare systems.

Pharmacogenomics

People's response to medications varies widely. Most respond within a statistical norm and thus benefit from a medication as expected. Some, however, can only benefit from a medication if given either a higher or lower dose than the general population requires. Even still, a few individuals suffer severe or even fatal adverse drug reactions because of genetic variations in genes involved in drug metabolism. The analysis and application of emerging knowledge about these genetic influences on drug metabolism is called **pharmacogenomics** (Edelmann and Hirschhorn 2009).

For example, 7 percent of the population lacks both copies of the gene CYP2D6, which is involved in metabolizing codeine and many other commonly prescribed medications. These individuals fail to benefit from treatment with codeine. Similarly, 1 in 300 people has a variation in the gene TPMT, which is involved in the response to mercaptopurine, a chemotherapeutic agent. These people can have potentially fatal reactions to mercaptopurine. Researchers at St. Jude hospital in Memphis, Tennessee, developed a genetic test that identifies persons with mutations in the TPMT gene (Krynetski et al. 1995). When the mutation is detected, physicians at St. Jude can adjust the dosage of mercaptopurine to prevent the risk of an adverse reaction.

Not all pharmacogenomics applications are based on hereditary variations. Early studies demonstrate that pharmacogenomics can be applied to (and yield exciting results for) the management of small-cell lung cancer. By determining whether somatic mutations are present in the EGFR gene, clinicians can predict whether a patient will respond to the drug gefitinib (Paez et al. 2004). Significantly, the 10 percent of patients with these mutations had a 100 percent response rate to the medication. Thus, screening for these EGFR mutations can be an important predictor of whether gefitinib, a costly medication, is likely to be successful.

Direct-to-Consumer Genetic Testing

A resource that provides well-curated information about drug–gene interactions is PharmGKB. Developed by a consortium led by Stanford University

(Hewett et al. 2002; Klein and Altman 2004), the PharmGKB website (www.pharmgkb.org) offers a rich collection of information that describes polymorphisms known to affect drug metabolism. The methods used to generate these findings are clearly indicated, allowing the informed user to determine how much weight to attach to a given finding. PharmGKB assumes that the user has a certain level of knowledge about genomics and the methods available to generate genomic findings. In addition, the general trend of PharmGKB is to support the requirements of the drug-development community rather than the delivery of patient care.

Another solution to the challenge of obtaining clear information about drug–gene interactions is extending the existing drug databases, such as the Multum database (www.multum.com), that already provide physicians with reference information describing drug–drug, drug–allergy, and drug–food interactions. The content of Multum is already tightly integrated with computerized physician-order entry (CPOE) applications; adding drug–gene interactions to this information is a natural extension and will expand the physician's readily available resources. Integrating pharmacogenomic information into medication-ordering capabilities has clear advantages over other approaches. It removes the burden of remembering to check whether a drug–gene interaction is likely, a step required by website-based resources.

Clinician Information

One of the most difficult issues in translating knowledge generated in the research setting into active clinical practice is educating the clinician in the conceptual basis of genomic medicine. Several studies, including the Biomedical Information Science and Technology Initiative, have proposed a high-level curriculum for interdisciplinary training (Friedman et al. 2004). The rapid pace of change in genomic information renders the specifics of genomic training perpetually out of date. Thus, the focus of such education should be on how to approach genomic questions and how to effectively and appropriately use genomic information in patient care.

Useful and growing online resources are an option for the clinician, including the following:

- *PharmGKB*. It assumes a certain level of knowledge, and its emphasis is on the needs of the pharmacogenomics researcher.
- *GeneTests*. Managed by the University of Washington in Seattle, the GeneTests directory (www.ncbi.nlm.nih.gov/sites/GeneTests/?db=GeneTests) enables the clinician to confirm or determine the disease or condition he or she suspects, to learn more about the condition, and to identify sites where testing for the condition is performed. This website delivers

content that uses accessible terminology and concepts but offers links to more technical information likely to be of interest to advanced clinicians.

- *Online Mendelian Inheritance in Man (OMIM)*. Developed by the NCBI, the website (www.ncbi.nlm.nih.gov/omim) offers detailed descriptions of hereditary and malignant conditions. OMIM, however, makes assumptions about the training of its users and contains a number of errors and inconsistencies.

The limitation of using website-based information is that clinicians must anticipate the need for such knowledge and then initiate and conduct the search. When a genetic finding has not been widely communicated to the practicing clinical community, clinicians likely will not recognize the need to run a query on any online resource or to feel a sense of ownership about its use. Because physicians are increasingly using CPOE, structured clinical documentation, and other health information technology (HIT) solutions to execute the administrative and clinical transactions involved in their daily activities, embedding genomic information in these systems is a logical means to deliver up-to-date genomic information. Embedding genomic information in an HIT system offers the following advantages:

- *Opportunity to reduce variance among users.* All users will be working in a system in which the same decision support capabilities are implemented.
- *Updates that are transparent to the user.* Other than the need for a small group of internal reviewers, who determine which decision support capabilities to adopt locally, the wider group of users does not need to be regularly trained in new findings. Some specific decision support capabilities may require brief training, however.
- *Ability to combine active and passive content.* Active content is delivered in the form of on-screen alerts, which require users to respond to be able to continue with their actions. These are appropriate for showing medication alerts related to drug–gene interactions. Passive content is encyclopedic in nature, easily accessible to users but requiring them to deliberately seek information.
- *Ability to reanalyze historical results.* By capturing all genetic test findings in an EMR, whether or not their clinical significance is understood at the time of capture, it becomes possible to re-examine previous results against newly generated knowledge and then to take action according to the newly identified associations.
- *Ability to generate and manage clinical pedigrees online.* Unlike standalone applications that generate clinical pedigrees, an integrated family medical information–clinical information system creates the opportunity

to infer results and estimate risks between patients. The risk that such associations could result in unintended disclosure of results that indicate paternity other than that currently believed to be true by the patient must be mitigated.

The combination of publicly accessible online information resources and genomic information embedded in clinical information systems offers clinicians new tools for integrating the advances of genomic medicine into their practice.

Genomic Health

The advent of low-cost single-nucleotide polymorphism (SNP) profiling systems has created a new market for direct-to-consumer genomic testing. Companies such as 23andMe, deCodeMe, and Navigenics, for example, offer consumers the opportunity to submit a saliva sample and then receive an online report that summarizes their disease risks. Conditions ranging from heart disease to restless-leg syndrome are assessed with statistical techniques, which compare the patient's SNP profile with profiles of a larger cohort and then summarize the relative risk for that condition. Included in the reports are suggestions for preventive measures, although there is widespread concern that the majority of the risk assessments are not actionable (Bloss, Schork, and Topol 2011). A recent study reports that few participants in a genomic analysis made changes in their lifestyle as a result of the testing (Bloss, Schork, and Topol 2011).

An important informatics opportunity will be the ability to integrate these results into the personal health record (PHR). PHR suppliers will need to determine whether to store only the interpretations, which may be updated over time, or both the interpretations and the raw genomic information (storage intensive). Likewise, through interoperability initiatives funded by the Meaningful Use section of the 2009 American Recovery and Reinvestment Act, the decisions about which information in the PHR should be exposed to providers and under what circumstances will pose challenging system-design and policy issues. Patients' access to genetic information can inform them and their families of health risks and might help enlist them in participating in the clinical process as co-producers.

While not yet available in practice, the $1,000 genome concept has stirred much discussion. This concept extends the approach currently applied in genomic health, which relies on SNP microarrays that sample the genome, and implies that in the near future the DNA sequence of an individual's genome can be obtained for a low cost—$1,000. The impact of this concept will be massive. First, storing the data in a manner that can be accessed in a clinical context will extend the storage requirements of the typical electronic health record by orders of magnitude. Second, information does not equal knowledge. The task of appropriately interpreting and applying the full genome sequence information will require new technologies in clinical data presentation and new policies related to the strength of evidence required before new information is applied in clinical practice.

Conclusion

The era of genomic health and medicine will transform healthcare. Genetic testing and analysis is already a significant part of clinical genetics, molecular pathology, and infectious disease management. Integrating clinical, family history, and genetic information into a common repository can offer many benefits both to research (McMahon et al. 1998) and to patient care delivery. The advent of pharmacogenomics-based clinical decision making and advanced diagnostic technologies, such as DNA microarrays, will contribute to the deepening use of genomic information in care delivery.

For health informatics, this transformation has major implications on the design and implementation of healthcare information systems, including the following:

- The need to support the expanding volume of the molecular diagnostics laboratory, including its unique workflow
- The challenge of clearly representing the precision and accuracy of the methods used to determine molecular diagnostic results
- The need to standardize genomic information to facilitate exchanges and communications between affiliated providers
- The need to develop or continue efforts to protect patient privacy and the security of EMRs
- The increasing need to offer clinicians useful and clear tools that help them interpret and apply genomic findings

These implications can be addressed by well-designed clinical information systems and can be transformed into significant opportunities, including the following:

- The ability to streamline and optimize workflow within the molecular diagnostic laboratory
- The opportunity to provide decision support capabilities that simplify the process of managing genomic information for the clinician

- The opportunity to support the personalization of medicine by hastening the adoption of pharmacogenomics technologies
- The opportunity to leverage the familial nature of genomic findings and support the type of inferencing described in the chapter

Recognizing these opportunities will require close collaboration among healthcare providers, developers of HIT, and academic researchers in medical informatics and genomics. A blend of embedded technology and user-friendly online information will support the rapid adoption of the many capabilities of genomic medicine.

Recommended Websites

- Clinical bioinformatics ontology: www.cerner.com/cbo
- GeneTests: www.genetests.org
- Genetics Home Reference: www.ghr.nlm.nih.gov
- National Center for Biotechnology Information: www.ncbi.nlm.nih.gov
- Online Mendelian Inheritance in Man: www.ncbi.nlm.nih.gov/entrez/query.fcgi?db=OMIM
- PharmGKB: www.pharmgkb.org

Chapter Discussion Questions

1. What are three key barriers to using genetic information in the delivery of personalized medicine?
2. Given enough genetic information, a precise identification of a person can be made. How can data warehouses that integrate clinical with genomic information be used to accomplish meaningful research while protecting patient privacy?
3. When non-clinically trained patients are able to order genetic tests directly, how can their right to informed consent be protected?
4. Describe some of the potential approaches to standardizing clinical genomic information. What are the benefits of standardizing these results?
5. What are some means by which clinicians can use information systems to manage and respond to advances in genomic medicine?

CASE STUDY   Whose Body?

Timothy B. Patrick, Peter J. Tonellato, and Mark A. Hoffman

Two health sciences graduate students, Sandy and Grace, are discussing their differences of opinion about the value of clinical uses of genetic and genomic patient information.

> Sandy: It's always the same story—the supposed trade-off between the benefits to society and the sacrificed rights of the individual! Just remember the case of Henrietta Lacks. HELA cells [cancer cells taken from Henrietta before she died] have been invaluable to medical science; they led to the polio vaccine and other medical "miracles." But Henrietta was never told what was going to be done with her cells; she never gave her permission—and, by the way, neither did her close relatives and family know or give their permission. It's a clear case of science overstepping its bounds to the detriment of the individual.

> Grace: Sandy, you yourself know that the scientific research's benefit to society really means the medical care benefit to the individual. Don't you remember the recent case that took place here in our own hospital—the case of Jean, a 17-year-old who was visiting at the home of a friend when she fell down, struck her head, and suffered serious injuries? She was raced to the ER where she required emergency surgery, and neither her parents nor relatives could be reached before the procedure. The mother of Jean's friend provided the hospital with Jean's name and home address, which allowed the ER personnel to associate Jean with her parents in the system. Using the hospital's healthcare information system, the surgeon entered an order for the protocol that she was planning to use to treat Jean. Among the details included in the protocol was the use of halothane [a type of anesthesia]. Jean had never been the subject of genetic testing, but her father had a genetic test, which found a mutation in the ryanodine receptor [RYR1] gene. When people with this mutation are exposed to halothane, they can experience malignant hyperthermia, an often-fatal reaction in which the core body temperature can reach 106°F.

> The hospital's information system used the demographic person–person relationship between the father and his daughter, and embedded pharmacogenomics decision support capabilities, to infer that Jean was at 50 percent risk of also possessing this rare mutation. The system flashed an interactive alert to the surgeon, who was unaware of this genetic association. The surgeon responded to the alert by activating

an alternative surgical plan that did not include the use of halothane. It was only by taking advantage of the genetic information about Jean's father that a potentially catastrophic clinical event was averted!

Sandy: But you make my case for me. The potential of abuse of the genetic data is magnified by the existence and use of sophisticated healthcare information systems. There's no mystery about the potential for abuse. Jean's father was the one who had the test, not Jean. Yet the information produced by the test was also about Jean. Sure, revealing that information happened to help Jean, but the principle is that the information was about Jean as much as it was about her father. And Jean never gave her permission for that information to be used or revealed! It's her body and her genome, not her father's, right? So it's her right to privacy that was violated.

Grace: It might be her body, Sandy, but given the genetic data and information, we are bound by our Hippocratic oath.[1] That includes "do no harm" [*primum nil nocere*, in latin]. In practice and in effect, Jean's life was ours to save. What other choice did we have?

Sandy: What about consent and protecting her privacy? And what about Jean's father? Did he give permission to release the information from his genetic test to be used in ways other than for his diagnosis and treatment? How is that different from the Havasupai Indians' lost-blood case? Arizona State University researchers asked the Havasupai if they would provide blood for studies to discover clues about the tribe's incredible rate of diabetes, presumably to help the Havasupai. Then the researchers used the collected blood for other purposes. They used the extracted DNA for studies on mental illness. The initial diabetes studies seem to have led nowhere, but even if that effort helped save lives, it would have been lives saved without the Havasupai's consent.

Grace: Sandy, for goodness sake, it was only blood!

Sandy: Not at all, Grace, not at all.

Note

1. Hippocratic oath (translated by and reprinted from North 2009):

   I swear by Apollo, the healer, Asclepius, Hygieia, and Panacea, and I take to witness all the gods, all the goddesses, to keep

(continued)

according to my ability and my judgment, the following Oath and agreement: To consider dear to me, as my parents, him who taught me this art; to live in common with him and, if necessary, to share my goods with him; To look upon his children as my own brothers, to teach them this art. I will prescribe regimens for the good of my patients according to my ability and my judgment and never do harm to anyone. I will not give a lethal drug to anyone if I am asked, nor will I advise such a plan; and similarly I will not give a woman a pessary to cause an abortion. But I will preserve the purity of my life and my arts. I will not cut for stone, even for patients in whom the disease is manifest; I will leave this operation to be performed by practitioners, specialists in this art. In every house where I come I will enter only for the good of my patients, keeping myself far from all intentional ill-doing and all seduction and especially from the pleasures of love with women or with men, be they free or slaves. All that may come to my knowledge in the exercise of my profession or in daily commerce with men, which ought not to be spread abroad, I will keep secret and will never reveal. If I keep this oath faithfully, may I enjoy my life and practice my art, respected by all men and in all times; but if I swerve from it or violate it, may the reverse be my lot.

Case Study Discussion Questions

1. Which perspective do you agree with, Sandy's or Grace's? Why?
2. Do you think there are important differences between the cases of Henrietta Lacks, Jean, and the Havasupai? Explain your answer.
3.
4. Are there cases of advances in medical knowledge that do not, at least potentially, threaten to violate the privacy of individual patients?
5. Does a patient have the right to use the genetic information on members of her direct-lineage family members? Information on members of her extended family or relatives? Information on patients with a similar condition?
6. What moral, ethical, and legal protocols can be considered in guiding clinicians in this case?
7. What moral, ethical, and legal protocols can be considered in guiding researchers in this case?

Further Readings

Harmon, A. 2010. "Where'd You Go with My DNA?" *New York Times Week in Review.* Accessed April 24. www.nytimes.com/2010/04/25/weekinreview/25harmon.html.

Skloot, R. 2010. *The Immortal Life of Henrietta Lacks.* New York: Random House, Inc.

HEALTH INFORMATION PRIVACY AND SECURITY

13

Dixie B. Baker

Learning Objectives

After reading this chapter, students will be able to

- Understand the principles of privacy and security applied to the use of information technology
- Conceptualize the logical relationship among privacy, security, and safety
- Identify and develop arguments to support the principles of fair information practices
- Identify the technical safeguards required by the HIPAA Security Rule and the risks each safeguard is designed to address
- Identify the security and privacy risks of applying data mining analytics

---

KEY CONCEPTS

- Privacy
- Security
- Risk
- Trust
- HIPAA Privacy and Security Rules

Introduction

The terms *privacy* and *security* are often used as if they were synonymous, but there are important distinctions. Indeed, security is necessary to protect individual privacy. More than that, it is also necessary to safeguard the integrity of data and the availability of critical information and services, to ensure the authenticity of identities and data, and to maintain accountability of system and user actions. Before we begin, we need to establish a common set of definitions for the four main components of our discussion: privacy, security, risk, and trust.

Defining Privacy, Security, Risk, and Trust

More than a century ago, Supreme Court Justice Louis Brandeis referred to privacy as "the right to be let alone" and characterized it as "the most comprehensive of rights and the right most valued by civilized men" (US Congress 1928). Essentially, privacy is the state of being free from intrusion or disturbance in one's private life or affairs and, in the United States, the constitutional right to such a state. The delivery of safe, high-quality healthcare necessarily involves the collection, use, retention, and sharing of individual consumers' most private information. Indeed, the safety and quality of care are dependent on the provider team's ability to access detailed, accurate, and complete information about an individual's medical and psychological state and lifestyle. Still, the individual has a right to expect that only the information required is collected, used, retained, and shared; that the information shared is used only for the intended purposes; and that privacy rights are respected and honored. In the healthcare context then, we can define privacy as follows:

> **Privacy** is the assurance that one's health information is collected, accessed, used, retained, and shared only when necessary and only to the extent necessary and that the information is protected throughout its life cycle using fair privacy practices consistent with applicable laws and regulations and the preferences of the individual.

Security is the state of being free from danger or harm, or the set of defensive measures that collectively ensures that state. Information security is a specialized area aimed at protecting the confidentiality of information, the integrity of data, and the availability of information and system services. These measures generally include mechanisms for validating that the people, software applications, and information systems seeking access are who and what they claim to be and for keeping a record of actions taken by users and the system. The administrative, physical, and technical standards and implementation specifications in the Health Insurance Portability and Accountability Act (HIPAA) Security Rule (HHS 2003) require such mechanisms. As health information is exchanged between organizations, consolidated in electronic health records (EHRs), and shared with personal health records (PHRs), security measures that ensure the integrity and provenance of data and metadata become increasingly important. In the healthcare context, security is defined as follows:

> **Security** is the protection of the confidentiality of private, sensitive, and safety-critical information; the integrity of health data and metadata; and the availability of information and services through measures that authenticate user and system identity and data provenance and that maintain an accounting of actions taken by users, software programs, and systems.

The relationship between privacy and security is evident. Security measures that protect the confidentiality of personal health information contribute to privacy protection. However, as we shall discuss later, protecting personal privacy involves more than securing confidential information. The importance of security to the safety and quality of care should also be apparent, as the availability of accurate, authenticated information and critical services at the point and time of care is essential to both patient safety and care quality.

Deciding what privacy and security protections are necessary and appropriate is a matter of assessing and managing risk. Risk is a probability function that involves three variables: (1) threat, (2) vulnerability, and (3) valued asset. **Risk**, then, is the probability that a threat will exploit a vulnerability to damage, destroy, or harm a valued asset. To identify and manage risk, a risk assessment is necessary. *Risk assessment* is a disciplined process of identifying valued assets (e.g., buildings, computers, information, people), threats (e.g., disgruntled employee, spyware), and vulnerabilities (e.g., storage of patient information on a laptop or flash drive) and determining the probability that the threat will exploit the vulnerability to cause harm (e.g., unauthorized access to patient information). Risk assessment provides the basis for deciding how to manage each risk—that is, whether to eliminate, moderate, or accept it (perhaps with insurance to reduce liability). Recognizing the importance of risk assessment in implementing appropriate security protections, the HIPAA Security Rule requires both risk analysis (to identify and assess potential risks and vulnerabilities) and risk management (to develop and execute security measures to counter the risks identified).

The final concept essential to privacy and security is trust—the level of comfort, belief, or assurance one senses on the basis of the evidence available. Trust lies at the heart of modern medicine. Providers must trust that the information and software services they need will be available when and where needed and that the decision support integrated with the EHR is accurate, reliable, and safe. In addition, clinicians must trust that the laboratory test result they receive is actually from the lab to which the test was sent for processing and that no modifications or corruptions occurred during the transmission. Conversely, individuals must trust that their providers keep their most private health information confidential and disclose and use the information only to the extent necessary and in ways that are legal, ethical, and authorized consistent with their personal expectations and preferences. Both providers and consumers must trust that the technology used to provide care will "do no harm." In this context, we can define trust as follows:

> **Trust** is the evidence-based confidence that the people, organizations, information and data, and information systems involved in healthcare delivery are what they claim to be and behave as expected.

As shown in Exhibit 13.1, trust involves a delicate balance among transparency, consent, technology, and laws and regulations. Transparency means that consumers and providers are told how their information is being used, protected, and shared. In some cases, the individual's consent must be (or should be) obtained before her information is collected, used, or disclosed. Technology guards against unauthorized disclosure, modification, and use of information and records how the information is used. Some laws and regulations, such as the HIPAA Security Rule and the Common Rule that protects human subjects (*Federal Register* 1991), mandate the implementation of certain policies and protective measures. Other laws, such as the Genetic Information Nondiscrimination Act (GINA 2008) and the Patient Protection and Affordable Care Act (US Congress 2010), protect consumers from unfair discrimination should their genetic or other health information be disclosed. Fair information practices serve as the foundation for trust and are the subject of the next section.

Fair Information Practices

Fair information practices (FIPs) are the foundation of information security and privacy law and regulations in the United States and throughout the world. FIPs constitute fair and responsible information stewardship, which is essential to establishing and maintaining public trust when collecting, using, disclosing, and sharing personal information. The heritage of FIPs is the *Code of Fair Information Practices*, published in 1973 by the Department of Health, Education, and Welfare (now the Department

EXHIBIT 13.1
Balance
Among the
Components of
Trust

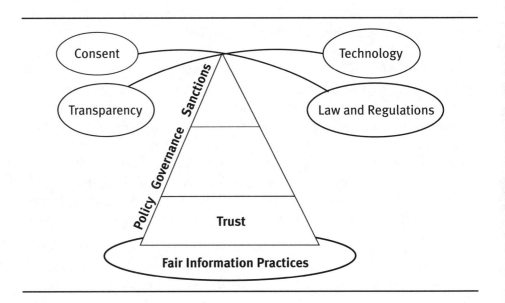

of Health and Human Services) and set forth the principles of openness, disclosure, secondary use, record correction, and security (HEW 1973). These original FIPs provided the framework for the Privacy Act of 1974, which protects certain personal information held by federal agencies (US Congress 1974). Further refinements and customizations to FIPs include the following:

- 1980: *Guidelines on the Protection of Privacy and Transborder Flows of Personal Data*, a consensus document published by the Organisation for Economic Co-operation and Development and involving 24 countries, including the United States (OECD 1980)
- 1998: *Privacy Online: A Report to Congress*, published by the Federal Trade Commission (FTC 1998)
- 2001: *Standards for Privacy of Individually Identifiable Health Information*, developed pursuant to HIPAA (US Congress 2001)
- 2007: *Fair Information Practice Principles*, published by the FTC (2007)

In 2008, the Office of the National Coordinator for Health Information Technology (2008) released *Nationwide Privacy and Security Framework for Electronic Exchange of Individually Identifiable Health Information*, which established FIPs specifically for electronic health information. The FIPs set forth in this document are shown in Exhibit 13.2, which also identifies how each principle is translated into healthcare laws and regulations.

HIPAA Technical Security Safeguards

HIPAA's Privacy and Security regulations (or "Rules"), further strengthened by the American Recovery and Reinvestment Act (ARRA), are the primary sources of standards and implementation specifications for health information security and privacy. Although technically the HIPAA Rules apply only to "protected health information" that is generated, used, and exchanged by specific entities covered under HIPAA, these standards are widely referenced and applied for protecting all individually identifiable health information.

The Privacy Rule essentially says that an individual's health information may be used or disclosed only as explicitly permitted by the law or as authorized by that individual. The Security Rule defines administrative, physical, and technical safeguards that a healthcare organization covered under HIPAA must implement to protect the confidentiality, integrity, and availability of health information. Enforcement of compliance with the HIPAA Privacy and Security Rules is the responsibility of the Office of Civil Rights

EXHIBIT 13.2
Fair Information
Practices for
Managing
Health
Information

Principle	Definition	Legal Codification
Individual Access	Individuals are given simple and timely means to access and obtain their individually identifiable health information in a readable form and format	• HIPAA Privacy Rule provides individuals the right to request and obtain a copy of their health information • ARRA[1] extends this to include the right to request and obtain an electronic copy
Correction	Individuals are given timely means to dispute the accuracy or integrity of their individually identifiable health information, to have erroneous information corrected, or to have a dispute documented if their requests are denied	• HIPAA Privacy Rule gives individuals the right to request that their health information be amended
Openness and Transparency	Uses of policies, procedures, and technologies that directly affect individuals and/or their health information are open and transparent	• HIPAA Privacy Rule requires that each covered entity provide individuals written notice of the organization's privacy practices, including uses and disclosures of health information, the individual's rights, and the entity's legal duties to protect health information
Individual Choice	Individuals should be provided a reasonable opportunity and capability to make informed decisions about the collection, use, and disclosure of their individually identifiable health information	• HIPAA Privacy Rule requires that covered entities obtain the individual's consent before using or disclosing that individual's identifiable health information for purposes other than treatment, payment, healthcare operations, or other uses permitted by law
Collection, Use, and Disclosure Limitation	Individually identifiable health information should be collected, used, and/or disclosed only to the extent necessary to accomplish a specified purpose(s) and never to discriminate inappropriately	• HIPAA Privacy Rule limits sharing of health information to the minimum necessary for the intended purpose • GINA[2] prohibits improper use of genetic information in health insurance and employment • PPACA[3] prohibits insurance companies from refusing to insure individuals with preexisting health conditions
Data Quality and Integrity	Persons and entities should take reasonable steps to ensure that individually identifiable health information is complete, accurate, and up to date to the extent necessary for the person's or entity's intended purposes and has not been altered or destroyed in an unauthorized manner	• HIPAA Privacy Rule gives individuals the right to review their health information and to request an amendment • HIPAA Security Rule requires integrity protection for health information transmissions
Safeguards	Individually identifiable health information should be protected with reasonable administrative, technical, and physical safeguards to ensure its confidentiality, integrity, and availability and to prevent unauthorized or inappropriate access, use, or disclosure	• HIPAA Privacy and Security Rule require administrative, technical, and physical safeguards to protect health information

Principle	Definition	Legal Codification
Accountability	These principles should be implemented and adherence to them should be assured through appropriate monitoring, and other means and methods should be in place to report and mitigate nonadherence and breaches	• HIPAA Privacy Rule requires an accounting of all disclosures between organizations other than those required for treatment, payment, and healthcare operations; ARRA eliminates this exception • HIPAA Security Rule requires collection of audit records and periodic audit review • ARRA requires notification of individuals whose health information may have been exposed through a breach incident

1. American Recovery and Reinvestment Act of 2009; 2. Genetic Information Nondiscrimination Act; 3. Patient Protection and Affordable Care Act

Source: Adapted from Office of the National Coordinator for Health Information Technology (2008).

EXHIBIT 13.2
Fair Information Practices for Managing Health Information (continued)

of the Department of Health and Human Services. In this section, we discuss each of the technical safeguards required by the HIPAA Security Rule and identify the risks the safeguards are designed to address.

Authentication

Essential to all security safeguards is authentication. Authentication is the verification that the true identity of a person or entity (such as a web server or a health clinic) attempting to perform a security-sensitive action (such as logging into a system) is the same as the asserted identity. Authentication addresses the risk that a person or entity masquerading as someone else will perform actions or access information that he or it is not authorized to do. After the person or entity has asserted an identity that is recognized by the system, the authentication process starts. For example, a person may type in a user name that is easily guessable, such as an actual name. Authentication then asks the user to prove her identity by providing something she "knows," such as a secret password; something she "has," such as a random number generated by a hardware token; or something she "is," such as a fingerprint.

If the action the user is attempting to perform carries a very high risk, should the person or entity be other than it claims, a "two-factor" authentication may be needed. In this case, to prove the user's identity, he must produce two pieces of evidence, such as a secret password and a fingerprint. For example, the Drug Enforcement Administration (DEA 2010) requires such two-factor authentication for electronically prescribing controlled substances. Authentication is "foundational" in that many other security safeguards depend on it. If authentication fails, any access-control decisions made on the basis of that identity, any documents that are digitally signed by that user, and any audit records of that user's actions will be based on a bogus identity.

Access Control

Access-control mechanisms mediate requests for access to protected resources and capabilities within a system to ensure that users are able to access all of and only the information they are authorized to access and to perform all of and only those actions they are authorized to perform. Access-control mechanisms generally make access decisions on the basis of the rules related to the identity and role of the requester or on the basis of a comparison between the trust attributes (for example, security clearance) of the requester and the sensitivity label of the resource being requested (for example, "SECRET"). Some access-control mechanisms also take into consideration context variables, such as the time the access is attempted and the location from which the request is received. Access-control mechanisms address the risk that an unauthorized person or entity is able to retrieve, read, write, or modify sensitive or safety-critical health information or to perform actions that person or entity is not authorized to perform.

The HIPAA Security Rule includes data encryption as an access control. Although closely related to access control, encryption is really a different protection mechanism. Whereas access control mediates attempts to access containers of data, such as files and database records, encryption garbles the data (bits) within those containers so that, even if the bits within the container are accessed, only authorized individuals are able to derive meaning ("information") from those bits. Encryption is discussed later in the chapter.

Security Auditing and Accounting for Disclosures

Security auditing is the process of recording security-relevant activities that occur within an information system, such as logging into the system, launching a software application, and opening a patient's health record. Recording an audit trail, along with an audit-record review process and technology, helps ensure that security safeguards are operating correctly. The audit trail enables an organization to monitor system actions and to detect potential misuse and intrusions so that appropriate actions can be taken. The audit trail also enables an organization to investigate breaches in security policy enforcement.

Security auditing addresses the risk that a system administrator is unable to ascertain whether security safeguards are operating correctly, whether authorized users are acting in accordance with the organization's security policy, and whether any unauthorized users have bypassed security safeguards to gain access to protected resources. Security auditing also can serve as a deterrent in that the mere knowledge that their actions are being recorded may discourage some potential intruders and misusers from taking unauthorized or inappropriate actions.

Closely aligned with auditing is the ARRA requirement to account for disclosures of health information. An accounting of disclosures is a record of every instance in which electronic health information is released, transferred, provided, given access to, or divulged in any other manner to an entity outside the entity holding the information. An audit trail may be useful in constructing an accounting of disclosures but is not intended to be such an accounting. Audit trails are system records that contain detailed information of activity within a system, including attempts to take actions that are not allowed. For example, an audit trail would include activities such as attempting to log on, attempting to open a file, running a software application, reading a database record, and creating a folder. An accounting of disclosures is a record of actual releases of health information to another entity. It addresses the risk that a trusted healthcare entity releases a patient's record to a third party without the patient's knowledge or consent.

Integrity Assurance

No security mechanism can prevent data from being damaged or corrupted. Access controls can help ensure that only authorized individuals and entities can write to, modify, or delete resources that contain protected data, but access control cannot prevent data from being accidentally corrupted or destroyed. Integrity assurance, or corroboration, guarantees that data that have been stored or transmitted are the same when they are used as when they were stored or transmitted. Integrity mechanisms address the risk that stored or transmitted data are corrupted or changed in an unauthorized manner and then later used without the user realizing that the data are not the same as when they were originally stored or transmitted. The most commonly used integrity-assurance mechanism is called a *hash function*, a mathematical formula executed against a block of data or a data stream to generate a number that represents that block or stream. Then before the data are used, the same hash function is executed again. If the number the function produces is different from the original number, the user knows that the data have been changed (but not what elements have changed).

Encryption

Another mathematical function used to protect data is encryption, which is simply the use of a mathematical algorithm (cipher) containing a secret variable (key) to scramble a block or stream of data such that the bits are no longer intelligible. The only way to make encrypted data intelligible again is to use the same mathematical algorithm and matching secret variable to decrypt them. Encryption algorithms are either symmetric (for which the same key is used to both encrypt and decrypt the data) or asymmetric (for which one key is used to encrypt and another to decrypt the data). *Asymmetric encryption* is also known as public key encryption because one of the keys is openly made public and the other is kept private. *Symmetric encryption* is used only to encrypt and decrypt data, and it does that efficiently no matter what amount of data is involved and regardless of whether the data are at rest or in motion.

Asymmetric encryption generally is used to secure exchanges between two parties, to whom we refer as Alice and Bob in the following scenarios. Which key is used to encrypt and which to decrypt depends on the objective to be achieved.

1. *Authenticate the identity of a person or entity.* In this scenario, to authenticate that Bob is in fact Bob, Alice encrypts some block of data using Bob's public key and Bob decrypts the data using his private key.
2. *Digitally sign a message or document.* Here, sender Alice signs her message to Bob using her private key, and Bob verifies that the message is actually from Alice by decrypting the signature using Alice's public key.
3. *Share a secret (symmetric) key to be used to exchange private or sensitive information.* In this case, sender Alice encrypts the secret key using Bob's public key, and receiver Bob decrypts the key using his own private key.

Secure e-mail brings these scenarios together along with an integrity hash. To send an encrypted and digitally signed message to Bob, Alice first constructs her message and digitally signs it by generating an integrity hash value on the message and encrypting that value using her private key. Then, Alice encrypts the message content using a secret key that she chooses. To keep the key secret, she encrypts it using Bob's public key so that only Bob can decrypt it using his private key that only he knows. Alice sends the encrypted message to Bob, along with her digital signature and the encrypted secret key. When Bob receives the message, he uses Alice's public key to decrypt the hash value, thus validating that the digital signature is hers. Bob uses his private key to decrypt the secret key and the hash value to verify that the message has not been changed.

Encryption is used to address a number of risks. Both symmetric and asymmetric encryption are used to help ensure that even if an unauthorized entity gets access to a container of data, such as a file or network transmission, the "information" represented by the "data" will not be intelligible to anyone not possessing the secret (or private) key. Asymmetric encryption also addresses the risk that someone claims an identity other than her own or that someone repudiates having taken some action (such as sending a message).

Security Implementation in EHR Technology

To be certified by an accredited certification body, EHR technology must be implemented according to standards and certification criteria specified in ARRA regulations (HHS 2010). A number of the standards and certification criteria ensure that certified EHR technology offers the technical security safeguards that the organization using that technology will need to comply with the HIPAA Security Rule. Exhibit 13.3 shows how each of the HIPAA technical security safeguards is implemented in certified EHR technology.

HIPAA Technical Security Safeguards	EHR Standards	EHR Certification Criteria
Implement procedures to verify that a person or entity seeking access to electronic protected health information (PHI) is the one claimed		Verify that a person or entity seeking access to electronic health information is the one claimed and is authorized to access such information
Implement technical policies and procedures that maintain electronic PHI to allow access only to those persons or software programs that have been granted access rights, including the following:		Establish controls that permit only authorized users to access electronic health information
• Unique user identification		Assign a unique name and/ or number for identifying and tracking user identity
• Emergency access procedure		Permit authorized users (who are authorized for emergency situations) to access electronic health information during an emergency
• Automatic logoff		Terminate an electronic session after a predetermined time of inactivity
• Encryption and decryption	Any encryption algorithm identified by the National Institute of Standards and Technology (NIST) as an approved security function in Annex A of the Federal Information Processing Standards (FIPS) Publication 140–42	Encrypt and decrypt electronic health information in accordance with the standard, unless the secretary determines that the use of such algorithm would pose a significant security risk for certified EHR technology

EXHIBIT 13.3
HIPAA Technical Security Safeguards for EHR Technology

(continued)

EXHIBIT 13.3
HIPAA Technical
Security
Safeguards for
EHR Technology
(continued)

HIPAA Technical Security Safeguards	EHR Standards	EHR Certification Criteria
Implement hardware, software, and/or procedural mechanisms that record and examine activity in information systems that contain or use electronic PHI	Record actions related to electronic health information; the date, time, patient identification, and user identification must be recorded when electronic health information is created, modified, accessed, or deleted, along with an indication of which action(s) occurred and by whom	1. Record actions related to electronic health information 2. Enable a user to generate an audit log for a specific time period and to sort entries in the audit log according to any of the elements specified in the standard
An individual has a right to receive an accounting of disclosures of PHI made by a covered entity in the six years before the date on which the accounting is requested, except for disclosures specifically listed in the regulation as exceptions, which include disclosures to carry out treatment, payment, and healthcare operations\n\n(Added by ARRA) If a covered entity uses or maintains an electronic health record, the HIPAA exceptions for treatment, payment, and healthcare operations do not apply; an accounting of disclosures for the previous three years must be made available to the individual	Record disclosures made for treatment, payment, and healthcare operations purposes; include the date, time, patient identification, user identification, and a description of the disclosure	*Optional.* Record disclosures made for treatment, payment, and healthcare operations in accordance with the standard
Implement policies and procedures to protect electronic PHI from improper alteration or destruction, including mechanism to corroborate that electronic PHI has not been altered or destroyed in an unauthorized manner (addressable)	A hashing algorithm with a security strength equal to or greater than SHA–1 (secure hash algorithm), as specified by the NIST in FIPS Publication 180–83, must be used to verify that electronic health information has not been altered in transit	1. Create a message digest in accordance with the standard 2. Upon receipt of electronically exchanged health information, verify that the information has not been altered 3. Detect the alteration of audit logs
Implement technical security measures to guard against unauthorized access to electronic PHI that is being transmitted over an electronic communications network, including\n• Integrity controls\n• Encryption	Any encrypted and integrity-protected link	Encrypt and decrypt electronic health information when it is exchanged

Source: Adapted from Office of the National Coordinator for Health Information Technology (2008).

Opportunities and Challenges

The standards specified in the HIPAA Privacy and Security Rules reflect principles that have been used for decades to protect the privacy of individuals, the confidentiality of information, the integrity of electronic data, and the availability of essential system resources and services. A healthcare organization that implements the fair information practices set forth in the Privacy Rule and the administrative, physical, and technical safeguards required by the Security Rule will have a solid foundation of policy, processes, and safeguards for effectively managing its privacy and security risks.

However, risk is a continually evolving construct. We observe the changing nature of threats over time, as former friends become foes and business partners become competitors. New technologies emerge almost daily, each with its own set of vulnerabilities to be exploited. Even our values change over time, sometimes driven by technology changes. For example, consider the pay phone, valued as essential in years past and now almost a relic. In this section, we explore some of the emerging technologies that pose new opportunities to improve healthcare as well as new challenges to personal privacy and information security.

Data Mining

As defined in an earlier chapter, data mining is the use of sophisticated search capabilities and analytical techniques on large databases to discover patterns, correlations, and trends that can be leveraged to produce new knowledge. The potential for applying data mining techniques to make new biomedical discoveries, support decision making, and improve health outcomes is tremendous. At the same time, data mining represents a new threat to individual privacy in that by aggregating and extracting inferences from large volumes of clinical information, even information that has been "de-identified" in accordance with the HIPAA Privacy Rule can become individually identifiable. One need only consider today's powerful search engines and personalized web services to realize that data mining makes remaining anonymous very difficult for any individual. New approaches to de-identification, as well as explicit privacy protections, are needed to enable healthcare to reap the benefits offered by data mining while protecting individual privacy.

Federated Identity

To increase efficiencies and lower the operational overhead attendant to forcing users to separately log into each system, application, and database, single sign-on has become common practice in healthcare organizations. Single sign-on enables a user to login once and then access all of the software applications and data she needs from across an enterprise. Single sign-on can be implemented in several ways, but the most common, standards-based approach is to pass a token called a *security assertion* to each system to which the user requests access. This approach also can be used to pass assertions between entities, allowing a user who has logged into a system in one organization to access resources in "federated" systems managed by other organizations. As discussed earlier, user authentication is the weakest link on which all security protections associated with individual users (e.g., access control, digital signature, audit) depend. This dependency poses a huge vulnerability for federated systems.

Virtualization

Virtualization is the creation and use of a virtual (rather than an actual) computing resource, such as a software application, operating system, or storage device. Just about anything can be virtualized, producing software-as-a-service (SaaS), platform-as-a-service (PaaS), or infrastructure-as-a-service (IaaS)—also known by the generic term "cloud" computing.

Virtualization offers significant security and privacy benefits because by virtualizing a resource, it is put under central control where security and privacy policies can be uniformly enforced. For example, installing an EHR software application on a workstation in a small health clinic may mean that the health information of all patients who come to that clinic for services is physically stored on that workstation, which may be protected by little more than the office door key and smoke detector. If the clinic chooses instead to use the same EHR software application, but subscribe to it as a service instead of installing and maintaining it locally, the clinic's data likely will reside in a large data center that is continuously protected at a high level explicitly defined in a service-level agreement. At the same time, cloud computing brings new risks because critical health data and essential applications are outside the physical and operational control of the subscriber. Organizations need to exercise due diligence, including carefully reviewing service-level agreements, in deciding which service providers are sufficiently reliable and trustworthy to provide virtualized services.

Social Technology

Social technology refers to technologies that encourage and facilitate web-based social interactions by providing individuals with tools and services that enable them to create and manage a personal web identity. Facebook, MySpace, YouTube, and Twitter are well-known examples of social technology. Social technology offers significant opportunities to engage consumers in keeping themselves and their families healthy and in supporting patients and families who are dealing with medical conditions. Social technology also offers benefits to medical researchers both in recruiting research participants and in supporting the research itself.

Personal privacy has been an ongoing concern in social media, and social networking sites have had to adjust their privacy practices in response to these public concerns. These concerns frequently relate to a lack of transparency—that is, a social networking site's practice of collecting or using private information without the user's knowledge or consent. Healthcare providers and medical researchers can capitalize on the potential of social technology but must be vigilant in adhering to the FIPs discussed earlier.

Smartphones

A smartphone is a wireless telephone that has computing capability and Internet connectivity. Smartphones are full-fledged computers that run operating systems (OSs) such as the Android open-source OS, BlackBerry OS, iPhone iOS, or Windows Phone OS. Smartphone applications (or apps) that help users manage their health—including medical-reminder apps to encourage compliance and apps to monitor medical conditions—are being developed at a rapid pace. Studies predict that by 2015, more than a third of the projected 1.4 billion smartphone users will be running at least one mobile healthcare app (Yahoo! 2011). Smartphones usually have integrated still and video cameras as well as geo-location technology. All of this capability offers tremendous value for improving health and health outcomes. At the same time, the ability to locate an individual who does not want to be located or to surreptitiously video (and potentially post to the web) an individual presents privacy risks that existing policy and fair practices have not anticipated.

Conclusion

In this chapter, we introduce the concepts associated with healthcare-related privacy and security, including risk, trust, fair information practices, and assurances necessary to attain and maintain information security and personal privacy. FIPs are shared throughout the world and serve as the framework for protecting individual privacy. We review the technical security safeguards required by the HIPAA Security Rule and the risks that each measure is designed to address, and we identify how these measures are supported by implemented standards and features in certified EHR technology. Finally, we discuss some leading-edge technologies that offer both opportunities and challenges to protecting electronic health information and individual privacy.

Chapter Discussion Questions

1. Draw a Venn diagram that represents the logical relationship among privacy, security, and safety. What risks might be representative of the overlap between privacy and safety?

2. Consider a physician practice that is transitioning from paper based to electronic. The receptionist area contains both hanging folders and the desktop computer on which the practice management system runs. During the transition, a patient's health information (valued asset) will exist in two states: on paper in a hanging folder and in an electronic record on a computer. Characterize the risks for each state in terms of threats, vulnerabilities, and probability of a breach (low, medium, or high).

3. Privacy is a human value that is somewhat dependent on context; for example, people who share private personal information with Facebook friends may not want to share that same information with their physician. As another example, an HIV/AIDS lab test result may be seen as more sensitive than a cholesterol test result. What factors do you think contribute to how an individual assigns a privacy value to health information?

4. Suppose a miscreant manages to capture the password of a physician in a hospital that is part of a large integrated delivery network (IDN) that shares identity assertions across all hospitals and clinics. Knowing that the IDN typically uses lastname_first-initial as user identifiers, the miscreant then remotely logs into the EHR system using the physician's user ID and captured password. Discuss the implications of this authentication failure on the access-control mechanisms, audit trail, and secure e-mail application in place.

CASE STUDY   Heinz Children's Health

Dixie B. Baker

Heinz Children's Health is a small pediatric practice serving the health-care needs of children in a small, rural community. Twenty-five years ago, Dr. Helen Heinz founded the practice, which now includes two physician assistants, two registered nurses, a home-health nurse, an office manager, and a receptionist. The practice has always used paper records, but when Dr. Heinz learns that, under the American Recovery and Reinvestment Act (ARRA) of 2009, the Centers for Medicare and Medicaid Services (CMS) is offering significant incentives to eligible professionals who adopt EHR technology and demonstrate its "meaningful use," she sees an opportunity to move her practice into the electronic age.

Once she decides to adopt an EHR system, Dr. Heinz is faced with another decision: which one to adopt. This is when she discovers that not only are there several EHRs from which to choose but also several ways to adopt them. The first option is to license the software and run it on a server that would be installed in her office. However, this would mean having to hire an information technology (IT) person to set up the system, configure it, install upgrades, and keep it running. The second option is to license the software and run it on a server that would be installed in a data center, but that is not much different from the first option except that the machine would be located somewhere else. She still would need to hire IT staff. The third option is to subscribe to an EHR software-as-a-service (SaaS), wherein Dr. Heinz and her staff would just log into the EHR over the Internet to get access to their patients' records. This option would not require Dr. Heinz to hire an IT person to install, configure, upgrade, or maintain any software and hardware. The SaaS provider would configure the software for Heinz Children's Health, create accounts for everyone in the office, provide 24/7 access, install updates, and keep it running smoothly. Plus, several SaaS vendors' salespeople have pointed out that by subscribing to an EHR service, Dr. Heinz would not have to worry about HIPAA compliance; the provider would take care of that for her. This sounds too good to be true (as it later turns out to be).

The SaaS vendor is Fleet Software, a small, local company that for the past ten years has been developing and implementing custom software for businesses in the area. The owner, Jake Fleet, is friends with Dr. Heinz's son, charming, and widely considered a "guru" in computers and software. When he reads about the ARRA incentives, his entrepreneurial mind sees a real opportunity to get into the EHR software business. He has developed a lot of business software, but has never developed EHR software. To avoid having to develop software for unfamiliar business processes and to enable him to get to the market soonest, he decides to license an EHR product and make it available through a SaaS subscription model.

Fleet checks out some of the leading EHR and practice-management commercial and open-source products designed for small practices. He hires his cousin, a retired physician, to help with product selection, training, and product. After calling several references who have done business with Fleet Software and were delighted with his work, Dr. Heinz

(continued)

signs up for Fleet's SaaS offering. Because Fleet Software will be providing a service involving protected health information (PHI), Heinz Children's Health signs a business associate agreement with Fleet, as required by HIPAA.

Fleet Software creates accounts for all of Heinz' staff and, using the existing paper records, sets up EHR records for patients with chronic conditions and patients with appointments scheduled over the next two months. Fleet and his cousin provide staff training in how to use the software, and he gives Dr. Heinz a number to call if her staff run into any problems with the software. Two months later, Heinz Children's Health goes "live" with its new EHR.

It takes some time for Dr. Heinz and her staff to get accustomed to using the EHR instead of the paper record, but they quickly see some real advantages. Information in the EHR is always easy to find and is organized. It provides reminders of when lab tests and vaccinations are due, and it is equipped with little pop-up calendars to help in scheduling a patient's next appointment. Graphs show the patient's growth in comparison with the mean growth patterns. Fleet and his cousin have done a good job selecting and customizing the EHR application for Dr. Heinz' practice.

Things are going smoothly until one morning Dr. Heinz and her staff discover that all of their patient records are gone from the EHR. They can log in, but no records are showing up. In a panic, Dr. Heinz calls Fleet. After doing some checking, he discovers that the system upgrade they rolled out the night before has inadvertently overwritten the storage partition containing the records. Fortunately, Fleet has backed up the records, and he promises to have the backup reloaded within a couple of hours. Meanwhile, Dr. Heinz and her staff revert back to paper until the EHR is restored.

Several months later, Dr. Heinz receives an irate phone call from the mother of a child who has been diagnosed with sickle cell disease. The mother's anger is triggered when a neighbor expresses her sympathy, although the mother has not discussed the diagnosis with anyone. Dr. Heinz questions her staff and learns that the receptionist, after seeing the child with his distraught mother, checked his medical record and saw the diagnosis. The receptionist became upset and discussed the information with the neighbor, who in turn approached the mother.

Dr. Heinz is surprised that the receptionist could even view the patient information, particularly given that the EHR is supposed to be HIPAA compliant, as promised by Fleet Software. She is also astounded that when she walks out into the reception area, she witnesses the receptionist's screen displaying another patient record and in full sight of those waiting for their appointments. After closing the exposed record and reprimanding the receptionist privately, Dr. Heinz calls Fleet. Fleet explains that the company just creates the accounts, but the responsibility for telling them about any restrictions on user access and privileges that should be set up for those accounts falls on Heinz Children's Health. Upon further discussion, Dr. Heinz learns that Fleet considers the clinic responsible for a number of other HIPAA requirements.

Later, Fleet Software's server suffers a malicious software attack. The attacker takes advantage of a known vulnerability in the server software, allowing the attacker to bypass user authentication and thus gain unauthorized access to all data stored on the server. Fleet reports the incident to Dr. Heinz and provides a list of patients whose information may have been exposed. When Dr. Heinz asks Fleet what the company is doing about the problem, he explains that they investigated the incident and found that the attacker had exploited a known vulnerability in the server-software vendor's critical security update. Then Fleet Software generated a list of individuals whose information could have been exposed and reported this information to its clients, including Heinz Children's Health. He declares that these steps complete the company's regulatory and contractual obligations as a business associate, leaving the clinic responsible for notifying the individuals whose information may have been exposed.

Dr. Heinz is now rethinking her decision to adopt an EHR to qualify for the incentive payment. The clinic may be better off using paper records until she retires.

Case Study Discussion Questions

1. Heinz Children's Health has experienced risks to information confidentiality, data integrity, service availability, and the business itself. Identify the consequences, the vulnerabilities exploited, the threats that exploited them, and the ways these risks could have been mitigated.

2. Thinking about a clinical practice that subscribes to an EHR service, rather than implementing its own system, how would you assign responsibility for the following HIPAA requirements?
   a. Deciding what access rights and privileges each user or user group should be assigned
   b. Configuring system accounts to restrict user access and privileges

(continued)

    c. Screening, supervising, and training personnel on appropriate use of patient information

    d. Installing, maintaining, testing, and configuration management of server security hardware and software

    e. Installing and updating malicious code–detection software

    f. Developing plans for emergency-mode operations and disaster recovery

    g. Security incident reporting and response

    h. Security and privacy awareness training and reminders

    i. Selecting and naming an individual to be responsible for HIPAA privacy and security compliance

    j. Secure data backup and online storage

    k. Securing paper copies of patient records

    l. Ensuring that user access devices are positioned so that the screens cannot easily be viewed by patients in the waiting room

    m. Securing the transport link between the system and users' browsers so that the integrity and confidentiality of all health information are protected

    n. Auditing system activities

    o. At the patient's (or patient representative's) request, providing an accounting of all disclosures of the patient's health information

    p. Notifying patients whose health information may have been exposed through a breach of the system security protections

3. What are some of the risks that are not addressed by HIPAA but a SaaS subscriber may need to consider?

STRATEGIC VALUATION OF ENTERPRISE INFORMATION TECHNOLOGY ARCHITECTURE

14

Gordon D. Brown and Ricky C. Leung

Learning Objectives

After reading this chapter, students should be able to

- Conceptualize the types of information technology (IT) architecture
- Demonstrate the interdependencies between enterprise strategy and IT architecture
- Develop a conceptual understanding of the transforming power of IT
- Compare and contrast how different types or stages of IT architecture relate to valuation
- Conceptualize IT valuation models and develop logical arguments for sources and levels of financing

---

KEY CONCEPTS

- Information infrastructure and architecture
- Range, richness, and reach of IT architecture
- Application silo architecture
- Standardized technology architecture
- Rationalized data architecture
- Modular architecture
- Interorganizational collaboration
- Dynamic capability
- Value measurement methodology

Introduction

The US healthcare system has lacked a coherent strategy on investment in information architecture. There has been overall underinvestment and it has been uneven across the system, with most initiatives put forth by academic health sciences centers and major health systems and the greatest reluctance displayed by small clinics. The federal government has increasingly encouraged the application of information technology (IT) and, with the HITECH Act of 2009, has included financial incentives to acquire and use IT (HHS 2009). Investment in IT must extend beyond the politics and discussion about the appropriate level of investment to explore how value of such investment would accrue, the level of value added, and the requisite properties of the information system at any level of investment. Currently, the US healthcare system is not only underinvesting in IT but also lacking a long-term vision and investment strategy.

The Strategic IT Architecture Perspective

IT architecture is applied in different contexts in the literature and is generally differentiated from information infrastructure (Ross 2003; Bradley 2006; Keen 1991; Bradley and Byrd 2009; Brown, Stone, and Patrick 2005). **Information infrastructure** is the set of properties of an information system viewed from the perspective of the IT function (department) and includes technology standards and the relationship between IT and business and clinical operations (Ross 2003; Brown, Stone, and Patrick 2005). This perspective casts IT as a support function to business and clinical operations, which then defines IT structure and assigns it a value. **Information architecture**, on the other hand, is a framework that takes the perspective of IT as a contributor to enterprise strategy. As such, it aligns IT with strategy from which it derives its value (Sauer and Willcocks 2002), and IT capability might alter the structure of the business and clinical functions. As Ross (2003, 5) states, at the enterprise level "IT architecture is the organizing logic for applications, data and infrastructure technologies, as captured in a set of policies and technical choices, intended to enable the firm's business strategy." This requires the organization to have an enterprise strategy first and an IT investment that is designed and valued in terms of meeting its strategic goals.

Ross emphasizes the concept of developing an IT architecture competency within the organization instead of developing an IT infrastructure, which entails establishing technology standards, vocabularies, data interface, and so on (see Chapter 2). IT architecture competency, meanwhile, focuses on three essential steps (Ross 2003, 2):

1. Define the firm's strategic objectives.
2. Define key IT capabilities for enabling strategic objectives.
3. Define the policies and technical choices for developing the IT capabilities.

Most healthcare organizations may not have a well-crafted enterprise strategy but instead may rely on platitudes (e.g., quality of care, patient-centered care, continuity of care) to focus and unite their workforce and to use in marketing and public relations. Currently, valuation of IT is assigned according to its contribution to operational issues such as reimbursement strategies and quality of clinical outcomes. While both are positive contributions, neither represents an enterprise strategy nor serves as an adequate basis for the valuation of IT architecture.

Valuation of IT architecture brings up the complexities of the strategic value of the clinical function to the organization and, by extension, how clinical processes are structured, how clinical decision support systems (CDSSs) are applied, and how organizational and interorganizational systems are designed (see Chapters 4 and 7). Medical informatics' traditional focus on IT, clinical knowledge, and information infrastructure provides a basis for valuation but is limited in that it does not include the exploration of how IT architecture contributes to the value of enterprise strategy and the design of the system to carry it out. This is an inadequate basis for discussing valuation and for developing arguments to support the level of investment and source of investment funds. The main requirement for developing IT competency is to focus on the enterprise and the value IT brings to enterprise strategy. This focus often necessitates a realignment of work processes and IT infrastructure that pose contradictory or difficult-to-meet demands. The driving force behind IT architecture is the enterprise strategy.

Enterprise Strategy as the Basis of Valuation

The purpose of this chapter is not to explore the vast and complex field of corporate strategy but to discuss the importance of strategy as the basis for conceptualizing and valuing IT architecture. To understand the relationship between IT architecture and corporate strategy, one has to know the concepts of reach, range, and richness (Segars and Grover 1998; Wells and Gobeli 2003). Reach, range, and richness describe the different strategic capabilities enabled by IT:

1. *Reach* is the degree to which an organization can manage its value-chain activities to connect its customers to an accessible product or service (Wells and Gobeli 2003). Simply, it is the number of individuals and families in a community who can be provided health services by a hospital or clinic (see Exhibit 14.1). Here, community might be defined as local, regional, national, or global. Historically, healthcare organizations thought locally, subscribing to the adage that all health services are local. Reach in the healthcare field was traditionally defined as the physical access to a clinical service, which de facto had limited the perspective to the local community. Even referrals

EXHIBIT 14.1
Strategic
Dimensions of
IT Architecture

	Reach	Richness	Range
Definition	The degree to which an organization can manage its value-chain activities to connect its customers to an accessible product or service	The degree to which an organization can facilitate the exchange of information to deliver products or services that match customers' exact wants and needs	The degree to which an organization can offer its customers a value proposition containing a breadth of products or services
Low	Offline physical products and services	Prebuilt, standardized products and services	Narrow set of projects and services
High	Online digital products and services	Segment of one, customized products and services	Broad set of products and services
E-business opportunities	Online digital products and services	Tailored customer-to-firm interaction	Strategic alliances

Source: Wells and Gobeli (2003). Reprinted with permission from *Business Horizons,* the journal of the Kelley School of Business, Indiana University.

to regional centers required patients to pass through local referring physicians. IT was deployed to support local physicians (such as decision support) and the administrative function (such as scheduling and insurance claims processing). While insurance, supplies, pharmaceuticals, and other such services were regional or national in nature, for patients and the clinical function the market was local. Reach, in this instance, reflected traditional measures of performance, such as market share. Telemedicine was an early application of IT to make selective, local medical services available within a region. In selective clinical services, such as dermatology and rehabilitation, IT application was based on the doctor-to-doctor referral relationship and not on the individual patient encounter. Telemedicine has evolved into e-health, covering a range of services distributed across broad spatial distances and provided directly to patients (as discussed in Chapter 11).

2. *Range* is the degree to which an organization can offer its customers a value proposition containing a breadth of products or services (Wells and Gobeli 2003). It refers to how well a healthcare provider brings to the patient a range of related services. Range might be narrowly defined as all services related to the care and treatment of a patient with a given illness (such as Type 2 diabetes) or broadly defined as a comprehensive health service for an individual or family. Most health centers that have a local reach (see previous discussion) state their commitment to the "health of the community" as a whole, but their services are primarily acute and geared toward a market with a given

illness (a population group) and do not include a broad range of well-ness or health maintenance care available within the community. IT can extend the range of services from merely acute and medical to preventive and maintenance. However, doing so might involve aligning financial incentives and removing regulatory restrictions consistent with the IT capability.

3. *Richness* is the degree to which an organization can facilitate the exchange of information to deliver products or services that match customers' exact wants and needs (Wells and Gobeli 2003). This refers to how a clinician or healthcare facility can deliver services that are tailored or customized to the patients, including how services are integrated to meet individual needs. IT architecture enables the richness of clinical services, which overcomes the institutional characteristics of large, centralized, and bureaucratic organizations and retains the traditional intimacy quality or approach of health professionals during a clinical encounter. Unlike the traditional model, however, service that is rich is integrated across professionals and organizations. Outside the healthcare field, individuals implement information customization all the time, such as setting up a personalized phone ringer, to make their experiences with the technology richer. Health professionals and institutions that tailor their services to individual patient preferences through IT architecture have a competitive advantage.

Futurists have predicted that most Americans will receive care from specialized chronic diseases centers (e.g., cancer, women's health, heart) (NCHL 2011). The question is the degree to which patients will demand these disparate specialized centers to function as (and have the feel of) an integrated and personalized system of care. Specialized centers need not take the form of a monolithic organization, but their services must be integrated and tailored through IT architecture. How will this architecture be designed, and who will make the necessary investment?

Strategy Related to IT Architecture

Ross (2003, 5) identifies four types or development stages of IT architecture that have different strategic capabilities (see Exhibit 14.2). She acknowledges that an organization might not desire or have the capacity to move from one stage to the next higher stage, as that is the nature of strategy. The four stages or types are application silo, standardized technology, rationalized data, and modular:

EXHIBIT 14.2
Development
Stages of IT
Architecture

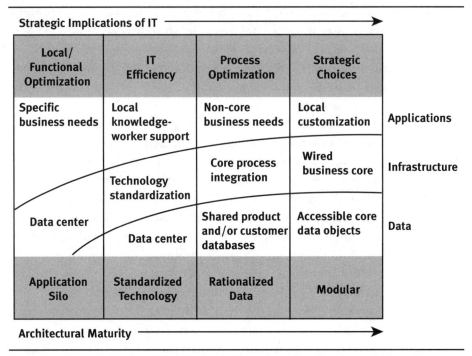

Source: Figure 1, page 7, from Ross (2003). Reprinted with permission from Massachusetts Institute of Technology, Cambridge, Massachusetts.

1. *Application silo.* At this stage, the IT architecture comprises individual applications rather than represents the whole enterprise. At this stage, the architecture is similar in concept to information infrastructure.
2. *Standardized technology.* At this stage, the IT architecture becomes enterprisewide and provides efficiencies through technology standardization and, in most cases, centralization.
3. *Rationalized data.* At this stage, the enterprisewide IT architecture expands to include standardization of data and processes.
4. *Modular.* At this stage, enterprisewide global standards with loosely coupled applications, data, and technology components are built into the IT architecture to preserve the global standards while enabling local differences.

Bradley and Byrd (2009) extend this IT architecture model to include interorganizational collaboration and communication, taking a systems orientation viewed from the perspective of the focal institution. The application of these IT architectures is a basis for determining the specific architecture needed to drive enterprise strategies and for estimating value and how (and to whom) it accrues within the enterprise. Exhibit 14.3 presents a summary of features and competencies of each type of IT architecture.

	Application Silo	Standardized Technology	Rationalized Data	Modular
IT Capability	IT applications serve isolated business needs	Firm-side technology standards	IT focused on wiring care process	Modules enable business-model extensions
Key Management Innovation	Technology-enabled change management	Firm-side technology standards	Recognition of essence of the business	Practices facilitating reusability
Business Case for IT	Return on investment of applications	Reduced IT costs, interoperability	Recognition of essence of the business	Speed to market, strategic agility
Locus of Control	Local control	Reduced IT costs, interoperability	Senior management, IT and process leadership	Senior management; IT, process, and local leadership
Key Governance Issues	Estimate, measure, communicate value	Establish (local/regional/national/global) standard setting, exception and funding processes	Determine core processes and funding priorities	Define boundaries for business experiments

EXHIBIT 14.3
Characteristics of the IT Architecture Development Stages

Source: Figure 2, page 13, from Ross (2003). Reprinted with permission from Massachusetts Institute of Technology, Cambridge, Massachusetts.

Application Silo Architecture

Most hospitals and large clinics are traditionally characterized as having **application silo architecture**, and small medical groups tend to retain this orientation. This type of architecture is designed for automating functional processes and delivering individual applications. It is characteristic of many clinical support departments, such as radiology and pharmacy, as well as business departments like finance and human resources. From the perspective of the overall organizational strategy, silo architecture might have negative value.

A hospital example is the automation of laboratory information to facilitate receiving, processing, recording, and reporting results. This architecture is designed for and responds to the needs of the laboratory alone, so it does not have to deal with other department's structure of information, interface system, cost, or vendor. Issues of vocabularies are of internal concern, and consensus is reached within the laboratory and not the institution. The selection of software to run the application is the responsibility of the laboratory. Value accrues to the laboratory, which secures and allocates funds with probably some unspecified value added to the institution.

The developers of IT were focused on the end users and functioned in operational silos (hence the name application silo). The results were independent applications that operated on multiple technology platforms. Ross (2003, 6) points out that such an IT architecture fosters innovation by individuals and departments but "innovation becomes offset by the difficulty of linking new applications to related systems." As healthcare institutions moved to the next stage of development, linking silo architecture to an integrated IT, institutions invested in writing interface programs. This presented complex problems such as developing a common vocabulary, determining the logic on which the system should be based, and changing processes and behaviors.

Estimating the value added and the allocation of funds for silo architecture is a simple process, as it is the responsibility of the one involved department. Value added is represented by the greater processing and reporting speed, reduction in staffing levels, accuracy of work and elimination of rework, and fewer redundancies in processes. The range of techniques used in value analysis includes cost–benefit analysis and is carried out by the department. We caution against using cost data that are based on allocated costs, instead of activity-based costing, as this technique introduces a systemic error in measurement that gets compounded as it is applied throughout the organization. The rapid development of application silo architecture in hospitals in the 1970s and 1980s created legacy systems that posed both technical and financing challenges that continue to plague the healthcare system today. The widespread implementation of this type of architecture represented not only the state of IT during that era but also the reluctance or inability of healthcare organizations to envision an enterprise strategy, which includes the clinical function. This reluctance is still present today but is quickly fading.

Standardized Technology Architecture

Advances in IT and changes in organizational capability and responsibility, such as increased accountability for quality and safety, have resulted in a shift from silo to **standardized technology architecture**. Such architecture is designed to integrate functions within the clinical domain and link clinical and business functions. The clinical side of healthcare puts much focus on the electronic medical record (EMR), including integrating laboratory, pharmacy, and radiology information with clinical information that serves as clinical decision support. The business side, on the other hand, focuses on coding clinical services and managing the revenue cycle. A standardized architecture is needed to integrate these functions, but standardization and centralization of IT are disruptive to both clinicians and department administrators.

Large hospitals and clinics are well under way in the standardized technology architecture process, but small facilities are just starting. In this stage, functions are linked through an integrated architecture, which entails establishing data and interface standards within the organization. New adopters will be helped by the increased standardization of vocabularies and data that has occurred in the field. Decisions on data and interface requirements, as well as decisions to purchase IT, are inherently centralized. Here, the position of chief information officer is created to manage the consolidation and integration process. One expectation from this process is that greater efficiencies can be obtained through reductions in redundant systems, a result that is difficult to appreciate because there is typically no decrease in IT investment. This phenomenon can be explained by two factors. First, under silo architecture, the organization typically does not have a good measure of its IT investment. Under standardized technology architecture, the department has an IT budget line (which is sometimes significant). Some managers justify this budget item to the board by presenting it as a capital cost that could be amortized over a number of years. This logic is flawed because the information system rapidly changes and much of the expenses are not incurred by the purchase of hardware and software but by the transformation process of the system itself. Second, a projection error is frequently introduced by underestimating future increases in aggregated (without consolidating) IT costs. Greater efficiencies will not necessarily be represented by decreased IT costs; the major value is integration of data and information to better support clinical and managerial decision making.

Standardized technology architecture makes estimating benefits and allocating costs more complex. Part of the difficulty is that value now accrues more directly to the organization as the unit of analysis and cannot be estimated only by compiling departmental estimates. Estimating relative value by a shared infrastructure is hard. The department might need to upgrade its system to meet the organization's IT requirements, even when the current system performs well and may be considered better than the upgrade. As a result, the department might incur added or upgrade costs for what it perceives to be lesser value. Valuation of standardized technology architecture must be viewed from the enterprise perspective. Currently, valuation is driven by reimbursement strategies linked to the quality of care provided. Meaningful use of IT is a current rubric for estimating the value contribution of IT to the clinical function. Reimbursement strategies, in turn, are increasingly driven by value-based reimbursement, which translates into payment for the actual clinical outcomes (compared with expected outcomes) achieved for a given case as measured by standardized metric. Value-based reimbursement characterizes the current investment strategy of the federal government and defines the healthcare organization's value justification for investing in IT. As such, IT is undervalued within the enterprise. Healthcare leaders must have a vision beyond this operational investment strategy, which means linking IT architecture to corporate strategy.

Rationalized Data Architecture

The IT architecture model submitted by Ross (2003) differentiates between the architecture needed to run the organization's overall operations and the architecture needed for the organization's core competency and strategy. The **rationalized data architecture** serves the core technology, which in healthcare is the clinical process. This stage or type is particularly powerful because clinical services are reliant on information and data. Ross (2003, 8) argues that data "must be unfailingly timely and accurate for the firm to consistently meet customer demands." In healthcare, patient and practice data and information offer decision support during clinical encounters and health and wellness information can be accessed directly by patients.

Moving to the rationalized data architecture stage requires the delineation of core processes that represent the enterprise strategy. What core clinical services will be provided? How will they be differentiated in terms of access, quality, continuity, and satisfaction? For its enterprise strategy, the organization examines outcomes and process–outcome relationships from the perspective of the patient and families who consume the services. Rationalized data architecture provides the IT capability to transform clinical processes, but the architecture itself does not transform them. Transforming clinical processes is the value-added contribution of the architecture, and if transformation is not accomplished the IT investment's value will not be realized. The IT architecture thus becomes fully integrated with and defined by the enterprise strategy. As Parton and Subbu (2012) state, "It is important to be able to integrate multiple data sources, including ambulatory and inpatient EHRs, labs, scheduling, billing, health information exchanges, insurance claims, remote monitoring, patient self-reports, research, demographic, administrative and financial data. Integrating population health IT with EHR functionality and workflow is a must." The locus of responsibility for IT and the structure of the clinical process shifts from the IT department and individual clinicians to the enterprise composed of overall strategy and integrated functions. Considerable complexity is introduced here because structuring clinical processes is more difficult than standardizing clinical data and guidelines. The ability of the organization to deploy this strategy is dependent on not only the IT architecture but also the ability of the organization to change clinical processes and behaviors (Chapters 4 and 7) and to integrate them with the business function. This suggests that the organization undertake a well-conceived, long-term process to introduce change that is transformational in nature.

Valuation and IT investment under the assumptions of a rationalized data architecture shift primarily to the enterprise level. The accumulative value that accrues from individual departments and functions undervalues this investment. The value-added potential is based more on volume and markets than on reimbursement formulas and assumptions under current and proposed reimbursement plans. Value-based reimbursement assumes a static or status quo market, while rationalized data architecture assumes a dynamic market strategy and enables market growth. Simply investing in rationalized data architecture does not position the enterprise for growth. Positioning is a broader strategic consideration, and not all organizations wish to or have the capability to pursue this potential. Investment in IT to expand markets and volume provides an advantage to larger institutions and those capable of transforming their clinical processes and establishing a competitive position on the basis of quality and service. Again, the future will depend not on how strong you are but how adaptable to change you are.

Valuation and investment in IT architecture under the assumptions of rationalized data architecture are not the decisions of the IT department or clinical services, but these departments must be involved and have the capacity to engage in setting the enterprise strategy. The costs associated with IT architecture investment extend beyond hardware and software purchases and decision support investments (such as a computerized physician order-entry system) and include structural change (such as in the clinical process) and enterprise leadership expenses. If strategic positioning is left to individual clinicians or departments and the business function, the development and execution of the strategy will likely be unsuccessful. Clinical as well as IT leadership must be part of the enterprise leadership team. If the skills of team members are limited to either clinical or technical, the IT architecture cannot achieve its full potential.

More information about valuation and investment related to rational data architecture may be gleaned from further study of strategy and finance. The finance emphasis should be on incurring and managing risks and should not be limited to reimbursement strategies or managerial accounting.

Modular Architecture and Interorganizational Collaboration

This section combines the interrelated concepts of modular architecture and interorganizational collaboration. **Modular architecture** entails the development of customized service modules. Two aspects of customization need to be considered: (1) standardized knowledge modules that can be distributed to individuals or to hospitals and clinics, and (2) the flexibility of the modules to be tailored to specific markets and individual patients. Knowledge-based services that can be extended into new markets by an enterprise or by linking through a loose-coupling architecture are strategies pursued by many tech-savvy firms in the commercial world. Web-based applications are examples of such a strategy and are gaining popularity as a strategy for healthcare organizations. Modules that consist of knowledge-based services can be transferred rapidly and applied throughout the enterprise or can be used as a strategy for rapidly extending the enterprise to new markets, based on all three concepts of reach; richness; and, through interorganizational collaborations, range. Modules are based on core competencies and processes of organizations, which distinguish them in the market. They leverage the distinctive competency of an organization that can be quickly and broadly distributed (Ross 2003, 12).

Customized knowledge modules have demonstrated their agility in the market as well as their considerable capacity to be upgraded and to maintain their distinctive competency. Agility in the market is demonstrated by the quickness to enter new markets through established organizations and to reach beyond the local market to regional, national, or international markets. Value of knowledge-based services is demonstrated by the ability to transcend distance. Web-based services can be developed and enabled by the focal organization and accessed in new markets. Embedding knowledge in the CDSS of other providers requires some type of *interorganizational collaboration* (see Bradley and Byrd 2009). Organizations will support collaboration through loosely configured structures such as franchising and mutual dependency, allowing rapid change and customization. Value based on the speed and reach of deployment is also dependent on the continued distinctive competency of the focal organization. For hospitals and clinics, this requires investing in their own rationalized data architecture as an internal institutional capacity and accessing (and, often, conducting) translational research and embedding that in knowledge modules. This suggests greater articulation between regional centers and distributed clinics and hospitals that are either too small or that choose a strategy to become informed users and not creators of knowledge modules.

Hospitals and clinics may potentially form interorganizational networks regardless of their respective enterprise strategy. These networks need not be consolidations or formal consortia, a strategy pursued by hospitals in the 1970s and 1980s. They can be loosely coupled and easily created and changed, and any given hospital or clinic might participate in more than one network. They enable nodal centers to rapidly and broadly expand their reach without the burden of forming new corporate structures or investing in their own institutional capacity. The value added to the distributed network includes both brand identification and a dynamic clinical knowledge base that (1) represents the best science and (2) is continuously updated. The valuation of such a service is based on the market impact of participating centers; availability of competing knowledge-based modules; and quality of clinical services as a result of the collaboration, which is important for maximizing both reimbursement and patient satisfaction. The value of a knowledge module is the ease with which it can be adapted to the specific desires of an organization and region or to the personal preferences and medical condition of a patient. The value of these features is assigned by the participating institutions and patients. Considering this value must be done within a given time frame because features that do not have value today might have value tomorrow, or vice versa.

The collaborating hospital or clinic likely has a basic type of IT architecture—for example, a standardized technology architecture such as an EMR. Importing modular architecture such as decision support protocols enables the collaborating institution to acquire access to a more advanced IT architecture without investing in its development. However, the imported architecture requires the participating institution to adapt its IT architecture and clinical processes according to that of its collaborating organizations. Transforming the structure of clinical processes is a much more complex and disruptive task than introducing a basic architecture such as the EMR. Changing the decision-making process of individual physicians is much less complex than changing the clinical processes that transcend health professionals and institutions. Changes in the structure of the decision process also involve patients and thus tailoring the process. If collaborating institutions are committed and able to transform the structure of clinical processes, considerable value added from the clinical modules might be realized. This value accrues to the collaborating institution and to the nodal organization through a franchising fee, shared reimbursement, or other types of fee structure. Changing the reimbursement structure is likely to be the major challenge to the clinical function or the IT structure that supports it. The ability of modular architecture to rapidly add collaborators may offset the cost of developing it.

Dynamic Capability of Organizations

The IT strategic planning process involves valuation related to two specific issues: (1) the appropriate level of IT investment and (2) the long-term pay-offs of IT investment. For both issues, the concept of **dynamic capability** offers a conceptual lens (Teece, Pisano, and Shuen 1997; Helfat and Peteraf 2003). This perspective builds on the resource-based view (Barney 1991; Barney and Clark 2007) but places more emphasis on the external environments of organizations. In particular, organizations are seen as situated in complex and constantly changing environments and need adaptive capacity to accommodate environmental pressures. This emphasis is applicable for building IT architecture in healthcare organizations (Leung 2012).

More specifically, dynamic capability is "the capacity of an organization to purposefully create, extend, or modify its resource base" for sustaining its competitive advantage (Helfat et al. 2007, 4). Resource base refers to all available tangible and intangible assets that the organization can deploy (through owning, renting, or hiring) to accomplish its purposes. Capacity, meanwhile, is the ability to accomplish defined tasks at some level of acceptability, reliability, and repeatability.

Following this perspective, first, healthcare administrators must define the organization's strategic objectives. For example, they may ask, does the organization seek to become the top provider with the best IT capability in the relevant markets? What level of health IT adoption should the organization attain in the next five years? Second, administrators must identify the necessary resource base (e.g., financial capital, human resources, computing equipment) for building the IT architecture and then evaluate if the organization has the adequate resource base. A related question is whether the organization possesses the managerial capacity to use resources effectively. For example, leadership and human resources are essential to implementing various health IT and building an integrated IT architecture. The organization needs to determine whether different staff members have developed complementary capabilities to provide mutual support (Khatri et al. 2010) and whether staff members are prepared to work with the IT architecture. Third, administrators must formulate policies and identify the specific technical components of the IT architecture. The technical choices made depend on the organization's capacity to determine what stage or type of IT architecture to invest in temporarily (see Exhibit 14.3).

Because the process of building IT architecture can take place while the organization is facing and adjusting to environmental pressures, conducting performance valuation over time is important. Performance valuation enables the organization to align IT with strategy (and strategic change) and to better understand the costs and benefits of the IT architecture. Consistent with the notion of dynamic capabilities, two concepts can be used to evaluate performance: (1) technical fitness and (2) evolutionary fitness (Teece 2007). Technical fitness depends on how well the organization produces its products or services "technically." For example, administrators can examine if the IT architecture has maximized the benefits of interorganizational collaboration with minimal computing and human resource costs. Both standardization and flexibility in a modular architecture can be evaluated according to the concept of technical fitness. Evolutionary fitness is a performance measure that goes beyond the organization itself. Administrators or the executive team need to compare the performance of the organization's IT architecture with that of comparable organizations in the relevant geographic or product market, assessing whether the IT architecture can increase reach, range, and richness (Segars and Grover 1998; Wells and Gobeli 2003). Note that technical fitness does not imply evolutionary fitness. That is, the IT architecture is not evolutionarily fit if customers cannot perceive its usefulness in comparison with other IT architectures in the market. Technical and evolutionary fitness can change over time, so administrators need to monitor performance improvement or degradation regularly.

At the estimation level, executive leaders can use one or more cost–benefit and valuation tools to assess technical and evolutionary fitness. In recent years, researchers have applied a quantitative technique called **data envelopment analysis** (DEA) to evaluate organizational performance (see Van de Ven et al. 2012; Leung and Pasupathy 2011). DEA is a technique for evaluating organizational performance, identifying exogenous and endogenous forces that affect that performance, and monitoring performance changes over time. Thus, this methodology is well suited to assess the technical and evolutionary fitness of different stages or types of IT architecture.

IT Valuation and Investment

Knowing the types of IT architecture is a foundation for understanding the relationship between IT architecture and enterprise strategy and estimating the value of an IT investment. A hospital, clinic, or long-term care facility must assess its capacity to deploy a strategy, given its market, competition, access to capital, structure, and culture. This assessment requires an awareness of the literature on enterprise strategy and organizational capability to pursue a given strategy. IT makes a value contribution to an organization in three ways: (1) It supports operations, (2) it is an essential resource for carrying out enterprise strategy, and (3) it is an enterprise strategy itself. Commercial industry has demonstrated the considerable capacity of IT as an enterprise strategy, and healthcare organizations are starting to draw from this body of science (Brown, Stone, and Patrick 2005; Davenport and Glaser 2002; Bradley et al. 2012; Weiss and Thorogood 2011; Greengard 2011). The US healthcare system relies on private nonprofit and investor-owned organizations to make this investment, and many other countries with national health systems are developing or increasing their private health sector to attract more capital for such an investment.

To understand the concept of value, one must learn the concepts of public and private goods and the perspectives each brings to valuing and investing in IT. This starts with knowing how value is defined and measured, as value is the motivating force for measuring and justifying investment. (Public and private goods are described further in a later section of this chapter.)

Theory of Value
The theory of value is a blend of economics, ethics, and political science, an in-depth discussion of which is beyond the scope of this book. Assigning

value to healthcare services is complex in all societies because it includes (in various degrees) the premise that an individual's health has intrinsic value. This intrinsic value supports the arguments for a service economy (as opposed to a pure market economy in which value is based on individual preferences and demand is based on price and ability to pay). In most countries, health services are primarily the responsibility of the public sector, but in the United States healthcare is provided by a combination of the public, private non-profit, and for-profit sectors. Each of these sectors brings different assumptions about value, making the valuation process more complex in the United States (as well as in other countries that are expanding their private-sector investments in health). The value premise in a service economy is achieved by public-sector regulations and controls, such as restrictions on risky behavior (e.g., wearing a seatbelt); direct provision of clean water, sanitation, and other services; investment in infrastructure such as IT; and reimbursement for clinical services. The United States has followed a somewhat unique course by providing social goods—particularly, hospital services—through the private nonprofit sector and generally allowing these private institutions to be exempt from taxes depending on their social contribution. The basis for IT investment includes decisions on what health services are to be made available and what value contribution IT can bring to these services.

Health services in the United States have been historically provided and paid for primarily by the private sector, and the public sector made considerable investment in facilities, research, manpower, and equipment. The market economy has defined and continues to influence the structure and culture of the healthcare system. Private hospitals and clinics that function under the assumptions of a market economy undervalue some services but respond to financial incentives and other controls from state and federal governments. The public sector, meanwhile, subsidizes and stimulates the private sector and has shifted its assumptions from a market economy to a service economy through the increasing level of direct financing of health services. The ongoing policy debate in the United States and other nations addresses how health services should be valued and how the health system (including IT) should be designed and financed. The responsibility for making insurance and thus health services available to citizens has shifted to the public sector through Medicare and Medicaid payments and most recently the Patient Protection and Affordable Care Act (US Congress 2010). In 2009, the federal government enacted the Health Information Technology for Economic and Clinical Health (HITECH) Act to stimulate and augment private-sector investment in IT.

As a major purchaser of health services, the public sector measures and takes accountability for the quality, continuity, and cost of health services because it is expending public funds. The private sector, on the other hand, engages in measurement and accountability for the purpose of the market and competition. The US healthcare system has always deployed a layered strategy of direct public-sector provision of services and public-sector purchase of services from the private sector, and it has operated under a robust market economy with private investment and consumption. Even with a strong market economy, however, many services are provided by nonprofit healthcare organizations and highly professionalized private clinicians dedicated to patients and communities and are balanced with profits. The healthcare system is thus a complex environment that negates any single set of assumptions about valuation and investment. Healthcare organizations and professionals function within this complexity, and so do IT systems. The integrated manner in which IT must operate further complicates how to make the optimal investment in IT capacity. The concept of dynamic capabilities of organizations is a framework for making such an investment decision from a market or modified market perspective.

Public or Private Good

IT valuation and investment in the US healthcare system are driven by whether it serves a private (market) good or a public (social) good. Market-driven investment in IT by hospitals and clinics varies across the healthcare system and has lagged because of the lack of incentives in most markets to achieve greater efficiency, increased quality, better integration, and more patient involvement. The desire to improve efficiency is offset by the ease with which providers and private insurers can pass on costs to corporations and patients in the form of higher premiums. Market demand for high quality, integrated, and patient-involved services enabled by IT is blunted by providers' general resistance to change and by insurance companies' reluctance to offer incentives for such a change. This situation then engenders a complacent market. The general principle of increased innovation and capital investment (including IT) through private-sector involvement is not currently demonstrated in the US healthcare system.

The policy interests of the federal government revolve around the government's role (1) as a public insurer that pays for medical services and thus demands providers to exercise sufficient accountability for quality and efficiency, and (2) as an investor in services, such as medical research and clean-air standards, that benefit the public at large. The private health insurance sector's lack of commitment to invest in greater efficiency and disease prevention (which results in overpayment for services) may be explained, in part, by the ability of these insurers to pass costs to patients and corporations. As a public insurer, the government has a policy objective to integrate clinical information so that patients can access their own medical records and other health information regardless of who is providing the health services. This integration has the potential to improve both effectiveness and efficiency, an interest of Medicare and Medicaid programs. In addition, access to patient records and other health information is valued in its own right, beyond that justified and verified by improved efficiency and quality. Access to information constitutes a new dimension of quality, valued in itself. This is the dominant logic that drives the IT investment of the federal government, which is focused on developing a standardized technology architecture consisting of an EMR and electronic exchange. It justifies the HITECH Act on the basis of private healthcare organizations' underinvestment in IT and has committed $27 million (disbursed over ten years) to stimulate and underwrite such investments. This underinvestment stems from the assumptions of a cottage industry filled with small, independent and market-driven clinics and hospitals (using standardized technology architecture). The IT investment by the federal government will likely galvanize the transition of the healthcare industry to a more integrated system focused on coordination of care, clinical quality, and patient centeredness.

Private-Sector Investment in IT

Leading healthcare organizations have created an IT investment strategy that incorporates IT into the institution's strategic plan and that recognizes information and knowledge as a valuable strategic asset, although the process has not been carefully examined in healthcare (Shortliffe 2005). Externally, the focus is on markets and competitors and the value assessment of services as the organization positions itself in the market. Internally, the focus is on the implications of strategy (including selecting the appropriate IT architecture and infrastructure) on governance and leadership functions, organizational structure, work processes, and operations. Enterprise strategy has been extensively researched in the business community with considerable knowledge and experience to guide the development of IT as a strategic resource (Bharadwaj 2000; Bradley et al. 2012; Chi, Ravichandran, and Andrevski 2010). Many models have evolved that can provide direction and can be used to test the effectiveness of IT valuation and strategy; some of these models are discussed here. Additional research by healthcare institutions is needed to reveal how these models value IT and guide investment strategy.

From the individual enterprise perspective, ISACA (2012) and other collaborations present models, such as the Information Technology Infrastructure Library (see www.itil-officialsite.com/home/home.aspx), that identify the dimensions of the problem, the methods of expressing elements within the enterprise, and the basis for assessing value contribution. These models introduce a disciplined approach to identifying the following:

- Domains within the organization involved in IT strategy and infrastructure
- Alignment of IT with the enterprise strategy
- IT architecture needed to support the business function
- Appropriate organizational structures, processes, and cultures that carry out the enterprise strategy

These are critical elements to consider to ensure that the organization and its professional staff are equipped to structure the clinical process and provide appropriate decision support tools. The integrated perspective that guides the development of the model and identifies the critical functions and players needed is more important than the precise measurement of value within any given unit or for the enterprise.

Once the appropriate levels and functions of the organization have been engaged and involved in developing the enterprise strategy, the essential IT architecture, and the structure of the organization and clinical processes, a more specific articulation of value and risk are then carried out. Rich experiential and research information is available to guide the process of conceptualizing value and risk down to the levels of measurement and management (Yokota and Thompson 2004). The focus is prospective and visionary and based on markets, competition, consumers and their wants, clinical knowledge (translational research), and IT technology. Valuation is not based on existing organizational or IT structures, professional domains, or reimbursement strategies; these are short-term considerations, which are probably obsolete and considered as constraints. Instead, valuation is based on the dynamic variables that position the organization for the future. The strategic vision of the organization is more critical to this process than technical or clinical knowledge or experience. ISACA has developed two modules—Val IT and Risk IT—that draw on best practices to guide valuation and risk decisions. Risk, in this instance, is not limited to traditional IT risk such as privacy and security (see Chapter 13); it refers to business risk. Val IT systematically addresses assumptions, costs, risks, and outcomes related to IT-enabled business investments and provides benchmarking capability to allow enterprises to exchange experiences on best practices for value management. The approach presents a structured analysis of IT investment represented by a decision matrix for a proposed investment in the following factors and measures (from ISACA at www.isaca.org/Pages/default.aspx):

- Calculated risks: Are calculated risks acceptable?
- Financial targets: Are financial targets met?

- Nonfinancial benefits: What are the nonfinancial benefits, are they explicit, and are they met?
- Alignment: Is there alignment between IT investment and enterprise strategy?

Private investment in IT will always involve risk, but risk must be managed by following a rigorous process with clearly stated goals and strategy, selecting the appropriate IT architecture, aligning all levels of the organization, and performing with operational efficiency. ISACA (2012) reports that two out of ten enterprise IT projects fail as a result of an avoidable breakdown in appropriately assessing value and estimating risk. If "failure to launch" is one of these breakdowns, the failure rate would be higher. The success rate in the healthcare field is not well documented.

Public-Sector Investment in IT

The government (or public sector) has many interests in IT, such as developing and maintaining national databases as instruments of surveillance, for both public health and national security purposes. Direct social good can be derived from such a national database, serving as a justification for this type of public investment, although little work has been done to estimate this benefit (Boles and Cook 2005; Ozdemir, Barron, and Bandyopadhyay 2011). The current investment in health registries and public-health surveillance reflects a strong commitment to install such a database. As mentioned, "health information as a public good" is a value that deserves public investment, and sufficient capital will be not allocated by the private sector or through reimbursement rates for medical services and will result in an underinvestment in this critical national resource.

Medicare and Medicaid programs and the provisions of the Patient Protection and Affordable Care Act are expressions of the public sector's investment in healthcare services for the public—specifically, the poor, elderly, young, uninsured, and high-risk populations. As the public sector provides access to medical care and ensures continuity and quality, it must also invest in information infrastructure to support that system. Public insurance differs from private insurance in that the expenditure of public funds requires provider accountability for quality, continuity, and efficiency. The government cannot allow the continued underinvestment in IT because IT is a critical resource of healthcare production. This investment is not a subsidy to private healthcare organizations and professionals but a factor cost of production to achieve the social (or public good) purpose.

The method the government uses to assess value and thus justify its IT investment is different from that used by the private sector. The government uses the **value measurement methodology** (VMM). Developed by the Federal Chief Information Officers Council (2012), the VMM is a framework and a toolkit for estimating values, costs, risks, and tangible and intangible returns of a given IT investment. It uses a scoring system to measure value using both quantitative and qualitative measures. It calculates return on investment (ROI), although ROI is not based solely on financial return but also includes factors such as social benefits, access and use of data by other agencies, and strategic/political goals. Public investment then relies on the valuation of IT investment related to the ROI of alternative public investments. VMM in itself does not differ substantially from the logic of private-sector IT investment, but the values differ, resulting in different decision choices. Both public and private investment processes start by defining and estimating value, risk, and cost parameters. If the logic of public-sector investment is limited to access, quality, efficiency, and continuity of medical services, underinvestment results because all social benefits are not included. The public sector should not expect the full investment to come from the private sector and its IT investment logic.

Coye and Bernstein (2003) offer an alternative model to estimating value and allocating public funds for private-sector IT investment that focuses on public infrastructure development. This approach is interesting in that it provides private organizations access to public capital through a revolving fund, which in turn stimulates private investment. The provision to repay the fund recognizes the importance of private-sector investment. Another provision is that "needy" organizations, such as safety net hospitals, receive funds in the form of grants for matching the public funds to stimulate IT investment. Such an approach has merit because it requires an organization to develop its own IT strategy and bring proposals to health IT corporations that have the authority to review and award grants or loans. In addition, it adds rigor to the concept of meaningful use as a basis for allocating IT investment.

Conclusion

Valuation of and investment in health services use a complex mix of public and private funds allocation. The valuation of and investment in IT architecture in healthcare are similarly complex in that different designs afford different capacities, each of which has a value basis. The logic of most IT architecture in healthcare organizations today reflects the tradition of independent clinicians and institutions, while the value of IT is derived primarily from integration of processes and services. Thus, deriving the value potential from an IT investment entails making a set of assumptions about how IT will be applied—that is, in many instances, how IT will enable an enterprise strategy, which includes redesigning the structure of clinical processes. For this reason, health IT and health informatics are considered to be a transformational science. Building IT capacity without using it to its full potential is certainly a failed strategy.

The increased role of the public sector in the US healthcare system will likely increase the pressure for structural change. The challenge is to stimulate private clinicians and organizations to change without adding to the significant costs required by regulations and public bureaucracy.

Chapter Discussion Questions

1. Discuss the importance of understanding the concept of strategic IT architecture as a basis for considering valuation in IT.
2. What type of IT architecture is needed for the EMR? Critically evaluate it in terms of IT value and investment.
3. Discuss the concept of dynamic capability in terms of the organizations it applies to and the factors for estimating the value of IT.
4. What areas of the organization should be involved in IT valuation, and what factors should be considered?
5. Discuss the logic of the HITECH Act in terms of how IT is valued and what impact it has on IT investment and on the healthcare system.

CASE STUDY   Metro Health's New Information System

Gordon D. Brown

Metro Health is an integrated health system comprising three urban hospitals that are strategically located in different neighborhoods. The original hospital is in the urban center, while the other two facilities (one of which is a local nonprofit hospital acquired when it incurred financial difficulties) are in growing suburbs. Each hospital has its own medical staff, chief operating officer, and EMR. Metro Health's governance includes the president and chief executive officer (CEO), chief medical officer (CMO), chief financial officer (CFO), and the board of directors. In the past several decades, the system developed an effective enterprise strategy under the leadership of a visionary and inspiring CEO.

In the 1980s and 1990s, the dominant strategy was to partner with individual members of the medical staff to develop a physician–hospital organization (PHO) to deliver health maintenance organization (HMO) contracts. The PHO was designed as an "open PHO" in which any member of the medical staff could participate. In addition, the system formed an open management services organization (MSO) and established a multispecialty clinic. The impetus for the MSO was to manage HMO contracts and implement an EMR for the clinic. Under this arrangement, the assets were owned and managed by the MSO, but the clinical practice remained the responsibility of the clinicians of the clinic. Metro Health's CEO and board also developed a strategy to purchase, partner with, or manage various primary care practices and clinics. The underlying motivation for this strategy was to funnel patients into these clinics and the system's hospitals, realizing the system's stated mission and vision to provide high-quality care through an integrated service network. None of the primary care clinics had an EMR and none was considered, even in the system-owned practices. The strategy was effective in increasing market share and access to capital, retaining patients within the system, and developing a brand image as an integrated delivery system (IDS). Metro Health was considered a model IDS, and the CEO received national recognition from the American College of Healthcare Executives. Because of his successes and newly acquired national stature, the CEO was aggressively recruited by Sun Valley Health Care, a larger system located in a nicer climate.

The new president and CEO of Metro Health, Catherine Kirk, was attracted to the job by the system's excellent reputation, strong market and financial position, and history of rapid growth, along with the high salary offer. Catherine found that the system's corporate strategy and culture fit her style and skills well. The high salary was a statement from the board that the system wants to recruit and retain leaders who would continue to expand the reputation of the system as a national leader in healthcare delivery. Catherine has closely followed the Institute of Medicine's reports on medical errors and patient safety as well as the revisions to the Medicare and Medicaid programs related to value-based reimbursement. Having previous experience in IT, Catherine is certain that patient access to information and participation in the clinical process are important to attracting and retaining patients. Such a strategy would serve as a way for the system to differentiate itself and strengthen its competitive advantage. In her first few months on the job, Catherine installed chief operating officers (COOs), a chief information officer (CIO), and a chief human resources officer (CHRO). She formed a strategic planning group made up of the CMO, CIO, CHRO, CFO, COOs, and medical directors of each of the three system hospitals and the MSO.

(continued)

She now brings to the board a preliminary proposal to invest in a new EHR, which has a price tag of more than $100 million, that would integrate the multiple institutions and include a clinical decision support system (CDSS). Even though Metro Health's financial position is strong with good reserves, the board hesitates to proceed with the investment of this scale because the cost exceeds the system's previous investments in IT. Catherine argues that an EHR with a CDSS is essential for carrying out the system's new bold strategy and that the investment would pay for itself by increasing patient volume, much as previous investments have brought in market growth and expansion. The board is concerned that the EHR would be disruptive to the clinical function and would be viewed by clinicians as corporate interference, much as the managed care contracts of the 1970s and 1980s were seen as an intrusion. The board thinks that Catherine is building a management empire instead of serving the best interests of the system. In private discussions, some medical directors express the reservations of their respective medical staffs. They reason that they are in the process of acquiring EMRs for all the clinics to meet the meaningful use standards mandated by the Patient Protection and Affordable Care Act.

The IT tactical plan is to migrate to common system architecture, including unique patient identifiers, a common patient database, a computerized physician order-entry system, and clinical guidelines and protocols. This database would allow physicians to access patient records anywhere in Metro Health, including results, orders, and other data from pathology, radiology, pharmacy, and other areas. Such a system would bring to physicians and other health professionals clinical information that is accurate, timely, integrated, and evidence based and may be used as the basis for clinical decision making. Catherine's and the strategic planning group's future plan includes making this information available to patients as part of an integrated personal health record.

You just started a two-year management and informatics residency at Metro Health. Catherine appoints you to help her and the strategic planning group. She wants you to analyze the changes that will occur in the locus of decision authority and responsibility of physicians and key managers within the system. You review various techniques, such as responsibility charting, for examining decision responsibility before and after the change. These techniques provide a systematic framework for identifying the possible changes to the roles and responsibilities of key players (i.e., individual physicians, clinical units, medical staffs, and hospital and system management). Catherine also asks that you work with the CIO and CFO to develop an investment plan for the new IT architecture to show its value-added contribution to the proposed corporate strategy.

Case Study Discussion Questions

1. Discuss alternative IT architectures, and develop arguments to support the architecture you would use to determine needed IT capacity.
2. What functions does the proposed IT architecture support, which serve as the basis for estimating value? (Be specific and provide as much detail as you can.)
3. Is the EHR investment decision driven by dollar amount or by the viability of the proposed corporate strategy?
4. Are proposed changes to the system technical, process, structural, or behavioral in nature?
5. How are the open PHO and MSO concepts consistent with the independent practice of physicians?

HEALTH SYSTEMS IN THE INFORMATION AGE

Gordon D. Brown

Learning Objectives

After reading this chapter, students should be able to

- Synthesize how information technology applications and new models can change the role of the patient
- Consider IT as a transformational science in healthcare
- Describe how information technology frames new business models and makes obsolete the old models
- Conceptualize the interface of clinical and business functions
- Assess the potential and limitations of applying clinical decision support to an international or global context

---

KEY CONCEPTS

- Transformational change in health systems
- Consumer-driven healthcare
- Regionalization
- Medical banking
- Cloud computing
- Globalization

Introduction

The rapid rate and the profound nature of change in the healthcare system and society are giving rise to both unprecedented threats to traditional healthcare structures and opportunities for innovation and leadership. Historically, change was viewed as an aberration and stability was considered the constant. Today, however, change has become the constant and stability the aberration. The growth in the number of health futurists reflects an awareness that more change is coming. These futurists consult with chief executive officers and other governance members, lead board retreats, train executives and administrators, and speak at professional meetings. Training programs for futurists and a futurist association have also emerged. As sources of information and vision guides, futurists are in high demand in national and international markets, public and private sectors, and business and service industries.

The following list of prognostications by a distinguished group of futurists spells out the current and future changes and trends in healthcare (NCHL 2011):

- Standard diagnostic health will largely be electronic, with people conducting their own "doctor visits" from home through miniature data collection and monitoring devices.
- The United States will be part of a global system that puts greater emphasis on wellness and preventive care. Patients worldwide will receive care from virtual or web-based centers of excellence.
- Deeper understanding of the human genome will create new drugs that can prevent disease from developing.
- As the rest of the baby boomers become senior citizens around 2020, rising costs, poor resource allocation, and improper health priorities will become bigger national issues.
- Fueled by the 24/7 access to information through the web, people will engage in more healthcare self-management, making personal health decisions and demanding to be treated as customers rather than users.
- Most Americans with chronic disease will receive care from specialized centers (e.g., cancer, women's health, heart).

This chapter addresses some of the implications of profound change on the healthcare system and the role of information technology (IT) in easing that impact or enabling the change. Changes in many areas, such as the aging of the population, will occur independently of IT but will create opportunities to apply IT. Bioinformatics science will enable genomics and, when applied to healthcare delivery, will be informed by health informatics. Nanocomputing will bring new technology that will alter clinical medicine and healthcare delivery organizations. Although IT itself does not cause the transformation of healthcare organizations, it does enable that change.

In this state of flux, how do health leaders adapt or cope? Different providers (clinicians and organizations) perceive and respond to change according and appropriate to their own markets, mission, strategy, and culture. Some cannot change and thus perish. Some are cautious and reactive, following what seems to have worked for others and only doing what is necessary for the time being. In a dynamic environment and future of healthcare, such a strategy may be categorized as a failure to respond. Some providers, however, are proactive and innovative, aspiring to greater levels of performance and outcomes. These clinicians and organizations are to whom this chapter is oriented.

Built to Change

As mentioned throughout this book, the design of many healthcare organizations and systems is based on the outmoded conditions and assumptions of healthcare delivery. The challenge is not one of modernizing but transforming the system based on the reality of the information age. In his 1984 book, Toffler recognized the need of society to shift from industrial revolution–based assumptions to the information and technology world in the design of organizations, communities, communications, work, and leisure. The hierarchical structure and independent functioning of organizations, the autonomy of professionals, and the institutionalization of services are outmoded concepts of the industrial age. Strong evidence exists for designing high-performance organizations, but it is not reflected in many of the current approaches to structuring clinical processes and communities of practice. Leaders must approach change as visionaries and innovators, not merely as adapters or reactors. Vision and innovation engender dialectic and are disruptive to the status quo. To appropriately respond to changing public expectations, organizations and professionals must prepare for rapid and continuous change characterized by services tailored to the wants and needs of individual patients and other consumers.

Change to the healthcare system is multifaceted, involving traditions, values, knowledge, behaviors, culture, and self-interests, and will not be easily accomplished. Etzioni (2010) correctly points out that these latent factors might override the demonstrated merits of change, such as increased efficiency and quality, and might slow the pace of implementation. In addition, the level of regulation and subsidization encourages resistance to change, even when there is a demonstrated need for that change. These factors, along with outdated design, make introducing, implementing, and sustaining change a challenge to healthcare leaders.

The need for and the nature of change in the healthcare system has been the subject of many studies and reports. Compelling arguments for this change have been made, but the basic structure of the system has remained unchanged. Of course, changes continue to occur in biomedical sciences, IT, sources and levels of financing, and regulations, but these developments occur within (and to a degree reinforce) the fundamental design and operation of the system. As dramatic as some of these innovations have been, however, they have not been transformational. Christensen

(1997) characterizes these changes as sustaining innovations. This reality calls into question society's capability to effect transformational change in the healthcare system. The balance of power and checks and balances suggest that internal change will be difficult. However, the system is not a closed system and thus is not immune to change.

We believe IT has the potential to enable (even initiate) significant transformation, which, to a degree, will be unstoppable. Some healthcare leaders will recognize this opportunity and lead the transformation. Reforms to and disruptive innovations in the structure and financing of healthcare services will initiate profound change (Christensen, Grossman, and Hwang 2008; Gianchandani 2011). The Patient Protection and Affordable Care Act might inhibit this change, however. Increased financing of or proper investment in health IT may not initiate the change but could facilitate it.

Change will likely emanate from several unrelated but equally information-driven sources. These sources include individuals and families who are accustomed to accessing needed and integrated information in other service industries and thus demand and expect the same kind of customer-focused, information orientation from the healthcare system. Sources may also be the integrated technologies themselves, such as cloud computing and mobile technology (such as the iPad and smartphones) with 4G, 5G, or higher communication standards. Other industries are also sources of change, such as telecommunications, banking, and retail—all of which have integrated previously isolated functions into a convenient, accessible, "one-stop-shopping" service. In addition, the perception that health services are local and thus dependent on local hospitals and doctors will be changed by regional, and potentially global, networks. These networks will bring to the local market knowledge-based information and will turn isolated hospitals and physicians into integrated systems of care. Most of the care will still be provided locally but within a transformed system that consists of communities of practice linked and informed by knowledge-based IT.

Given that the healthcare system in the near future will be more dynamic, organizational structures and functions will be built to change. Structures will be less hierarchical, more loosely coupled and nimble, more integrated, and more responsive to changing markets and individual demands—all of which will be enabled by electronic information systems (Kocharekar 2004; Hillard 2010). New markets will be defined for health professionals and organizations on the basis of not only the quality or cost of services but also how services are accessed, integrated, and customized for the individual. These will be the value-added features of health services and will likely not be provided by the traditional hospital and specialist-dominated system. Successful organizations will be horizontally structured to manage the value-added continuum of services, where each organization is committed to the collaboration and its effective functioning. These services will have rapid response times, be improvisational, and be tailored to individual customers and markets (Pavlou and El Sawy 2010). Corporate orientation will shift to commitment-based cultures enabled by virtual socialization or social networks (Ahuja and Galvin 2003; Briggs, Nunamaker, and Sprague 2006; Raghuram, Tuertscher, and Garud 2010; Shu-Mei 2010; Liu, Raahemi, and Benyoucef 2011; Rajnish 2011; Gianchandani 2011). Shared mental models will facilitate the processes and performance of team members who work across organizational boundaries (Mathieu et al. 2000; Vaccaro, Veloso, and Brusoni 2009; Borzillo and Kaminska-Labbé 2011).

Consumer-driven Healthcare and Technology

Change enabled by health informatics is empowering consumers to play a major role in managing their care; that is, patients are becoming consumers and co-producers of healthcare, sharing power and control with those who give care (Brown, Bopp, and Boren 2005; Berwick 2009). IT will continue to have an impact on how individuals communicate (e.g., through social media and through computing technology that enables information exchange). Administrative as well as clinical functions will be more unified, easing scheduling appointments, monitoring health status, accessing information from distributed knowledge bases, and integrating many health functions into health social networks. Health-specific information will be combined with personal data and communications systems.

The US government's goal of establishing a national health information system must be developed around the context of a consumer-driven system that is nimble, integrated (open), and based on information exchange of medical records and meaningful use by physicians. A study of access to and integration of medical services among wheelchair-bound individuals reveals that among this population's priority concerns are getting a retrofitted van, obtaining medical authorization for a driver's license and handicapped parking permit, and locating services accessible to people with disability (Schopp et al. 2004). These findings indicate that the patient-centered care orientation needs to shift from the clinical encounter as the unit of analysis to the integration of services provided in disparate but related domains. Again, IT enables this integration as well as the transfer or sharing of information across various sectors. This task is not technical but conceptual.

The question of whether individuals are patients or customers will be settled for health professionals and organizations in the future. Information and communications technology empower individuals as customers, and those who insist on treating them as patients subject to the logic of the traditional healthcare design are at a disadvantage. Organizations have an opportunity to lead change by moving beyond the personal health record (PHR) to an information and communications system that is consumer-centric and well integrated with other personal services and communications technologies. In other words, we should not build information systems based on an old logic and then later change them; rather, we should build them on a consumer-centric logic from the start and ensure that they are built to accommodate change.

Technologies that enable an integrated consumer-based system are wide-ranging, such as sensors for monitoring health conditions and health risks. Sensors have been tested in institutions to support "aging-in-place," allowing the elderly and home-bound patients to stay and be cared for in their homes rather than be sent to nursing homes (Reich, Zhao, and Shin 2002). Miniature, integrated data collection and monitoring devices empower individuals to access information and make decisions about health and medical care, recreation, transportation, finances, and other services. The processing power and speed of computer technology have increased exponentially, extending a user's capacity beyond personal computing to more sophisticated embedded technology and faster connectivity. Medical devices have become smaller but faster and more powerful, which then allows devices to be attached to or embedded in clothing, furniture, other appliances, and the human body in a way that they are less obtrusive but always available. In addition, these devices use network technologies, such as wireless computing, voice recognition, Internet capability, and artificial intelligence.

The development and use of miniature monitoring and data collection devices will change values and behaviors of individuals and bring new expectations and demands (opportunities) to healthcare institutions. Similar to Gladwell's (2000) concept of the power of context, the miniature information phenomenon will be the "little thing that makes a big difference" and soon create a "tipping point" that causes organizations to transition from clinician-centered to patient-centered to individual-centered services. Change will be slow at the start but will rapidly accelerate. Some will lead, others will follow, and those who cannot change will disappear.

Wellness, Prevention, and Community Health

Wellness and prevention have always made good sense from economic, social, and medical perspectives, although actually fostering healthy behaviors in individuals has been complex. Individuals are caught at the confluence of research-based, rational information and behaviors derived from the mass marketing of unhealthy (fast) foods and lifestyles. However, health behaviors are changing in some areas, as represented by smoking bans in public places, laws to wear seatbelts, better family and school nutrition, and (in some states) prohibition of driving and texting. Health status of a population reflects the nature and values of a community or society. In the past, hospitals (which were primarily nonprofit) contributed to their communities by providing the poor and uninsured with medical care and access to emergency services. Today, community orientation is broadly interpreted by institutions to mean decentralized clinics within neighborhoods, clinics in retail malls to improve access to medical services, clinics in schools to increase access to primary care, and even centralized medical pavilions to provide "convenient access" to physicians (e.g., see Community Health Network at www.ecommunity.com). Simply, community health has been defined as making medical services more accessible and convenient. The challenge to healthcare institutions to exercise greater accountability and transparency is encouraging and could increase organizations' commitment to wellness (AHA 2007).

Increasing access to medical care is important to community health, but better access alone does not address the essential elements of prevention, wellness, integration of services, and integration of human service information—all of which are value-added qualities in the consumer-driven market. The medical model focuses on curative services, and one could justifiably argue that medical centers should maintain focus on what they do best. However, we can also argue that these centers' value-added contributions to communities are not limited to clinical services; they also have organizational capacity to develop and integrate IT and support community-based personal health and social services. Hospitals and clinics should redefine their role in the community and move beyond traditional community service approaches, such as giving money to United Way Campaigns and Feeding America and volunteering at various local agencies. Such programs are positive and engender good public relations, but they do not bring high-value resources to institutions that need the help. Hospitals and clinics that are dedicated to expanding their community service role broaden their reach and strengthen their institutional identity and capacity. They may do this through providing the institution's technical and managerial expertise to community agencies and offering services external to the core medical function (Duke University 2012). Human services (provided to needy individuals and families) in most communities are categorical in nature and lack service integration and coordination, a structure similar to that of healthcare systems. Clinics and hospitals have the opportunity to invest their knowledge of IT and their organizational and management competencies to improve the human service agencies' infrastructure and help them provide wellness and preventive programs that are integrated with the institution's clinical services.

Applying IT to wellness, prevention, and community health enables communities and institutional leaders to reconceptualize systems to increase effectiveness and efficiency. They have to understand, first of all, that the health of a population is not dependent (solely or even primarily) on either medical care or traditional public health services. Nutrition, sanitation, water and food quality, and personal and environmental safety are traditional services of the public health system but are interdependent on housing, employment, transportation, education, law enforcement, and human rights. Health status depends on multiple interrelated services that are managed by social welfare, human services, and public health programs and agencies. As new human or medical conditions and needs are identified, the typical response is to establish programs or an agency dedicated to addressing the specific condition or need. The result is a myriad of different programs and agencies, each with its own eligibility criteria, processing forms, service networks, and staff. Navigating this matrix of agencies and services is very difficult, and most individuals and families are ill-equipped to do so.

The vertical and hierarchical structure of community services is similar to that of a typical healthcare organization, because both are designed from traditional assumptions. A community health service provider can be increased in size and scope of services, relocated, or housed in the same building, all of which might have some marginal impact on meeting needs but fail to address problems of coordination and integration and the conditions that led to these core problems. Integration and coordination are viewed merely as a consumer convenience, not as fundamental elements to delivering health and human services. Leaders of both the community health provider and the healthcare organization must realize that success must be defined from a systems perspective, not on the basis of the exemplary performance and outcomes of a single agency, program, or department. The coordination of health and human services is a health systems problem that cannot be solved within a given program, profession, or agency.

The literature on how a community collaboration should be structured and managed is extensive but shows a lack of consensus on the relationship between structure and performance (Lasker and Weiss 2003; Camarinha-Matos et al. 2009; Ell et al. 2011; Kirkman et al. 2011). Interest in studying collaborative models is increasing, and the results show an improved knowledge of how effective collaborations are structured and managed (Hovmand et al. 2012). Many studies conclude that collaborative arrangements do not work (White and Wehlage 1995), and some cite the reasons for this failure is that these collaboratives "get organized" by following traditional models of formal management and governance structures (Mitchell and Shortell 2000). Such a strategy simply creates a new and frequently more complex hierarchy with more rules and politics, which will likely conflict with the existing hierarchies and agency function. Such a structure compromises the concept of collaboration among a confederation of agencies. Among the many involved agencies, the medical center is likely to possess the greatest cache of knowledge and capacity for designing the structure of collaborative programs. It must guard against the temptation of trying to own or manage them directly.

Integrating services across independent organizations is a capacity already being developed by medical centers and can provide a significant value-added contribution to the community. An investment in coordinating human and social services is also consistent with (and, in fact, is the essence of) individual health, enlisting patients as co-producers of health and the design of the PHR. Such a strategy does not take medical institutions out of their core competency but builds on their essential core competency (in addition to clinical expertise) of structuring and managing virtual networks. Developing information networks to structure and coordinate disparate health and human services complements the clinical strategy of medical centers by creating and sustaining markets for clinical services. However, developing new clinical markets should not serve as the primary focus of strategy, as that distorts the overall enterprise strategy. Such a strategy requires new mental models and new analytics that are information based and that link the clinical to a broader health function, both within a new business model. Informatics thus becomes a new enterprise strategy and places medical centers in a major and meaningful way in the business of wellness, prevention, and community health (Brown, Stone, and Patrick 2005). The potential contribution of this value-added service is considerable, but the probability that it will be accomplished is small. New organizations will then arise, and traditional institutions will be marginalized.

Regionalization and Globalization

The concept of geographic space has historically been viewed from the perspective of physical space, related to distance and time. Early marketing concepts and principles were built around these assumptions. IT changes the assumptions about markets, potential competitors, and strategic partners. IT has facilitated the globalization of many commercial industries and will affect the major components of the healthcare system (such as IT and insurance vendors and the education of health and other professionals) and the way patients consume health services. Local hospitals and healthcare organizations will be the first transformed and become regionalized. Similarly, the global healthcare landscape will change as major medical centers in many regions demonstrate high clinical outcomes, accessibility, and patient satisfaction achieved at a lower cost. These factors are the ingredients of change.

Regionalized Systems

Regionalization, a concept that has been applied in the health system in the past 60 years, describes how organizations within a geographic area relate to each other in the market. The tradition of health systems is steeped in regionalization—from the Hill Burton Program in the 1950s to 1970s (see www .hrsa.gov/gethealthcare/affordable/hillburton), to the Regional Medical Programs in the 1960s (see http://profiles.nlm.nih.gov/ps/retrieve/Narrative/RM/p-nid/154), to the Comprehensive Health Planning programs of the 1960s and 1970s, to the integrated delivery systems of the past two decades. The concept of region as geographic space continues to frame the current policy debate on accountable care organizations.

Regionalization of health services is based on the logic of patient access to a full range of clinical services through referrals—upward to centralized specialty institutions and downward to distributed primary care. Referral patterns create a pyramid of clinical services, with few tertiary clinics and hospitals at the top supporting regional and small local clinics and hospitals. Although interdependent in the market, organizations have retained considerable independence in operations, ownership, and control. Procedures and consults are provided primarily on-site, making distance an important determinant of where patients go for care. Telemedicine programs allow the patient to be treated at a local facility for selective diseases by a specialist located in the centralized medical center. As markets became more competitively integrated, formalized structures (including mergers and acquisitions) became more prominent, linking hospitals and clinics vertically as a means of controlling the market and ensuring a steady flow of patients to sustain the specialized services.

In the information age, regionalization will increase but will be radically transformed. The new regionalization will be characterized by *knowledge work,* shared information systems that support professional staff interactions from which knowledge is extracted for the mutual benefit of all engaged, including patients and their families. Clinical decision support systems (CDSSs) become valued knowledge systems and serve as the corporate strategy for hospitals and clinics. Specialty clinics leverage knowledge across cyberspace (which is not geographically bounded and is available 24 hours a day) and become collaborating institutions that are not owned or managed by the regional center. Specialty services that are procedural (e.g., surgery, dialysis) will require the patient to be physically present at the center (although technology such as robotics will redefine physical presence), and cyberspace will continue to have a spatial dimension. Specialty centers are able to rapidly form collaborations with other centers to serve multiple regional systems. For example, Banner Health in Phoenix, Arizona, quickly positioned itself as a major regional provider of oncology services by collaborating with

MD Anderson Cancer Center in Houston, Texas, to form the Banner MD Anderson Cancer Center (see www.bannerhealth.com/Locations/Arizona/ Banner+MD+Anderson+Cancer+Center/About+Us/_About+Us.htm). Such collaborations bring the mission, culture, and knowledge of a major, highly regarded specialty center into the market of a large, regional general medical and surgical system. The two organizations jointly provide a range of specialty services but still maintain their own identities and core competencies.

Specialty, full-service medical centers are developing subspecialty institutes that conduct the clinical research in the specialty and embed clinical knowledge in decision support systems available to collaborating communities of practice. Patients and families who seek specialized procedures likely will select and travel to a regional center that has a reputation for providing high-quality care. At the same time, they will expect that this center has a continuum of care that is fully integrated with local primary care networks. In other words, consumers will select specialty centers on the basis of the value of both the clinical quality and the integrated network. Centers structured as such are knowledge systems. They have the capacity to integrate clinical services, clinical information, insurance claims, and other functions, making them to be of value and the basis of competitive strategy.

In the near future, such systems will not be monolithic, hierarchical, or geographically bounded. They will consist of an interdependent network of institutions that draw on their distinctive identities and core competencies and have the capacity, dedication, and culture to apply the best science to select, integrate, and coordinate services. If one organization becomes self-serving, it will be uncoupled from the network. The types of organization structures will vary depending on mission, market, financing system, and strategy. These structures will be enabled (and, in part, defined) but not initiated by or designed around IT. Such systems will be characterized by interdisciplinary leadership teams who are visionary; are risk taking; and build a strong culture that is committed, has integrity, and earns and gives respect. The current locus of corporate power will likely shift from relatively independent hospitals and systems to large but loosely structured integrated systems to better align organizations with the clinical enterprise, but the clinics themselves will be transformed (Enthoven and Tollen 2005; Quadagno 2010; Miller and Wechsler 2011). Prominent clinics are starting to demonstrate new information-enabled designs, which inform decisions; coordinate and integrate care; manage for consumers a seamless process for accessing clinical information, making appointments, and coordinating referrals inside and outside the system; and manage reimbursement functions. These systems will be large in size, capacity, and distributed markets—just like Mayo, Geisinger, Cleveland Clinic, MD Anderson, and Kaiser. As Sachs (2005, 3) states, the systems of the future will not be driven by the bricks-and-mortar operations but by their ability to move "petabyes of data to the right people at the right time."

Globalization

Globalization evokes images of great spatial distances and different cultures, customs, languages, and politics. IT has brought geographically dispersed people and institutions closer, transforming how financial, transportation, business, communication, politics, trade, and other commerce-related functions are conducted and how consumers are served. Social media, the Internet, and web-based technologies affect the politics, individual rights, and social fabric of the world's communities. Health systems across the globe are similarly influenced by this IT-enabled globalization.

The traditional perspective that all healthcare is local will be greatly countered with the argument that healthcare is global. Any notion that knowledge work in healthcare ends at or is limited by regional and national borders is an artifact of thinking within the framework of the physical world (p-world) instead of the information/electronic world (e-world). For clinics and hospitals in many countries, including many in the United States, "region" has international or global context. Scientific knowledge embedded in CDSSs can be generalized, adapted, and easily moved to other populations—beyond national boundaries. Health problems across populations differ considerably, and cultural, religious, and other preferences regarding treatment must be taken into account. Such features already exist or can be developed in CDSSs. Knowledge systems that link organizations can be adapted to fit local cultures, organizational control, and work styles (Magnier-Watanabe, Benton, and Senoo 2011). Other regional strategies pursued by prestigious clinics include establishing centers in other countries supported by the focal organization's reputation, brand name, clinical knowledge, and information capacity. Health systems in many countries are developing privatized insurance, clinics, and hospitals, in part because of limited public funding and the growth of the middle class, which has higher expectations from the healthcare and human service sectors. One of the strengths of traditional American healthcare organizations is that they can support sophisticated technology and deliver high-quality technical services, but that strength might be undermined by their inability to respond to changing values and markets. Health centers in other countries may more easily adapt to or develop around modern and innovative models, which exposes the limitations of the US healthcare system. This does not suggest that foreign-based health centers will establish deep markets in the United States, but their acceptance of new care models and demonstrations that these models are effective could bring disruptive innovations to American healthcare.

The direct provision of healthcare services in the global market will have a winnowing effect on clinics and hospitals that have strong regional facilities in the United States but limited reach internationally. For example, medical tourism, which used to be a windfall for US-based specialty systems, is starting to share the global market with centers of excellence in Dubai, India, Thailand, and Singapore. Local systems in the United States might pursue a limited global strategy by partnering with major international specialty systems that provide referrals and by managing the continuity of care in local acute and minimal care facilities. Continuity of care includes both clinical care and coordination of transportation, accommodations, financing, and personal health information. Depending on the nature of the illness, accommodations might include personalized trips or cultural events. The reality is that in the transformed global healthcare system, services will remain local but will be provided by local organizations that are integrated and have international reach.

New Business Models

Business models will consist of knowledge-based services from established and new organizations within and outside the healthcare system. In the e-world, many of the healthcare delivery innovations will likely originate outside of the industry or at least outside hospitals and clinics. In this section, we discuss new business models created as a result of consumers' knowledge demands and new knowledge assets in the industry. Predicting who the new entrants might be or how they will contribute is difficult, although some notable trends have emerged that serve as our basis.

Cloud Computing

Cloud computing, a representation of the systems concept, is a means of unifying health information across clinicians and organizations and integrating it with consumer services to make the information truly consumer based. Cloud computing providers offer to individuals or corporations high-capacity networks, which include private storage capacity, shared capacity (federated or community clouds), public clouds (open access) application software, and computing capacity. Security and privacy issues, which are discussed in Chapter 13, are compounded by cloud computing.

The core functions of IT in an organization are to store, retrieve, integrate, analyze, transmit, and make available data and information. The traditional health system is characterized by a culture of distinctiveness and separation, owing to the highly professionalized nature of clinical services and the intimacy of the clinician–patient relationship. This individual-centric system is often viewed as being patient centered, which justifies the bias toward the clinician and the organization that although flexible (allows variation) is disaggregated. In the information age, however, the concept of patient centeredness is broader, with services that are fully integrated, accessible, and enabled by IT and with patients as co-producers of care. Even the current mandate to developing an integrated, national health information infrastructure presupposes that the healthcare organization has its own information system (which supports the traditional perspective). The concepts of uniqueness and separation violate the important knowledge-based principles of integration, accessibility, and leverage (Giniat 2011).

In the information age, clinicians, healthcare organizations, and IT vendors do not have the option of protecting their markets by treating health information and information systems as closed and proprietary. In a consumer-driven world, individuals choose to communicate on web-based integrated platforms. One such platform is cloud computing, which has been applied to healthcare purposes, such as the Microsoft Health Vault (see www.microsoft.com/en-us/healthvault/). Because of the risk of privacy and security violations, cloud computing environments might not be suitable for highly sensitive patient information, which is protected by the Health Insurance Portability and Accountability Act (HIPAA). This has led to the development of the more restrictive hCloud technology, which can still interface with other cloud applications. The announcement by Dell of its collaboration with Microsoft to provide secure information sharing for physicians and hospitals is a measure of the potential of this disruptive technology (Business Wire 2011).

The short tenure of Google Health, another cloud-based healthcare-interface platform, might reflect people's continued reluctance to manage their personal health and wellness, a possible latent and tacit response to the traditional mind-set that clinicians and healthcare organizations are in charge of the provision of care. As discussed in Chapter 8, another factor that may give individuals pause in using cloud computing and other web-based tools is the degree of difficulty of entering data, managing access, navigating the site, and so on. Clunky systems will be refined in the future. If the healthcare system as a whole shifts risks and costs to consumers, interest in wellness, prevention, and self-management will likely increase. The now-defunct Google Health represents the unpredictable nature of technological innovation in healthcare, but most importantly it identified the management of personal health information as a new business opportunity. However, the cloud is a significant strategic technology and is highly likely to be a disruptive technology (Sinnett 2012).

Medical Banking

Like clinical services, healthcare financing has suffered from a lack of common nomenclature that standardizes health plan enrollment, eligibility, benefits, claims and reporting, and payment structure. The wide differences have been perpetuated by the insurance industry as a competitive strategy. The federal government strongly encourages the health insurance industry to shift from paper to electronic and to set forth standards for electronic transactions. Managing reimbursement and the revenue process has been complex and costly (in terms of processing claims and days in accounts receivable) for hospitals, healthcare systems, clinics, and individual practitioners and has been a source of considerable confusion and frustration for patients and families.

The establishment of standard nomenclature and the transition of information to digital format present an opportunity to address another major issue in financing: the lack of connectivity among healthcare providers, patients, and payers. This connectivity will likely improve the financial function and align it with the clinical function. Such change is transformational but disruptive to the current business and clinical functions, and the pitfall of merely automating the system is always present. New business models will usher in this transformation.

In the past few years, medical banking has entered the market. It is an electronic system for processing and managing financial transactions, including billing and collections, making payments, accounts reconciliation, and investing account balances. The goal of medical banking is to integrate financial transactions with information on the patient's condition and treatment outcomes and to verify that billed procedures were satisfactorily completed and the billing and receivables transactions were managed. Banks bring considerable potential value to the healthcare system in that they can integrate financial information, manage collections, and provide customers a portal for managing transactions (Casillas 2009).

Medical banks may take over the control of claims processing and reconciliation from hospitals, clinics, and insurance companies on behalf of patients (see www.mbproject.org). This shift is consistent with the movement to consumer-oriented healthcare, and finance will facilitate this reorientation. Part of a patient's PHR will include health-insurance benefit status, claims processing, and reconciliation, and payments for services are linked with information on whether the service was delivered as well as the cost and quality of the service. Patients will have access to alternative service providers, cost structures, and quality measures. The business and clinical functions will become more formally linked, and that will transfer control to the consumer who has information to manage the care and finance processes.

Medical banks, which are customer service oriented, may become the portal for patients to access their PHR (Parente 2009). The banking industry will now be involved in managing transactions on behalf of patients and family to whom they are accountable. Revenue cycle management will shift substantially from hospitals and clinics to medical banks. Accounts receivable might be reduced from weeks to days. Banks will also be well positioned to receive, manage, and distribute funds from medical savings accounts (which might dramatically increase if Medicare and Medicaid beneficiaries become eligible for private medical savings accounts). Medical savings accounts enable an individual to invest her health insurance reserves in a range of different financial products, such as bonds or money market accounts (Parente 2009). Finally, medical banking will link payment and clinical services to the global healthcare network.

Analytics and Other Value-Added Services

Healthcare boundaries will become less distinct. Businesses not previously directly involved in delivering medical services (such as suppliers, financial institutions, and insurance brokers that perform risk analysis) are analyzing and extracting value from big data and will approach the industry to offer value-added services. Many of these services have been around for a long time, and some have been adopted, but mostly health systems have given lip service to them or have tried and failed to make changes (see Chapter 1). However, the industry is now in an information- and knowledge-based era, and now is the time to adopt these analytics-supported services.

Pharmaceutical

The pharmaceutical industry can make a value-added contribution by providing analytic tools to patients, especially those who are noncompliant and nonadherent to their prescriptions. Drug information can be embedded in the PHR with medication alerts and reminders to patients. Changing adherence and noncompliance can positively affect patient health and can offset costs for health plans and pharmacy benefit managers. In addition, pharmaceutical companies are exploring value-based contracting, where the companies assume the risk for effectively managing disease protocols, including medications. Under this model, the firms would become not only developers and sellers of medications but also managers of drug regimens for both chronic care and prevention purposes. Pharmaceutical companies that do not offer such value-added services might become disadvantaged in the market. All firms involved in health and wellness must consider and, in many instances, develop patient-oriented models and explore new ways of adding value to clinical quality and efficiency. The greatest challenge to the pharmaceutical industry is the relentless marketing of prescription and nonprescription drugs whose claims exceed the evidence.

Enterprise Risk

As more healthcare organizations develop regional and global strategies and new service delivery models, they will be exposed to new types of and possibly greater risks. Corporate officers might sense a need to innovate more and develop new strategies but not understand the culture or the fact that the enterprise's risk exposure must stay close to its risk tolerance (Shaw 2005). Historically, risk in healthcare organizations has been managed within functional silos. For example, health and retirement risk is managed by human resources, liability risk is managed by the legal department, and revenue cycle risk is managed by finance; intellectual property and strategic risks are implicit but vaguely understood and thus not quantified. In addition, innovative enterprises must consider the risks in these and many other areas:

- Information security
- Collaborative arrangements (in both domestic and global markets)
- Knowledge embedded in proprietary clinical decision support tools
- Loss of key knowledge workers
- Equipment failure

Future risks might include health risk of population (when or if capitation-based financing, or bundling, increases) and new forms of business risk. For an enterprise that is implementing or considering a global strategy (such as destination medical centers and medical center collaboration), risk exposures are numerous, varied, and significant.

Enterprise risk assessment and management is complex and dynamic and requires the use of large databases and sophisticated analytics. It is not an area that medical, insurance, or legal firms have sufficient capacity and presence to manage. However, risk management corporations and insurance brokerages are abundant and use complex analytical models that can examine world health systems and global health (see, for example, www.aon.com). One study indicates that the first reason that healthcare organizations do not engage in enterprise risk management is the lack of analytical tools (Zolkos 2000). The second reason cited is organizational turf mentality. Few studies of enterprise risk have been done that include all elements of risk in hospitals and health systems. The health insurance sector is the one area in healthcare that has deployed sophisticated risk management tools but includes only the health risks of enrolled populations and has a vested interest in the outcomes of the models (Violino 2009). As repeated throughout this book, healthcare organizations must develop an enterprise perspective and abandon their silo mentality.

Core Competencies in Clinical, Management, and Informatics Education

Educational preparation of health professionals must be changed to include core content in systems theory, change management, systems engineering, informatics, and relationship-centered care. This recommendation is not new; it was proposed by several clinical, informatics, and policy leaders in the Pew Health Professions Commission reports published in the 1990s (see O'Neil and the Pew Health Professions Commission 1998). Furthermore, the *Health Professions Education and Relationship-Centered Care* provides the following justification for relationship-centered care (Tresolini and the Pew-Fetzer Task Force 1994, 25):

> Within a community of practitioners, members must be able to interpret one another's work, resolve conflicts related to the care of the patient, allow responsibilities and leadership to shift as the patient's needs change, and provide support for one another.

Thinking that relationship-centered care can be effectively carried out within an environment characterized by institutional, financial, professional, cultural, and regulatory barriers is unrealistic. Change must extend beyond building communications skills of students in the health professions. They must undergo training programs on how to build relationship-centered teams as they work up clinical cases. Health professionals must understand the impediments to relationship-centered caregiving and must have both the knowledge and commitment to effect changes.

In the healthcare practice, education that is science based, relationship centered, and knowledge and systems oriented frequently gets translated into platitudes about patient-centered care, interdisciplinary teams, evidence-based practice, and quality improvement that are not supported by the science of how complex systems are analyzed, structured, and changed (Greiner and Knebel 2003). Change typically focuses on restructuring the existing clinical training models, such as clerkships, apprenticeships, or shortened core rotations, but such models are themselves isolated and restrictive (Cooke et al. 2006). Leaders in biomedical informatics, meanwhile, have proposed to broaden the science to include many of the competencies in systems and process design, management, and organization behavior (Staggers, Gassert, and Skiba 2000). However, little progress in this respect has been made by most health professional training programs, and the prospects are not hopeful as the field moves further toward professionalization through accreditation and education based on clinical competency. The BISTI Report (see Chapter 1) on competencies in biomedical informatics should be expanded to add competencies from health informatics.

How health informatics content is structured and taught will vary, but it should be conceived as a set of competencies rather than as a separate profession or belonging to the biomedical informatics profession. As an academic program, health informatics might be better structured as a multidisciplinary science taught by an interdisciplinary team of doctoral-trained faculty members who maintain competency in their own disciplines but engage primarily in interdisciplinary research. This is difficult to design and maintain in universities, where resources are limited and power and control reside in the core disciplines.

Curriculum change can be implemented in various health professions programs. Specifically, health informatics courses should be taught by the core faculty in disciplines such as biostatistics, computer and information science, systems engineering, organization behavior and theory, and so on. Members of the faculty should be prepared at the doctoral level of their core disciplines and should maintain competency in and contribute to their core's body of science through publishing peer-reviewed articles and engaging in collaborative health informatics research. Courses should draw on the latest and best science from these core disciplines, and this science should not be diluted and taught separately from the clinical sciences.

Each health professional would need not only to adapt the science in other disciplines to his clinical core knowledge but also train to work in multiprofessional teams to develop his skills in communications and collaborative decision making. The traditional approach of training professionals in isolation might be sustainable in entrenched university programs but is not defensible. Degree programs should find an important market filled with clinically trained individuals who want to develop sufficient depth and competency in a specialized area in order to enter and advance in a clinical, informatics, or management profession. In some instances, achieving specialized competency might require earning a dual degree. The best science in all disciplines and professions must be engaged to solve the most complex problems in society.

Conclusion

This chapter discusses the multiple areas that need and might undergo transformational change in the information age. It demonstrates that the traditional independence of the clinical and business functions in healthcare organizations is fallacious. In the near future, health and wellness services will be provided by professionals who work in complex organizations that leverage IT to structure, manage, and collaborate and who will be held accountable for outcomes and processes. The increased availability of large databases will spawn new products and business models that bring or add value to current service offerings.

Chapter Discussion Questions

1. Differentiate between horizontally and vertically integrated health systems and describe how IT might change regional strategies.
2. What is the relationship between the market for services and freedom of choice, minimal delays, integration of services, and patient involvement? How might electronic linkages among or between healthcare organizations affect markets?
3. How might medical banking change the way healthcare institutions, insurance firms, and patients process, manage, and control healthcare finances?
4. How will IT change the role of the patient?
5. What competencies will be needed by informatics professionals to engage in leading change?
6. How has IT changed the concept of patient-centered information from individual, disaggregated information to integrated cloud computing?

CASE STUDY | **Medical Banking: The Next Frontier of Health Information Technology and Financing**

Gordon D. Brown

The Past

Mid-Atlantic Health System comprises a medical center and 12 primary care and specialty clinics and serves as a major referral site in its region. It considers itself a leader in IT development, having just upgraded its electronic medical record (EMR) to include computerized physician order entry (CPOE) and adopted the use of clinical guidelines in most clinical areas. Mid-Atlantic is facing the challenge of developing an IT architecture that links the medical center's EMR with the EMRs of local physician practices and other hospitals in the region. Installing such an integrated architecture is difficult, not from a technical perspective but from an economic and behavioral perspective.

For small clinics and hospitals, the cost of implementing an EMR is steep, especially with the interface properties needed to run the EMR. From a behavioral perspective, hospital-based physicians and management find it difficult to support an IT investment, which they may perceive to contribute or add limited value to the work performed at Mid-Atlantic.

They may view the US mandate for IT interconnectivity as another form of regulation that does not serve the local community well.

The medical community in the region consists primarily of physicians who practice in or run small offices with shared space and administrative staff. All of these clinics, including those owned by Mid-Atlantic, manage their finances alongside their other administrative responsibilities. Financial management, which is the most complex administrative function, consists of coding, billing, reconciliation of changes, accounts payable, and collections (which constitute the revenue cycle). Despite this complexity, much of management's and staff's time is taken up by developing the clinical IT system. As a result, administrative costs are rapidly increasing, much to the chagrin of the physicians who are paid on the basis of their clinic's net income.

The Future

Mid-Atlantic's chief financial officer, Joe Sanford, attends a roundtable conference on medical banking and learns strategies on how the EMR might be used to better manage the revenue cycle (*Healthcare Financial Management* 2007). Currently, Mid-Atlantic uses a claims processing software for managing the revenue cycle, including the reconciliation process. Joe thinks that collaborating with a bank to institute a medical lockbox would enable remittances from insurance companies to go directly to the bank. This, in turn, would reduce the delay in deposits by at least a day and increase Mid-Atlantic's cash position. He understands that direct payments from patients who send checks by mail and from walk-ins as well as payments from the state Medicaid office (which does not have an electronic capability to transmit payment) would be hand processed by the accounting department. An optical character recognition (OCR) scanner would increase the processing efficiency because staff would not have to key in the data.

Joe approaches Jackie Green, a senior vice president of the local bank, to discuss the possibility of a medical lockbox. Jackie emphasizes that the core competency of the bank is to manage and account for financial transactions across a range of industries. She explains that the electronic age has brought about a considerable, worldwide integration of financing and investment functions. This integration transcends currencies and industries and is consumer focused, which means not

(continued)

merely having friendly and knowledgeable banking personnel but also (perhaps most important) offering services and value tailored to the needs, wants, and goals of the customer. She addresses the need for the healthcare system to fully adopt this customer perspective and argues that integrating clinical information is only a rudimentary start. With medical banking, health insurance companies can provide incentives and rewards for healthy behaviors and for the efficient use of healthcare services. It also provides the incentives of capitation financing but based on individual choice. According to Jackie, Mid-Atlantic's process of accessing and managing financial transactions is institution centric. Medical records and payment systems that have been automated are still designed according to the logic of the clinical practice and not the patient as consumer. She also points out that retirement plans and health insurance are based on the concept of defined contribution, which gives rise to medical savings accounts (including Medicare). This, in her mind, further justifies a healthcare organization's use of a financial institution to manage investment accounts.

Jackie recommends that Mid-Atlantic allow the integration of financial function with the medical lockbox and give the bank the responsibility for all financial transactions (including insurance and other payments and investments) and thus serve as the critical link for patients who manage their own PHR. Specifically, the bank would receive payments in any form (including paper), process payments immediately, perform the accounting function, and serve as a data warehouse. Data would be mined to better understand insurance payment plans and the relationship between the financial and clinical functions. The bank uses advanced OCR equipment, which is costly but is part of banking functions.

Joe is impressed with Jackie's presentation and arguments. She is knowledgeable about the reconciliation process and has some insights about the healthcare industry, and she challenges Joe to think beyond banks' traditional role. He knows that Mid-Atlantic on its own cannot conceptualize such a future, let alone develop the institutional capacity to support it.

The Present

Although Joe is convinced that Jackie did her homework, he knows she has limited understanding of healthcare financing and the operational difficulties of managing it. Reconciliation of claims alone is a complicated process, because the benefit structure of claims is different for each insurance carrier and supplemental payments and contractual adjustments vary. In addition, the claims processing system of insurance companies and payers uses either electronic or paper format or a combination of the two. In other words, there is no standardization, which is opposite to how banking services function.

Mid-Atlantic has launched a major patient satisfaction initiative, and has asked all departments to submit innovative ideas on how to better serve patients and their families. Joe believes that installing a friendly cashier's office that gladly provides various personal-finance services and answers questions about charges or fees and related concerns would go a long way toward improving customer satisfaction. Patients and their families want face-to-face interaction and a welcoming staff to help them deal with their issues. The cashier's office would depend on the accounting office to provide explanations of benefits (EOBs), which vary by insurance carrier. Accounting has the responsibility of converting EOB formats into standardized HIPAA-compliant 835 forms. A major concern Joe has about medical banking is its ability to abide by HIPAA regulations for privacy and security. He does not want Mid-Atlantic's finance function to be solely dependent on the bank to meet HIPAA requirements.

Joe acknowledges Jackie's summation that the EMR/EHR design, investment, and assessment are based primarily on the logic of the clinical function. However, as Jackie emphasized, the IT architecture for the PHR should be patient oriented, and the banking industry has learned and mastered this design. Making clinical quality the basis for value-based reimbursement would increase demands on coding and reconciliation, but these demands could extend far beyond the reimbursement function. Joe remembers the days when IT operated under the finance department, and losing that function decreased the size of his staff by 30 percent. He is not interested in further reducing the staff or the department's responsibility by outsourcing financial services to the bank. A medical lockbox, however, seems to be the most solid strategy.

Case Study Discussion Questions

1. Who is the community that Mid-Atlantic serves and government regulations (like HIPAA) protect?
2. Critically assess Joe's plan to improve patient satisfaction in the future through better financial services.

(continued)

3. In what ways has the banking industry become customer oriented? Contrast this with the orientation in the healthcare industry.

4. Make a case for the importance of patient-centered care in the future. How might medical banking facilitate this process by providing incentives to patients to maintain their health and use health services efficiently? Can you envision other or alternative effective solutions?

5. Differentiate the clinical logic vs. the patient-centered logic basis of IT architecture and the financial programs that support them.

GLOSSARY

Accountable care organization (ACO): A designation that offers financial incentives to institutions that provide quality, safe, and effective care to Medicare and Medicaid beneficiaries while keeping down operational costs.

Agent-based (AB) modeling: Used to study the behavior of systems on the basis of the interactions between agents or entities.

American Health Information Management Association (AHIMA): An association of health information management professionals whose areas of interest include procedural coding and data standards in a national and global environment.

Application silo architecture: IT architecture that comprises individual applications rather than represents the whole enterprise.

Big data: Large databases, which in healthcare contain considerable information on behaviors; individuals; or small population sectors, such as a physician's panel of patients or a subpanel made up of a specific meaningful pattern of individuals.

Bioinformatics: Discipline that combines the biological sciences (microbiology, biochemistry, physiology, and genetics) with computational fields (such as statistics and computer science).

Certification Commission for Health Information Technology (CCHIT): Organization that issues Complete EHR certification to systems that meet all of the current criteria adopted by the secretary of the US Department of Health and Human Services and EHR Modules certification to systems that meet one or more (but not all) of these criteria.

Clinical decision support system (CDSS): Computer software that presents users with a knowledge base, patient-specific data, and related information at the point of care to enhance healthcare provision and management.

Clinical guidelines: Evidence-based clinical information that guides clinicians during clinical encounters; also used to represent alerts and reminders embedded within the EMR.

Clinical protocols: Evidence-based clinical information that informs clinicians in a clinical process, as opposed to a clinical encounter; similar to critical pathways, a concept developed in industrial engineering.

Communication mechanism or interface: Part of the CDSS that allows decision makers to see the computational results and that supports input through direct or indirect methods.

Community of practice: A clinical team that is structured and that functions around the needs of the patient and thus transcends individual clinicians, organizations, or systems.

Complex adaptive system: Organization with a large number of interdependent parts or agents that have their own schemata (pattern relationships), present interaction complexity, and are self-organizing but can adapt to their environments and help create those environments (coevolution).

Computerized physician-order entry (CPOE): A software system that enables a clinician to enter an order for patient treatment.

Consumer health informatics: Area of health informatics that focuses on the implementation and evaluation of system design to ensure that it interacts directly with the consumer, with or without the involvement of healthcare providers.

Controlled vocabulary (concept-based controlled biomedical vocabulary): A set of multiword terms and relationships purposely selected to express thematically related concepts and the associations among them; also known as *standardized terminology*.

Current procedural terminology (CPT): Standard codes of clinical procedures developed by the American Medical Association for the purpose of insurance reimbursement for care provided by hospitals, clinics, and other providers.

Data envelopment analysis (DEA): Technique for evaluating organizational performance, identifying exogenous and endogenous forces that affect that performance, and monitoring performance changes over time.

Data mining: Use of sophisticated search capabilities and analytical techniques on large databases to discover patterns, correlations, and trends that can be leveraged to produce knowledge.

Discrete event (DE) modeling: Used primarily to study processes, streamline them, and reduce bottlenecks through better resource allocation, capacity utilization or standardization, and mechanization of routine processes.

Dynamic capability: An organization's ability to integrate, build, and reconfigure internal and external competencies to address rapidly changing environments.

E-health: Use of telecommunication platforms, mobile and ubiquitous hardware and software, and advanced information systems to support and facilitate healthcare delivery and education.

Electronic health record (EHR): Based on the EMR and includes documentation of the clinical workflow and provides alerts, reminders, therapy plans, and medication orders.

Electronic medical record (EMR): An individual's electronic clinical information created, integrated, managed, and accessed by authorized clinicians, nurses, coders, and other health professionals within a healthcare organization.

Electronic personal health record (e-PHR): An individual's digital medical record that conforms to nationally recognized interoperability standards and is managed, shared, and controlled by the individual (patient); also known simply as PHR.

Fair information practices (FIPs): The foundation of information security and privacy law and regulations in the United States and throughout the world, FIPs constitute fair and responsible information stewardship, which is essential to establishing and maintaining public trust when collecting, using, disclosing, and sharing personal information.

Free text: Method of entering and reporting data and information into the CDSS using natural language; also known as *unstructured data*.

Genetic medicine: Practice in which clinical decisions are made on the basis of information about a single gene.

Health informatics: The application of multidisciplinary sciences to transform (not just automate) the structure and behavior of health-related systems, organizations, and individuals (including patients, professionals, and support personnel) who interact to provide personalized care. This systems concept draws on biological, clinical, engineering, social, and behavioral sciences.

Health information exchange (HIE): A framework that enables the movement of patient health data and information across organizations that are geographically dispersed by using nationally recognized standards.

Health Insurance Portability and Accountability Act of 1996 (HIPAA): Established by the US Department of Health and Human Services, HIPAA sets the standards for privacy of individually identifiable health information (or "Privacy Rule").

Inference engine: Part of the CDSS that combines rules from the knowledge base with patient-specific information to draw conclusions or recommend actions.

Informatics: The study of linguistics applied broadly to scientific language. Informatics applies the study of morphology (the formation and composition of words) and syntax (the rules that determine how words combine into meaning) to analyze biological and clinical databases. As such, informatics combines basic and clinical sciences with computational science, particularly computer science. The concept has expanded to include modeling of enterprise decision processes.

Information architecture: Framework of information system that takes the perspective of IT as a contributor to enterprise strategy; different from *information infrastructure*.

Information infrastructure: Set of properties of an information system viewed from the perspective of the IT function (department) and includes technology standards and the relationship between IT and business and clinical operations.

International Classification of Diseases (ICD): A common vocabulary developed by the International Statistical Congress in 1853 and maintained by the World Health Organization. It classifies diseases and causes of death to enable countries to establish surveillance programs.

Knowledge-based CDSS: Loaded with and offers recommendations from a large body of expert and science-based information.

Knowledge management: Concept that "promotes an integrated approach to identifying, managing, and sharing all of an enterprise's information needs" (Lee 2000).

Locally preferred synonym: Expression of a concept that is commonly used in a particular healthcare practice environment.

Meaningful use: Concept generated by Public Law 111-148 (Patient Protection and Affordable Care Act) as a measure of the level of application of information technology in clinical decision support.

Medical informatics: The discipline that deals with the structure and properties of clinical information generated from clinical trials and medical records; generally includes imaging informatics and clinical informatics.

Medical knowledge base: Systematically organized collection of medical knowledge that is accessible electronically and interpretable by computer.

Metadata: Data about data and information.

Metadata schema: Collection of fields or data elements, names for the fields, definitions for the fields, and specifications of what constitute permissible values for the fields; also known as *data dictionary*.

Modeling: Method of studying, understanding, and then replicating the complexities of the real world in order to design, change, and improve information systems.

Modular architecture: Enterprisewide IT architecture with loosely coupled applications, data, and technology components that preserve global standards while enabling local differences.

Non–knowledge-based CDSS: Developed from the learning or experiential knowledge of clinical decision makers and builds patterns out of this learning to make recommendations.

Organized environment: Formal organization with structure, purpose, and integrated functions.

Pharmacogenomics: Analysis and application of emerging knowledge about genetic influences on drug metabolism.

Postcoordinated concept: An expression that combines precoordinated concepts and semantic relationships.

Precoordinated concepts: Basis of the vocabulary and are the building blocks of more complicated expressions of meaning.

Privacy: In the healthcare information context, assurance that one's health information is collected, accessed, used, retained, and shared only when necessary and only to the extent necessary and that the information is protected throughout its life cycle using fair privacy practices consistent with applicable laws and regulations and the preferences of the individual.

Production rule: Conditional statement used in CDSS that has the general form "IF some condition is true, THEN the following inference can be made or action taken."

Rationalized data architecture: Enterprisewide IT architecture that includes standardization of data and processes.

Risk: Probability that a threat will exploit a vulnerability to damage, destroy, or harm a valued asset.

Security: Protection of the confidentiality of private, sensitive, and safety-critical information; the integrity of health data and metadata; and the availability of information and services through measures that authenticate user and system identity and data provenance and that maintains an accounting of actions taken by users, software programs, and systems.

Standardized technology architecture: Enterprisewide IT architecture that provides efficiencies through technology standardization and, in most cases, centralization.

System documentation problem: Lack of documentation of the features, changes, or activities related to the information system.

System drift problem: Changes to a science-based recommendation as a result of the seemingly minor adjustments to the content and expression of the original evidence when it is implemented in the local environment.

System dynamics (SD) modeling: Used to model complex nonlinear relationships between components and to study the dynamics of the system over time.

Translational research: Translation of healthcare evidence into healthcare practice.

Trust: In the healthcare context, evidence-based confidence that the people, organizations, information and data, and information systems involved in healthcare delivery are what they claim to be and behave as expected.

Value measurement methodology (VMM): Developed by the Federal Chief Information Officers Council, VMM is a framework and a toolkit for estimating values, costs, risks, and tangible and intangible returns of a given IT investment.

Vocabulary mapping: A scheme for matching concept expressions among controlled vocabularies by meaning.

Vocabulary problem: The clash of opposing forces of control and decentralization, or the basic problem of maintaining control of a scheme for expressing concepts and the need to support integration and interoperability of information.

REFERENCES

AAPHelp. 2011. "Education and Decision Support for Junior Doctors." *AAPHelp.* Accessed January 1. www.aaphelp.leeds.ac.uk/aaphelp/background.asp.

Ackerson, L. K., and K. Viswanath. 2009. "The Social Context of Interpersonal Communication and Health." *Journal of Health Communication* 14 (1 Suppl): 5–17.

Ackoff, R. L., J. Magidson, and H. J. Addison. 2006. *Idealized Design: Creating an Organization's Future.* Upper Saddle River, NJ: Wharton School Publication.

Adams, S. A. 2010. "Revisiting the Online Health Information Reliability Debate in the Wake of 'Web 2.0': An Inter-Disciplinary Literature and Website Review." *International Journal of Medical Informatics* 79 (6): 391–400.

Adler-Milstein, J., J. Landefeld, and A. C. Jha. 2010. "Characteristics Associated with Regional Health Information Organization Viability." *Journal of the American Medical Informatics Association* 17 (1): 61–65.

Agency for Healthcare Research and Quality (AHRQ). 2012. *National Guideline Clearinghouse.* Accessed March 16. www.guideline.gov.

———. 2011. *United States Health Information Knowledgebase.* Accessed June 7. http://ushik.ahrq.gov.

Ahuja, M. K., and J. E. Galvin. 2003. "Socialization in Virtual Groups." *Journal of Management* 29 (2): 161–85.

Alomaim, N., M. Sihini Tunca, and M. Zairi. 2003. "Customer Satisfaction @ Virtual Organizations." *Management Decision* 41 (7): 666–70.

Alonso-Coello, P., A. Irfan, I. Sola, I. Gich, M. Delgado-Noguera, and D. Rigau. 2010. "The Quality of Clinical Practice Guidelines Over the Last Two Decades: A Systematic Review of Guideline Appraisal Studies." *Quality and Safety in Health Care* 19 (6): 1–7.

American Board of Medical Specialties. 2011. "How Specialists Stay Current in Their Knowledge and Skills." *Maintenance of Certification: Ten Years Strong and Growing,* 42. Chicago: American Board of Medical Specialties.

American Hospital Association (AHA). 2007. "Community Accountability and Transparency." Accessed March 1, 2012. www.aha.org/aha/content/2007/pdf/07nov-communityaccountability.pdf.

American Medical Association. 2011. *Current Procedural Terminology (CPT).* Chicago: American Medical Association.

American Nurses Association (ANA). 2012. "Florence Nightingale Pledge." *American Nurses Association*. Accessed March 16. www.nursingworld.org/FunctionalMenuCategories/AboutANA/WhereWeComeFrom/FlorenceNightingalePledge.aspx.

———. 2010. *ANA Recognized Terminologies That Support Nursing Practice*. Accessed June 6, 2011. www.nursingworld.org/MainMenuCategories/ThePracticeofProfessionalNursing/NursingStandards/Recognized-Nursing-Practice-Terminologies.aspx.

Ancker, J., K. Carpenter, P. Greene, R. Hoffman, R. Kukafka, L. Marlow, H. Prigerson, and J. Quillin. 2009. "Peer-to-Peer Communication, Cancer Prevention, and the Internet." *Journal of Health Communication* 14 (1): 38–46.

Anderson, C., T. Brock, I. Bates, M. Rouse, J. Marriott, and H. Manasse. 2011. "Transforming Health Professional Education." *American Journal of Pharmaceutical Education* 75 (2): 1.

Arndt, M., and B. Bigelow. 2000. "Presenting Structural Innovation in an Institutional Environment: Hospitals Use of Impression Management." *Administrative Science Quarterly* 45 (3): 494–552.

Audet, A. J., M. Doty, J. Shamasdin, and S. Schoenbaum. 2005. "Measure, Learn, and Improve: Physicians' Involvement in Quality Improvement." *Health Affairs* 24 (3): 843–53.

Avery, S. L., and P. M. Swafford. 2009. "Social Capital Impact on Service Supply Chains." *Journal of Service Science* 2 (2): 9.

Axelrod, R. C., and D. Vogel. 2003. "Predictive Modeling in Health Plans." *Disease Management and Health Outcomes* 11 (12): 779–87.

Bacigalupe, G. 2011. "Is There a Role for Social Technologies in Collaborative Healthcare?" *Families, Systems, and Health* 29 (1): 1–14.

Baker, A. M., J. E. Lafata, R. E. Ward, F. Whitehouse, and G. Divine. 2001. "A Web-based Diabetes Care Management Support System." *The Joint Commission Journal on Quality Improvement* 27 (4): 179–90.

Bakken, S., S. Hyun, C. Friedman, and S. Johnson. 2004. "A Comparison of Semantic Categories of the ISO Reference Terminology Models for Nursing and the MedLEE Natural Language Processing System." *Studies in Health Technology and Informatics* 107 (Pt 1): 472–76.

Balas, A. E., S. M. Austin, J. A. Mitchell, B. G. Ewigman, K. D. Bopp, and G. D. Brown. 1996. "The Clinical Value of Computerized Information Services." *Archives of Family Medicine* 5 (5): 271–78.

Balas, E. A., and S. A. Boren. 2000. "Managing Critical Knowledge for Health Care Improvement." In *Yearbook of Medical Informatics 2000: Patient-Centered System*s, 65–70. Stuttgart, Germany: Schattauer.

Banaszak-Holl, J., L. T. Nembhard, and E. H. Bradley. 2012. "Leadership and Management: A Framework for Action." In *Health Care Management*, by R. Burns, E. Bradley, and B. Weiner, 33–62. Albany, NY: Delmar.

Barnett, G. O., J. J. Cimino, J. A. Hupp, and E. P. Hoffer. 1987. "DXplain. An Evolving Diagnostic Decision-Support System." *JAMA* 258 (1): 67–74.

Barney, J. 1991. "Firm Resources and Sustained Competitive Advantage." *Journal of Management* 17 (1): 99–120.

Barney, J. B., and D. N. Clark. 2007. *Resource-based Theory: Creating and Sustaining Competitive Advantage*. Oxford, UK: Oxford University Press.

Baron, R., E. Fabens, M. Schiffman, and E. Wolf. 2005. "Electronic Health Records: Just Around the Corner? Or Over the Cliff?" *Annals of Internal Medicine* 143 (3): 222–26.

Basch, E., D. Artz, D. Dulko, K. Scher, P. Sabbatini, M. Hensley, N. Mitra, J. Speakman, M. McCabe, and D. Schrag. 2005. "Patient Online Self-Reporting of Toxicity Symptoms During Chemotherapy." *Journal of Clinical Oncology* 23 (15): 3552–61.

Bashshur, R. L. 1995. "On the Definition and Evaluation of Telemedicine." *Telemedicine Journal* 1 (1): 19–30.

Bebow, G. L. 2011. "The CEO's Role in Small and Rural Hospitals' EMR Implementation." *Frontiers of Health Services Management* 28 (1): 31–34.

Beer, M. 1993. "The Transformation of the Human Resource Function: Resolving the Tension Between a Traditional Administrative and a New Strategic Role." *Human Resource Management* 36 (1): 49–56.

Bellazzi, R., C. Larizza, S. Montani, A. Riva, M. Stefanelli, G. d'Annunzio, R. Lorini, E. J. Gomez, E. Hernando, E. Brugues, J. Cermeno, R. Corcoy, A. de Leiva, C. Cobelli, G. Nucci, S. Del Prato, A. Maran, E. Kilkki, and J. Tuominen. 2002. "A Telemedicine Support for Diabetes Management: The T-IDDM Project." *Computer Methods and Programs in Biomedicine* 69 (2): 147–61.

Bergeson, S. C., and J. D. Dean. 2006. "A Systems Approach to Patient-Centered Care." *JAMA* 296 (23): 2848–51.

Bergmo, T. S. 2010. "Economic Evaluation in Telemedicine: Still Room for Improvement." *Journal of Telemedicine and Telecare* 16 (5): 229–31.

Berkman, L. F. 1984. "Assessing the Physical Health Effects of Social Networks and Social Support." *Annual Review of Public Health* 5 (1): 413–32.

Berkman, L. F., T. Glass, I. Brissette, and T. E. Seeman. 2000. "From Social Integration to Health: Durkheim in the New Millennium." *Social Science and Medicine* 51 (6): 843–57.

Bernd, D. L., and P. S. Fine. 2011. "Electronic Medical Records: A Path Forward." *Frontiers of Health Services Management* 28 (1): 3–13.

Berner, E. S. 2007. *Clinical Decision Support Systems: Theory and Practice*. New York: Springer.

Berwick, D. M. 2009. "What 'Patient-Centered' Should Mean: Confessions of an Extremist." *Health Affairs* 28 (4): 555–66.

Bharadwaj, A. S. 2000. "A Resource-based Perspective on Information Technology Capability and Firm Performance: An Empirical Investigation." *MIS Quarterly* 24 (1): 169–96.

Bloss, C., N. Schork, and E. Topol. 2011. "Effect of Direct-to-Consumer Genomewide Profiling to Assess Disease Risk." *New England Journal of Medicine* 364: 524–34.

Blount, Y., T. Castleman, and P. M. C. Swatman. 2005. "E-Commerce, Human Resource Strategies, and Competitive Advantage: Two Australian Case Studies." *International Journal of Electronic Commerce* 9 (3): 73–89.

Blumenthal, D. 2009. "Stimulating the Adoption of Health Information Technology." *New England Journal of Medicine* 360 (15): 1477–79.

Boles, K. E., and M. J. Cook. 2005. "Investing in Information Technology." In *Strategic Management of Information Systems in Healthcare*, by G. D. Brown, T. T. Stone, and T. B. Patrick, 195–221. Chicago: Health Administration Press.

Bøllingtoft, A., D. D. Hakonsson, J. F. Nielsen, C. C. Snow, and J. P. Ulhoi. 2009. *New Approaches to Organization Design: Theory and Practice of Adaptive Enterprises.* New York: Springer Science Business Media.

Bonias, D., T. Bartram, S. G. Leggat, and P. Stanton. 2010. "Does Psychological Empowerment Mediate the Relationship Between High Performance Work Systems and Patient Care Quality in Hospitals?" *Asia Pacific Journal of Human Resources* 48 (3): 319–37.

Borghoff, U. M., and J. H. Schlichter. 2000. *Computer-Supported Cooperative Work: Introduction to Distributed Applications.* Heidelberg, NY: Springer.

Borzillo, S., and R. Kaminska-Labbé. 2011. "Unravelling the Dynamics of Knowledge Creation in Communities of Practice Though Complexity Theory Lenses." *Knowledge Management Research and Practice* 9 (4): 353–66.

Bott, E. 1957. *Family and Social Network: Roles, Norms, and External Relationships in Ordinary Urban Families.* London: Tavistock Publications.

boyd, D. M., and N. B. Ellison. 2007. "Social Network Sites: Definition, History, and Scholarship." *Journal of Computer-Mediated Communication* 13 (1): 210–30.

boyd, D. M., and E. Hargittai. 2010. "Facebook Privacy Settings: Who Cares?" *First Monday* 15 (8): 13–23.

Bradley, V. 2006. "Strategic Valuation of Enterprise Information Technology Architecture in Healthcare Organizations." Unpublished doctoral dissertation, Auburn University.

Bradley, R. V., and T. A. Byrd. 2009. "A Theoretical Investigation and Extension of a Model of Information Technology Architecture Maturity." *Journal of Organizational and End User Computing* 21 (4): 41–62.

Bradley, R. V., R. M. E. Pratt. T. A. Byrd, C. N. Outlay, and D. E. Wynn, Jr. 2012. "Enterprise Architecture, IT Effectiveness, and the Mediating Role of IT Alignment in US Hospitals." *Information Systems Journal* 22 (2): 97–127.

Brahman, R. J., and H. J. Levesque. 2004. *Knowledge Representation and Reasoning.* San Francisco: Elsevier.

Brandeau, M. L. 2004. "Allocating Resources to Control Infectious Diseases." In *Operations Research and Health Care: A Handbook of Methods and Applications,* edited by M. L. Brandeau, F. Sainfort, and W. P. Pierskalla, 443–64. Boston: Kluwer Academic Publishers.

Briggs, R. O., J. F. Nunamaker, and R. H. Sprague. 2006. "Crossing Boundaries in Information Systems." *Journal of Management Information Systems* 22 (4): 7–11.

Brown, G. D., K. D. Bopp, and S. A. Boren. 2005. "Assessing Communications Effectiveness in Meeting Corporate Goals of Public Health Organizations." *Journal of Health and Human Services* 28 (2): 159–88.

Brown, G. D., T. T. Stone, and T. B. Patrick. 2005. *Strategic Management of Information Systems in Healthcare.* Chicago: Health Administration Press.

Brown, G. D., and T. T. Stone. 2005. "Introduction: The Role of Information Technology in Transforming Health Systems." In *Strategic Management of Information Systems in Healthcare,* by G. D. Brown, T. T. Stone, and T. B. Patrick. Chicago: Health Administration Press.

Bruck, L. 2008. "Virtual Health, Second Life: Virtual Test Drive for the Real World." *Hospitals & Health Networks* 82 (10): 50–56.

Brynjolfsson, E., and L. M. Hitt. 2000. "Beyond Computation: Information Technology, Organizational Transformation and Business Performance." *Journal of Economic Perspectives* 14 (4): 23–48.

Brynko, B. 2007. "A Revolution in Online Healthcare." *Information Today* 24 (6): 46.

Buchan, J. 2004. "What Difference Does ('Good') HRM Make?" *Human Resources for Health* 2 (6): 1–7.

Buchanan, E. C. 2003. "Computer Simulation as a Basis for Pharmacy Reengineering." *Nursing Administration Quarterly* 27 (1): 33–40.

Buntin, M. B., M. F. Burke, M. C. Hoaglin, and D. Blumenthal. 2011. "The Benefits of Health Information Technology: A Review of the Recent Literature Shows Predominantly Positive Results." *Health Affairs* 30 (3): 464–71.

Burt, R. S., and T. Schøtt, T. 1985. "Relation Contents in Multiple Networks." *Social Science Research* 14 (4): 287–308.

Bushe, G. R., and R. J. Marshak. 2009. "Revisioning Organization Development: Diagnostic and Dialogic Premises and Patterns of Practice." *Journal of Applied Behavioral Science* 45 (3): 348–68.

Business Wire. 2011. "Dell Launches New Cloud-Based Services for Hospitals and Physician Practices." *Business Wire.* Accessed May 15, 2012. www.businesswire.com/news/home/20110221005126/en/Dell-Launches-Cloud-Based-Services-Hospitals-Physician-Practices.

Cabrera, E. F., and A. Cabrera. 2005. "Fostering Knowledge Sharing Through People Management Practices." *International Journal of Human Resource Management* 16 (5): 720–35.

Camarinha-Matos, L. M., H. Afsarmanesh, N. Galeano, and A. Molina. 2009. "Collaborative Networked Organizations: Concepts and Practice in Manufacturing Enterprises." *Computers & Industrial Engineering* 57 (1): 46–60.

Carlucci, D., and G. Schiuma. 2007. "Knowledge Assets Value Creation Map: Assessing Knowledge Assets Value Drivers Using AHP." *Expert Systems with Applications* 32 (3): 814–21.

Carter, J. 2008. "From Process Analysis to Product Evaluation." In *Electronic Health Records: A Guide for Clinicians and Administrators,* 2nd edition, by J. Carter, 345–55. Philadelphia: ACP Press.

Casillas, J. 2009. "Measuring ROI of Medical Banking on the Healthcare Revenue Cycle." *Healthcare Financial Management* 63 (4): 114–16.

Center for IT Innovations in Healthcare (CITIH). 2012. *Wexler Medical Center.* Accessed April 3. http://citih.osumc.edu/.

Centers for Medicare and Medicaid Services (CMS). 2011. "Medicare Resource Use Measurement Plan." Accessed March 18. www.cms.gov/QualityInitiatives GenInfo/downloads/ResourceUse_Roadmap_OEA_1-15_508.pdf.

Cerner Corporation. 2012. "The Clinical Bioinformatics Ontology™ (CBO)." *Cerner Corporation.* Accessed May 15. www.cerner.com/about_cerner/clinical_bioinformatics_ontology.

Certification Commission for Health Information Technology (CCHIT). 2011. *Certification Commission for Health Information Technology.* Accessed June 10. www.cchit.org.

Charns, M., and G. Young. 2010. "Organization Design and Coordination." In *Health Care Management: Organization Design and Behavior,* 6th edition, by L. Burns, E. Bradley, and B. Weiner. Independence, KY: Delmar Cengage Learning.

Chaudhry, B., J. Wang, S. Wu, M. Maglione, W. Mojica, E. Roth, S. C. Morton, and P. G. Shekelle. 2006. "Systematic Review: Impact of Health Information Technology on Quality, Efficiency, and Costs of Medical Care." *Annals of Internal Medicine* 144 (10): 742–52.

Chi, L., T. Ravichandran, and G. Andrevski. 2010. "Information Technology, Network, Structure and Competitive Action." *Information Systems Research* 21 (3): 543–70.

Chin, T. 2004. "Health Information Networks: A Growing Trend." *American Medical News,* September 14.

Chou, W. Y., Y. M. Hunt, E. B. Beckjord, R. P. Moser, and B. W. Hesse. 2009. "Social Media Use in the United States: Implications for Health Communication." *Journal of Medical Internet Research* 11 (4): e48.

Christensen, C. M. 1997. *The Innovators Dilemma: When New Technologies Cause Great Firms to Fail.* New York: HarperBusiness.

Christensen, C. M., R. Bohmer, and J. Kenagy. 2000. "Will Disruptive Innovations Cure Health Care?" *Harvard Business Review* 78 (5): 102–17.

Christensen, C. M., J. H. Grossman, and J. Hwang. 2008. *The Innovator's Prescription: A Disruptive Solution for Health Care.* New York: McGraw Hill.

Cimino, J. J. 1998. "Desiderata for Controlled Medical Vocabularies in the Twenty-First Century." *Methods of Information in Medicine* 37 (4–5): 394–403.

Civan, A., and W. Pratt. 2007. "Threading Together Patient Expertise." In *AMIA Annual Symposium Proceedings, Volume 2007*, 140–44. Bethesda, MD: AMIA.

Civan, A., M. M. Skeels, A. Stolyar, and W. Pratt. 2006. "Personal Health Information Management: Consumers' Perspectives." In *AMIA Annual Symposium Proceedings, Volume 2006*, 156–60. Bethesda, MD: AMIA.

Coates, E., G. Lloyd, and D. Simandl. 1979. *The BSO Manual: The Development, Rationale, and Use of the Broad System of Ordering.* The Hague, Netherlands: Federation Internationale de Documentation.

Coenan, A., and C. Bartz. 2010. "ICNP: Nursing Terminology to Improve Healthcare Worldwide." In *Nursing and Informatics for the 21st Century: An International Look at Practice, Education and EHR Trends*, 2nd ed., by C. A. Weaver, C. W. Delaney, P. Weber, and R. L. Carr, 207–16. Chicago: Healthcare Information and Management Systems Society.

Coenan, A., and T. Y. Kim. 2010. "Development of Terminology Subsets Using ICNP." *International Journal of Medical Informatics* 79 (7): 530–38.

Cohen, J. T., and P. J. Neumann. 2008. "Using Decision Analysis to Better Evaluate Pediatric Clinical Guidelines." *Health Affairs* 27 (5): 1467–76.

Collen, M. F. 1995. *A History of Medical Informatics in the United States, 1950 to 1990.* Indianapolis, IN: American Medical Informatics Association.

Collins, F. S., J. Rogers, R. H. Waterston, and the International Human Genome Sequencing Consortium. 2004. "Finishing the Euchromatic Sequence of the Human Genome." *Nature* 431 (7011): 931–45.

Cooke, M., D. M. Irby, W. Sullivan, and K. M. Ludmerer. 2006. "American Medical Education 100 Years After the Flexner Report." *New England Journal of Medicine* 355 (13): 1339–44.

Corley, S. 2008. "Creating a Request for Proposal and Negotiating a Contract." In *Electronic Health Records: A Guide for Clinicians and Administrators*, 2nd edition, by J. Carter, 383–92. Philadelphia: ACP Press.

Coye, M. J., and W. S. Bernstein. 2003. "Improving America's Health Care System by Investing in Information Technology." *Health Affairs* 22 (4): 56–58.

Cross, S. S., F. C. Hamby, J. R. Goepel, and R. F. Harrison. 2008. "Prostate Cancer: A Systems Approach Overview." *Diagnostic Histopathology* 14 (3): 122–33.

Currie, G., R. Finn, and G. Martin. 2010. "Role Transition and the Interaction of Relational and Social Identity: New Nursing Roles in the English NHS." *Organization Studies* 31: 941–61.

Curry, A., and G. Knowles. 2005. "Strategic Information Management in Health Care: Myth or Reality?" *Health Services Management Research* 18 (1): 53–62.

Dartmouth Atlas of Health Care. 2012. Accessed March 21. www.dartmouthatlas.org.

Davenport, T., and J. Glaser. 2002. "Just-in-Time-Delivery Comes to Knowledge Management." *Harvard Business Review* 80 (7): 107–11.

Davenport, T. H., J. G. Harrison, and R. Morrison. 2010. *Analytics at Work: Smarter Decisions, Better Results.* Cambridge, MA: Harvard Business School Publishing Corporation.

Davenport, T. H., J. G. Harris, D. W. De Long, and A. L. Jacobson. 2002. "Data to Knowledge to Results: Building an Analytic Capability." *California Management Review* 43 (2): 117–38.

Davis, S. M. 1983. "Management Models for the Future." *New Management* 1 (Spring): 12–15.

Day, M. 2002. *Metadata: Mapping Between Metadata Formats.* Accessed June 6, 2011. www.ukoln.ac.uk/metadata/interoperability/.

Dean, B., A. V. Ackere, S. Gallivan, and N. Barber. 1999. "When Should Pharmacists Visit Their Wards? An Application of Simulation to Planning Hospital Pharmacy Services." *Health Care Management Science* 2 (1): 35.

Demiris, G., S. Finkelstein, and S. M. Speedie. 2001. "Considerations for the Design of a Web-based Clinical Monitoring and Educational System for Elderly Patients. *Journal of American Medical Informatics Association* 8 (5): 468–72.

Demiris, G., S. M. Speedie, and S. Finkelstein. 2001a. "Change of Patients' Perceptions of TeleHomeCare." *Telemedicine Journal and E-Health* 7 (3): 241–48.

———. 2001b. "The Nature of Communication in Virtual Home Care Visits." In *AMIA Annual Symposium Proceedings, Volume 2001*, 135–38. Bethesda, MD: AMIA.

———. 2000. "A Questionnaire for the Assessment of Patients' Impressions of the Risks and Benefits of Home Telecare." *Journal of Telemedicine and Telecare* 6 (5): 278–84.

Demner-Fushman, D., W. W. Chapman, and C. J. McDonald. 2009. "What Can Natural Language Processing Do for Clinical Decision Support?" *Journal of Biomedical Informatics* 42 (5): 760–72.

DesRoches, C. M., E. G. Campbell, C. Vogeli, J. Zheng, S. R. Rao, A. E. Shields, K. Donelan, S. Rosenbaum, S. J. Bristol, and A. K. Jha. 2010. "Electronic Health Records' Limited Successes Suggest More Targeted Use." *Health Affairs* 29 (4): 639–46.

DeVore, S. D., and K. Figlioli. 2010. "Lessons Premier Hospitals Learned About Implementing Electronic Health Records." *Health Affairs* 29 (4): 664–67.

Dewett, T., and G. R. Jones. 2001. "The Role of Information Technology in the Organization: A Review, Model, and Assessment." *Journal of Management* 27 (3): 313–46.

Dewing, M. 2010. "Social Media 2: Who Uses Them?" Accessed March 27, 2011. www.parl.gc.ca/Content/LOP/ResearchPublications/2010-05-e.htm.

Digwell, R. 2009. *Essays on Professions*. Hampshire, UK/Burlington, VT: Ashgate Publishing Company.

Dilts, D., and Y. Zhang. 2004. "System Dynamics of Supply Chain Network Organization Structure." *Information Systems and e-Business Management* 2 (2): 187–206.

Doherty, I. 2008. "Web 2.0: A Movement Within the Health Community." *Health Care and Informatics Review Online* 12 (2): 49–57.

Drucker, P. F. 1999. "Knowledge-Worker Productivity: The Biggest Challenge." *California Management Review* 41 (20): 79–94.

Drug Enforcement Agency (DEA), US Department of Justice. 2010. "Electronic Prescriptions for Controlled Substances; Final Rule." 21 CFR Parts 1300, 1304, 1306, and 1311. *Federal Register,* March 31.

Dublin Core Metadata Initiative Limited. 2011. *The Dublin Core Metadata Initiative.* Accessed June 7. http://dublincore.org/.

Duggal, R., and D. B. Menkes. 2011. "Evidence-based Medicine in Practice." *International Journal of Clinical Practice* 65 (6): 639–44.

Duke University and Duke University Health System. 2012. "Doing Good in the Neighborhood." Accessed March 1. http://doinggood.duke.edu/.

Dussault, G., and C. Dubois. 2003. "Human Resources for Health Policies: A Critical Component in Health Policies." *Human Resources for Health* 1 (1). Accessed January 1, 2012. www.human-resourceshealth.com/content/1/1/1.

Dye, J. 2006. "Folksonomy: A Game of High-Tech (and High-Stakes) Tag." *DTB EContent* 29 (3): 38–43.

Edelmann, L., and K. Hirschhorn. 2009. "Clinical Utility of Array CGH for the Detection of Chromosomal Imbalances Associated with Mental Retardation and Multiple Congenital Anomalies." *New York Academy of Science* 11 (51): 157–66.

Eli, K., L. Cabassa, M. Hansen, L. A. Palinkas, and A. Wells. 2011. "Sustainability of Collaborative Care Interventions in Primary Care Settings." *Journal of Social Work* 11 (1): 99–117.

Ellison, N. B., C. Lampe, and C. Steinfield. 2009. "Social Network Sites and Society: Current Trends and Future Possibilities." *Interactions* 16 (1): 6–9.

Elsa, S. E., N. M. Lang, and S. P. Lundeen. 2006. "Time for a Nursing Legacy: Ensuring Excellence Through Actionable Knowledge." *Nurse Leader* 4 (6): 42–44, 55.

Ende, J., L. Kazis, A. Ash, and M. A. Moskowitz. 1989. "Measuring Patients' Desire for Autonomy: Decision Making and Information-Seeking Preferences Among Medical Patients." *Journal of General Internal Medicine* 4 (1): 23–30.

Enes, J. E. 2011. "A Patient-Centered Care Model." *Radiologic Technology* 82 (3): 212.

Enthoven, A. C., and L. A. Tollen. 2005. "Competition in Health Care: It Takes Systems to Pursue Quality and Efficiency." *Health Affairs* 24 (5): 420–33.

Etzioni, A. 2010. "Personal Health Records: Why Good Ideas Sometimes Languish." *Issues in Science & Technology* (Summer): 59–67.

Eysenbach, G. 2008. "Medicine 2.0: Social Networking, Collaboration, Participation, Apomediation, and Openness." *Journal of Medical Internet Research* 10 (3): e22.

———. 2007. "From Intermediation to Disintermediation and Apomediation: New models for Consumers to Access and Assess the Credibility of Health Information in the Age of Web 2.0." *Studies in Health Technology and Informatics* 129 (Pt 1): 162–66.

———. 2000. "Consumer Health Informatics." *British Medical Journal* 320 (7251): 1713–16.

Faraj, S., S. L. Jarvenpaa, and A. Majchrzak. 2011. "Knowledge Collaboration in Online Communities." *Organization Science* 22 (5): 1224–39.

Farand, L., and J. Arocha. 2004. "A Cognitive Science Perspective on Evidence-Based Decision-Making in Medicine." In *Using Knowledge and Evidence in Health Care: Multidisciplinary Perspectives,* by L. Lemieux-Charles and F. Champagne. Toronto: University of Toronto Press.

Faulconbridge, J., D. Muzio, S. Hall, D. Hodgson, and J. Beaverstock. 2011. "Towards Corporate Professionalization: The Case of Project Management, Management Consultancy, and Executive Search." *Current Sociology* 59 (4): 443–64.

Federal Chief Information Officers Council, Best Practices Committee. 2012. "The Value of IT Investments, It's Not Just Return on Investment." *Federal Chief Information Officers Council.* Accessed March 2, 2012. www.cio.gov/Documents/TheValueof_IT_Investments.pdf.

Federal Register. 1991. "Federal Policy for the Protection of Human Subjects; Notices and Rules." *Federal Register* 56 (117).

Feld, C. S., and D. B. Stoddard. 2004. "Getting IT Right." *Harvard Business Review* 82 (2): 72–79.

Fenstermacher, D. 2005. "Introduction to Bioinformatics." *Journal of the American Society for Information Science and Technology* 56 (5): 440–46.

Fernandopulle, R., and N. Patel. 2010. "How the Electronic Health Record Did Not Measure Up to the Demands of Our Medical Home Practice." *Health Affairs* 29 (4): 622–28.

Feste, C., and R. M. Anderson. 1995. "Empowerment: From Philosophy to Practice." *Patient Education and Counseling* 26 (1–3): 139–44.

Finkelstein, J., G. O'Connor, and R. H. Friedmann. 2001. "Development and Implementation of the Home Asthma Telemonitoring (HAT) System to Facilitate Asthma Self-Care." *Studies in Health Technology and Informatics* 84 (Pt 1): 810–14.

Fisher, K. E., J. C. Durrance, and K. T. Unruh. 2003. "Information Communities: Characteristics Gleaned from Studies of Three Online Networks." *Proceedings of the ASIST Annual Meeting* 40: 298–305.

Fjeldstad, Ø. D., C. Snow, R. E. Miles, and C. Lettl. 2012. "The Architecture of Collaboration." *Strategic Management Journal* 33 (6): 734–50.

Flexner, A. 1910. *Medical Education in the United States and Canada: A Report to the Carnegie Foundation for the Advancement of Teaching*, Bulletin No. 4, 346. New York City: The Carnegie Foundation for the Advancement of Teaching.

Fogel, J., and E. Nehmad. 2009. "Internet Social Network Communities: Risk Taking, Trust, and Privacy Concerns." *Computers in Human Behavior* 25 (1): 153–60.

Ford, E. W., N. Menachemi, T. R. Huerta, and F. Yu. 2010. "Hospital IT Adoption Strategies Associated with Implementation Success: Implications for Achieving Meaningful Use." *Journal of Healthcare Management* 55 (3): 175–88.

Fowler, A. 2003. "Systems Modeling, Simulation, and the Dynamics of Strategy." *Journal of Business Research* 56 (2): 135–44.

Fowler, J. H., and N. A. Christakis. 2010. "Cooperative Behavior Cascades in Human Social Networks." *Proceedings of the National Academy of Sciences of the United States of America* 107 (12): 5334–38.

Frampton, S. B., and S. Guastello. 2010. "Patient-Centered Care: More than the Sum of Its Parts." *American Journal of Nursing* 1 (9): 49–53.

Franzini, L., K. R. Sail, E. J. Thomas, and L. Wueste. 2011. "Costs and Cost-Effectiveness of a Telemedicine Intensive Care Unit Program in Six Intensive Care Units in a Large Health Care System." *Journal of Critical Care* 26 (3): 329.e321–329.e326.

Friedman, C. P., R. B. Altman, I. S. Kohane, K. A. McCormick, P. L. Miller, J. G. Ozbolt, E. H. Shortliffe, G. D. Stormo, M. C. Szczepaniak, D. Tuck, and

J. Williamson. 2004. "Training the Next Generation of Informaticians: The Impact of 'BISTI' and Bioinformatics: A Report from the American College of Medical Informatics." *Journal of the American Medical Informatics Association* 11 (3): 167–72.

Friedson, E. 2001. *The Third Logic.* Chicago: University of Chicago Press.

———. 1994. *Professionalism Reborn: Theory, Prophecy, and Policy.* Chicago: University of Chicago Press.

Fung, K. W., and O. Bodenreider. 2005. "Utilizing the UMLS for Semantic Mapping Between Terminologies." In *AMIA Annual Symposium Proceedings, Volume 2005,* 266–70. Bethesda, MD: AMIA.

Gale, K. 2009. "What's Next for Revenue Cycle Technology?" *Healthcare Financial Management* 63 (3): 80–84.

Geisler, E., and N. Wickramasinghe. 2009. *Principles of Knowledge Management: Theory, Practice and Cases,* 28–52. Armonk, New York: M.E. Sharpe, Inc.

Genetic Information Non-Discrimination Act of 2008 (GINA). *Public Law 110-233.* May 21, 2008.

Gera, S., and W. Gu. 2004. "The Effect of Organizational Innovation and Information Technology on Firm Performance." *International Productivity Monitor* 9 (Fall): 37.

Ghandforoush, P. 1993. "Optimal Allocation of Time in a Hospital Pharmacy Using Goal Programming." *European Journal of Operational Research* 70 (2): 191–98.

Gianchandani, E. P. 2011. "Toward Smarter Health and Well-Being: An Implicit Role for Networking and Information Technology." *Journal of Information Technology* 6 (22): 120–29.

Giniat, E. J. 2011. "Cloud Computing: Innovating the Business of Health Care." *Healthcare Financial Management* 65 (5): 130–32.

Gladwell, M. 2000. *The Tipping Point: How Little Things Make a Big Difference.* New York: Little Brown.

Glaser, J. 2009. "Implementing Electronic Health Records: 10 Factors for Success." *Healthcare Financial Management* 63 (1): 50–52, 54.

———. 2008. "Clinical Decision Support: The Power Behind the Electronic Health Record." *Healthcare Financial Management* 62 (7): 46–48, 50–51.

Goedert, J. 2011. "Tackling the Health I.T. Workforce Shortage." *Health Data Management* 19 (2): 40–42, 44–47.

Goldstein, S. M. 2003. "Employee Development: An Examination of Service Strategy in a High-Contact Service Environment." *Production and Operations Management* 12 (2): 186–203.

Gong, Y., and J. Zhang. 2005. "A Human-Centered Design and Evaluation Framework for Information Search." In *AMIA Annual Symposium Proceedings, Volume 2005,* 281–85. Bethesda, MD: AMIA.

Grant, R. M. 1996. "Prospering in Dynamically-Competitive Environments: Organizational Capability as Knowledge Integration." *Organization Science* 7 (4): 375–87.

Grant, A., A. Kushniruk, A. Villeneuve, N. Bolduc, and A. Moshyk. 2004. "An Informatics Perspective on Decision Support and the Process of Decision-Making in Health Care." In *Using Knowledge and Evidence in Health Care: Multidisciplinary Perspectives,* by L. Lemieux-Charles and F. Champagne, 199–226. Toronto: University of Toronto Press.

Greengard, S. 2011. "The Future of IT Infrastructure." *CIO Insight* 119: 26–29.

Greenhalgh, T., and R. Stones. 2010. "Theorising Big IT Programmes in Healthcare: Strong Structuration Theory Meets Actor–Network Theory." *Social Science and Medicine* 70 (9): 1285–94.

Greiner, A. C., and E. Knebel, eds. 2003. *Health Professions Education: A Bridge to Quality.* Washington, DC: National Academies Press.

Grimmelmann, J. 2009. "Saving Facebook." *Iowa Law Review* 94 (4): 1137–206.

Grimshaw, D., and M. Miozzo. 2009. "New Human Resource Management Practices in Knowledge-Intensive Business Service Firms: The Case of Outsourcing with Staff Transfer." *Human Relations* 62 (10): 1521–50.

Grizzle, A. J., M. H. Mahmood, Y. Ko, J. E. Murphy, E. P. Armstrong, G. H. Skrepnek, and D. C. Malone. 2007. "Reasons Provided by Prescribers When Overriding Drug–Drug Interaction Alerts." *The American Journal of Managed Care* 13 (10): 573–78.

Grossman, J. M., A. Gerland, M. C. Reed, and C. Fahlman. 2007. "Physicians' Experience Using Commercial E-Prescribing Systems." *Health Affairs* 26 (3): w393–w404.

Gupta, V., and M. B. Murtaza. 2009. "Approaches to Electronic Health Record Implementation." *The Review of Business Information Systems* 13 (4): 21–28.

Hafferty, W., and D. Levinson. 2008. "Moving Beyond Nostalgia and Motives: Towards a Complexity Science View of Medical Professionalism." *Perspectives in Biology and Medicine* 51 (4): 599–615.

Hagland, M. 2011. "Revenue Cycle Management Automation." *Healthcare Informatics* 28 (1): 36–39.

Hagle, M. E., and P. Senk. 2009. "Evidence-based Practice." In *Infusion Nursing: An Evidence-based Approach,* by A. C. M. Alexander, 10–21. St. Louis, MO: Mosby Elsevier.

Halvorsen, L., S. Garolis, A. Wallace-Scroggs, J. Stenstrom, and R. Maunder. 2007. "Building a Rapid Response Team." *AACN Advanced Critical Care* 18 (2): 129–40.

Halvorson, G. 2007. *Healthcare Reform Now: A Prescription for Change.* San Francisco: John Wiley & Sons.

Hansen, J. I., and C. A. Thompson. 2002. "Knowledge Management: When People, Process, and Technology Converge." *LIMRA's Market Facts Quarterly* 2 (2): 14–21.

Hanson, W. R., and R. Ford. 2010. "Complexity Leadership in Healthcare: Leader Network Awareness." *ScienceDirect* 2: 6587–96.

Harris, C. 2006. *Hyperinnovation and Building Innovative Teams.* New York: Palgrave MacMillan.

Hassol, A., J. M. Walker, D. Kidder, K. Rokita, D. Young, S. Pierdon, D. Deitz, S. Kuck, and E. Ortiz. 2004. "Patient Experiences and Attitudes About Access to a Patient Electronic Health Care Record and Linked Web Messaging." *Journal of the American Medical Informatics Association* 11 (6): 505–13.

Havighurst, C. C. 2008. "Disruptive Innovation: The Demand Side." *Health Affairs* 27 (5): 1341–44.

Hawn, C. 2009. "Take Two Aspirin and Tweet Me in the Morning: How Twitter, Facebook, and Other Social Media Are Reshaping Health Care." *Health Affairs* 28 (2): 361–68.

Haynes, A.B., T. G. Weiser, W. R. Berry, S. R. Lipsitz, A. S. Breizat, E. P. Dellinger, T. Herbosa, S. Joseph, P. L. Kibatala, M. C. Lapitan, A. F. Merry, K. Moorthy, R. K. Reznick, B. Taylor, and A. Gawande. 2009. "Safe Surgery Saves Lives Study Group: A Surgical Safety Checklist to Reduce Morbidity and Mortality in a Global Population." *New England Journal of Medicine* 360 (5): 491–99.

Healthcare Financial Management. 2007. "Paving the Way for Medical Banking." *Healthcare Financial Management* 61 (5): 1–4.

Heckathorn, D. 1979. "The Anatomy of Social Network Linkages." *Social Science Research* 8 (3): 222–52.

Helfat, C. E., S. Finkelstein, W. Mitchell, M. A. Peteraf, H. Singh, D. Teece, and S. Winter. 2007. *Dynamic Capabilities: Understanding Strategic Change in Organizations.* Malden, MA: Blackwell Publishing.

Helfat, C. E., and M. A. Peteraf. 2003. "The Dynamic Resource-based View: Capability Lifecycles." *Strategic Management Journal* 24 (10): 997–1010.

Hempel, P. S. 2004. "Preparing the HR Profession for Technology and Information Work." *Human Resource Management* 43 (2/3): 163–77.

Herzenberg, S. A., J. A. Alic, and H. Wial. 1998. *New Rules for a New Economy: Employment and Opportunity in Postindustrial America.* Ithaca, NY: Cornell University Press.

Herzlinger, R. E. 2006. "Why Innovation in Health Care Is So Hard." *Harvard Business Review* 84 (5): 58–66, 156.

Heskett, J., W. E. Sasser, and L. Schlesinger. 1997. *The Service Profit Chain.* New York: The Free Press.

Hewett, M., D. E. Oliver, D. L. Rubin, K. L., Easton, J. M. Stuart, R. B. Altman, and T. E. Klein. 2002. "PharmGKB: The Pharmacogenetics Knowledge Base." *Nucleic Acids Research* 30 (1): 163–65.

Hillard, R. 2010. *Information-Driven Business: How to Manage Data and Information for Maximum Advantage.* New York: John Wiley & Sons.

Hillstad, R., J. Bigelow, A. Bower, F. Girosi, R. Meili, R. Scoville, and R. Taylor. 2005. "Can Electronic Medical Record Systems Transform Health Care? Potential Health Benefits, Savings, and Costs." *Health Affairs* 24 (5): 1103–17.

Hirsch, G. B. 1979. "System Dynamic Modeling in Health Care." *ACM SIGSIM Simulation Digest* 10 (4): 38–42.

Hoffman, M., C. Arnoldi, and I. Chuang. 2005. "The Clinical Bioinformatics Ontology: A Curated Semantic Network Utilizing RefSeq Information." Pacific Symposium on Biocomputing 2005, 139–50.

Hook, M. L., L. J. Burke, and J. Murphy. 2009. "An IT Innovation for Individualizing Care: Success with Clinicians Leading the Way." *Studies in Health Technology and Informatics* 46: 493–97.

Hook, M. L., E. C. Devine, and N. M. Lang. 2008. "Using a Computerized Fall-Risk Assessment Process to Tailor Interventions in Acute Care." In *Advances in Patient Safety: New Directions and Alternative Approaches,* by K. Henriksen, J. B. Battles, M. A. Keyes, and D. I. Lewin, 387–405. Washington, DC: Agency for Healthcare Research and Quality.

Hook, M. L., and C. Winchel. 2006. "Fall-Related Injuries in Acute Care: Reducing the Risk of Harm." *MEDSURG Nursing* 15 (6): 370–77, 381.

Hoomans, T., A. Ament, S. Evers, and J. L. Severens. 2011. "Implementing Guidelines into Clinical Practice: What Is the Value?" *Journal of Evaluation in Clinical Practice* 17 (4): 606–14.

Horn, S. D. 2006. "Performance Measures and Clinical Outcomes." *JAMA* 296 (22): 2731–32.

Horrocks, J. C., A. P. McCann, J. R. Staniland, D. J. Leaper, and F. T. de Dombal. 1972. "Computer-Aided Diagnosis: Description of an Adaptable System and Operational Experience with 2,034 Cases." *British Medical Journal* 2: 5.

Hovman, P. S., D. F. Andersen, F. Rouwette, G. P. Richardson, K. Rux, and A. Calhoun. 2012. "Group Model-Building 'Scripts' as a Collaborative Planning Tool." *Systems Research and Behavioral Science* 29 (2): 179–93.

Hudon, C., M. Fortin, J. L. Haggerty, M. Lambert, and M-E. Poitras. 2011. "Measuring Patient Perceptions of Patient-Centered Care: A Systematic Review of Tools for Family Medicine." *Annals of Family Medicine* 9 (2): 155–64.

IBM. 2011. *Analytics: The New Path to Value.* Armonk, NY: IBM Institute for Business Value.

————. 2006. "Dialogue for AIX 5L on IBM POWER Processor-Based Systems." Accessed March 30, 2012. www-07.ibm.com/systems/includes/pdf/PSS01840USEN.pdf.

Ichniowski, C., and K. Shaw. 2003. "Beyond Incentive Pay: Insiders' Estimates of the Value of Complementary Human Resource Management Practices." *Journal of Economic Perspectives* 17 (1): 155–80.

IDX Systems Corporation. 2012. Accessed March 21. www.enotes.com/company-histories/idx-systems-corporation.

Ilie, V., C. Van Slyke, M. A. Parikh, and J. F. Courney. 2009. "Paper Versus Electronic Medical Records: The Effects of Access on Physicians' Decisions to Use Complex Information Technologies." *Decision Science* 40 (2): 213–41.

Institute for Healthcare Improvement (IHI). 2006. *100,000 Lives Campaign: How-to Guide. Getting Started Kit: Rapid Response Teams.* Accessed November, 2006. www.ihi.org/IHI/Programs/Campaign/.

Institute of Medicine (IOM). 2001. *Crossing the Quality Chasm: A New Health System for the 21st Century.* Committee on Quality of Health Care in America. Washington, DC: National Academies Press.

Institute of Translational Health Sciences. 2010. "About Translational Research." Accessed June 8, 2011. www.iths.org/about/translational.

International Health Terminology Standards Development Organisation. 2010. *SNOMED Clinical Terms User Guide.* Copenhagen, Denmark: The International Health Terminology Standards Development Organisation.

International Organization for Standardization and the International Electrotechnical Commission. 2004. *Information Technology—Metadata Registries (MDR).* Geneva, Switzerland: The International Organization for Standardization and the International Electrotechnical Commission.

Internetworldstats.com. 2012. "World Internet Usage Statistics News and World Population Stats." Accessed May 17. www.internetworldstats.com/stats.htm.

Isaac, R. G., I. M. Herremans, and T. J. B. Kline. 2009. "Intellectual Capital Management: Pathways to Wealth Creation." *Journal of Intellectual Capital* 10 (1): 81–92.

ISACA. 2012. "Val IT Framework 2.0." *ISACA.* Accessed May 21. www.isaca.org/Knowledge-Center/Research/ResearchDeliverables/Pages/Val-IT-Framework-2.0.aspx.

Israel, B. A. 1982. "Social Networks and Health Status: Linking Theory, Research, and Practice." *Patient Counselling and Health Education* 4 (2): 65–79.

Jacobs, L. 2009. "Interview with Lawrence Weed, MD, The Father of the Problem-Oriented Medical Record Looks Ahead." *The Permanente Journal* 13 (3): 84–89.

Jagatic, T. N., N. A. Johnson, M. Jakobsson, and F. Menczer. 2007. "Social Phishing." *Communications of the ACM* 50 (10): 94–100.

Janz, B. D., and P. Prasarnphanich. 2003. "Understanding the Antecedents of Effective Knowledge Management: The Importance of a Knowledge-Centered Culture." *Decision Sciences* 34 (2): 351–84.

Jatem, M. E. P., K. Casey, and A. L. Kushner. 2011. "Can Twitter Campaigns Increase Awareness About Health Issues?" *Bulletin of the American College of Surgeons* 96 (2): 44.

Jaw, B. S., and W. Liu. 2003. "Promoting Organizational Learning and Self-Renewal in Taiwanese Companies: The Role of HRM." *Human Resource Management* 42 (3): 223–41.

Jerant, A. F., R. Azari, and T. S. Nesbitt. 2001. "Reducing the Cost of Frequent Hospital Admissions for Congestive Heart Failure: A Randomized Trial of a Home Telecare Intervention." *Medical Care* 39 (11): 1234–45.

Johnston, B., L. Wheeler, J. Deuser, and K. H. Sousa. 2000. "Outcomes of the Kaiser Permanente Tele-Home Health Research Project." *Archives of Family Medicine* 9 (1): 40–45.

Jones, J. H. 1982. *Bad Blood*. New York: The Free Press.

Kaba, R., and P. Sooriakumaran. 2007. "The Evolution of the Doctor–Patient Relationship." *International Journal of Surgery* 5 (1): 57–65.

Kahn, J. S., V. Aulakh, and A. Bosworth. 2009. "What It Takes: Characteristics of the Ideal Personal Health Record." *Health Affairs* 28 (2): 369–76.

Kahn, M. G., S. A. Steib, V. J. Fraser, and W. C. Dunagan. 1993. "An Expert System for Culture-based Infection Control Surveillance." *Proceedings of the Annual Symposium on Computer Application in Medical Care*, 171–75.

Kaiser Permanente, Sidney R. Garfield Health Care Innovation Center. 2012. Accessed March 18. http://xnet.kp.org/innovationcenter/?kp_shortcut_referrer=kp.org/innovationcenter/.

Kaplan, B. 2001. "Evaluating Informatics Applications—Clinical Decision Support Systems Literature Review." *International Journal of Medical Informatics* 64 (1): 15–37.

Kaplan, R. M., and D. L. Frosch. 2005. "Decision Making in Medicine and Health Care." *Annual Review of Clinical Psychology* 1: 525–556.

Kaplan, S. H., S. Greenfield, and J. E. Ware. 1989. "Assessing the Effects of Physician-Patient Interactions on the Outcomes of Chronic Disease." *Medical Care* 27 (3, Suppl): S110–S127.

Kaplan, A. M., and M. Haenlein. 2010. "Users of the World, Unite! The Challenges and Opportunities of Social Media." *Business Horizons* 53 (1): 59–68.

Kappelman, L., R. McKeeman, and L. Zhang. 2006. "Early Warning Signs of IT Project Failure: The Dominant Dozen." *Information Systems Management* 23 (4): 31–36.

Karreman, D., and M. Alvesson. 2004. "Cages in Tandem: Management Control, Social Identity, and Identification in a Knowledge-Intensive Firm." *Organization* 11 (1): 149–75.

Karsh, B., M. Weinger, P. A. Abbot, and R. Wears. 2010. "Health Information Technology: Fallacies and Sober Realities." *Journal of the American Medical Informatics Association* 17 (6): 617–23.

Keen, P. G. W. 1991. *Shaping the Future: Business Design Through Information Technology.* Cambridge, MA: Harvard Business School Press.

Kerfoot, K. M., S. P. Lundeen, E. Harper, N. M. Lang, L. J. Burke, and M. L. Hook. 2010. "Building an Intelligent Clinical Information System for Nursing: The Aurora, Cerner, and University of Wisconsin, Milwaukee Knowledge-Based Nursing Initiative, Part II." In *Nursing and Informatics for the 21st Century: An International Look at Practice, Education and EHR Trends,* 2nd ed., by C. A. Weaver, C. W. Delaney, P. Weber, and R. L. Carr, 225–41. Chicago: Healthcare Information and Management Systems Society.

Khatri, N. 2006a. "Building HR Capability in Health Care Organizations." *Health Care Management Review* 31 (1): 45–54.

———. 2006b. "Building IT Capability in Health Care Organizations." *Health Services Management Research* 19 (2): 73–79.

Khatri, N., A. Baveja, N. M. Agrawal, and G. D. Brown. 2010. "HR and IT Capabilities and Complementarities in Knowledge-Intensive Services." *The International Journal of Human Resource Management* 21 (15): 2889–909.

Khatri, N., A. Baveja, S. Boren, and A. Mammo. 2006. "Medical Errors and Quality of Care: From Control to Commitment." *California Management Review* 48 (3): 115–41.

Kidd, M. R. 2008. "Personal Electronic Health Records: MySpace or Health-Space?" *British Medical Journal* 336 (7652): 1029–30.

Kim, T. Y., N. M. Lang, K. S. Berg, C. Weaver, J. Murphy, and S. E. Ela. 2007. "Clinical Adoption Patterns and Patient Outcome Results in Use of Evidence-based Nursing Plans of Care." In *AMIA Annual Symposium Proceedings: Biomedical and Health Informatics: From Foundations to Applications to Policy,* 423–27. Chicago: Curran Associates, Inc.

King, W. R. 2002. "IT Capabilities, Business Processes, and Impact on the Bottom Line." *Information Systems Management* Spring 19 (2): 85–87.

Kingsland, L. C, III. 1985. "The Evaluation of Medical Expert Systems: Experience with the AI/RHEUM Knowledge-based Consultant System in Rheumatology, Proceedings: Annual Symposium on Computing Applications." *Medical Care* (November 13): 292–95.

Kinney, W. C. 2003. "Web-based Clinical Decision Support Systems for Triage of Vestibular Patients." *Ontolaryngology Head and Neck Surgery* 128 (1): 48–53.

Kirkman, B. L., J. E. Mathieu, J. L. Cordery, B. Rosen, and M. Kukenberger. 2011. "Managing a New Collaborative Entity in Business Organizations: Understanding Organizational Communities of Practice Effectiveness." *The Journal of Applied Psychology* 96 (6): 1234–45.

Klein, T. E., and R. B. Altman. 2004. "PharmGKB: The Pharmacogenetics and Pharmacogenomics Knowledge Base." *Pharmacogenomics Journal* 4 (1): 1.

Kocharekar, R. 2004. "An IT Architecture for Nimble Organizations: Managing Access from Cyberspace." *Information Systems Management* 21 (2): 22–30.

Kohn, L. T., J. M. Corrigan, and M. S. Donaldson (eds.). 2000. *To Err Is Human.* Institute of Medicine Committee on Quality of Health Care in America. Washington, DC: National Academies Press.

Kolfschoten, G. L., G. deVreede, R. O. Briggs, and H. G. Sol. 2010. "Collaboration Engineerability." *Group Decision and Negotiation* 19 (3): 301–21.

Korczynski, M. 2002. *Human Resource Management in Service Work.* New York: Palgrave MacMillan.

Krynetski, E. Y., J. D. Schuetz, A. J. Galpin, C. H. Pui, M. V. Relling, and W. E. Evans. 1995. "A Single Point Mutation Leading to Loss of Catalytic Activity in Human Thiopurine S-Methyltransferase." *Proceedings of the National Academy of Science* 92 (4): 949–53.

Kubick, W. R. 2009. "Applying the Supply Chain Model." *Applied Clinical Trials* 18 (2): 34.

Lakhno, V. D. 2010. "Mathematical Biology and Bioinformatics." *Herald of the Russian Academy of Sciences* 81 (5): 539–45.

Lander, E. S., et al. 2001. "Initial Sequencing and Analysis of the Human Genome." *Nature* 409 (6822): 860–921.

Landro, L. 2006. "The Informed Patient: Social Networking Comes to Health Care; Online Tools Give Patients Better Access to Information and Help Build Communities." *Wall Street Journal*, December 27.

Lang, N. M. 2008. "The Promise of Simultaneous Transformation of Practice and Research with the Use of Clinical Information Systems." *Nursing Outlook* 56 (5): 232–36.

Lang, N. M., M. L. Hook, M. E. Akre, T. Y. Kim, K. S. Berg, and S. P. Lundeen. 2006. "Translating Knowledge-based Nursing into Referential and Executable Application in an Intelligent Clinical Information System." In *Nursing and Informatics for the 21st Century: An International Look at Practice, Education and EHR Trends,* 2nd ed., by C. A. Weaver, C. W. Delaney, P. Weber, and R. L. Carr, 291–303. Chicago: Healthcare Information and Management Systems Society.

Lasker, R. D., and E. S. Weiss. 2003. "Broadening Participation in Community Problem Solving: A Multidisciplinary Model to Support Collaborative Practice and Research." *Journal of Urban Health: Bulletin of the New York Academy of Medicine* 80 (1): 14–47.

Latoszek-Berendsen, A., H. Tange, H. J. van den Herik, and A. Hasman. 2010. "From Clinical Practice Guidelines to Computer-Interpretable Guidelines." *Methods of Information in Medicine* 49 (6): 550–70.

Lattimer, V., S. Brailsford, J. Turnbull, P. Tarnaras, H. Smith, S. George, and S. Maslin-Prothero. 2004. "Reviewing Emergency Care Systems I: Insights from System Dynamics Modeling." *Emergency Medicine Journal* 21 (6): 685–91.

Laurent, M. R., and T. J. Vickers. 2009. "Seeking Health Information Online: Does Wikipedia Matter?" *Journal of the American Medical Informatics Association* 16 (4): 471–79.

Law, A. M., and W. D. Kelton. 1991. *Simulation Modeling and Analysis.* New York: McGraw-Hill, Inc.

Lawler, E. E. III, and S. A. Mohrman. 2003. *Creating a Strategic Human Resource Organization: An Assessment of Trends and New Directions.* Stanford, CA: Stanford University Press.

Ledley, R. S., and L. B. Lusted. 1959a. "Probability, Logic and Medical Diagnosis." *Science* 130 (3380): 892–930.

———. 1959b. "Reasoning Foundations of Medical Diagnosis. Symbolic Logic, Probability, and Value Theory Aid Our Understanding of How Physicians Reason." *Science* 130 (3366): 9–21.

Lee, J., Sr. 2000. "Knowledge Management: The Intellectual Revolution." *HE Solutions* 32 (10): 34–37.

Leggat, S. G., T. Bartram, G. Casimir, and P. Stanton. 2010. "Nurse Perceptions of the Quality of Patient Care: Confirming the Importance of Empowerment and Job Satisfaction." *Health Care Management Review* 35 (4): 355–64.

Lemieux-Charles, L., and F. Champagne. 2004. *Using Knowledge and Evidence in Health Care: Multidisciplinary Perspectives.* Toronto: University of Toronto Press.

Lenhart, A. 2009. "Adults and Social Network Websites." *Pew Internet & American Life Project.* Accessed March 27, 2011. www.pewinternet.org/~/media//Files/Reports/2009/PIP_Adult_social_networking_data_memo_FINAL.pdf.pdf.

———. 2007. "Social Networking Websites and Teens: An Overview." *Pew Internet & American Life Project.* Accessed March 27, 2011. www.pewinternet.org/~/media/Files/Reports/2007/PIP_SNS_Data_Memo_Jan_2007.pdf.pdf.

Lerman, C. E., D. S. Brody, G. C. Caputo, D. G. Smith, C. G. Lazaro, and H. G. Wolfson. 1990. "Patients' Perceived Involvement in Care Scale: Relationship to Attitudes About Illness and Medical Care." *Journal of General Internal Medicine* 5 (1): 29–33.

Leung, R. C. 2012. "Health Information Technology and Dynamic Capabilities." *Health Care Management and Review* 37 (1): 43–53.

Leung, R. C., and K. S. Pasupathy. 2011. "The Economics of Social Computing: Some Preliminary Findings on Healthcare Organizations." *Journal of Computational Science* 2 (3): 253–61.

Library of Congress. 2008. "MARC to Dublin Core Crosswalk." Accessed March 18, 2012. http://loc.gov/marc/marc2dc.html.

Lichtenstein, B. B., and D. A. Plowman. 2009. "The Leadership of Emergence: A Complex Systems Leadership Theory of Emergence at Successive Organizational Levels." *The Leadership Quarterly* 20 (4): 617–30.

Liu, P., B. Raahemi, and M. Benyoucef. 2011. "Knowledge Sharing in Dynamic Virtual Enterprises: A Socio-Technological Perspective." *Knowledge-Based Systems* 24 (3): 427–43.

Lundeen, S., E. Harper, and K. Kerfoot. 2009. "Translating Nursing Knowledge into Practice: An Uncommon Partnership." *Nursing Outlook* 57 (3): 173–75.

Maccoby, M. 2011. "Constructing Collaboration." *Research Technology Management* 54 (1): 59.

Maglio, P. P., and P. L. Mabry. 2011. "Agent-based Models and Systems Science Approaches to Public Health." *American Journal of Preventive Medicine* 40 (3): 392–94.

Maglott, D. R., K. S. Katz, H. Sicotte, and K. D. Pruitt. 2000. "NCBI's LocusLink and RefSeq." *Nucleic Acids Research* 28 (1): 126–28.

Magnier-Watanabe, R., C. Benton, and D. Senoo. 2011. "A Study of Knowledge Management Enablers Across Countries." *Knowledge Management Research and Practice* 9 (1): 17–28.

Maguire, S., and T. Redman. 2007. "The Role of Human Resource Management in Information Systems Development." *Management Decision* 45 (2): 252–64.

Mahesh, K., and J. K. Suresh. 2009. "Knowledge Criteria for Organization Design." *Journal of Knowledge Management* 13 (4): 41–51.

Maiga, A. S., and F. A. Jacobs. 2009. "Performance Impacts of Extent of Information Technology Usage." *Journal of International Technology and Information Management* 18 (3/4): 277–98.

Manolio, T. A., and F. S. Collins. 2009. "The HapMap and Genome-Wide Association Studies in Diagnosis and Therapy." *Annual Review of Medicine* 60: 443–56.

Margolis, P., L. Provost, P. J. Schoettker, and M. T. Britto. 2009. "Quality Improvement, Clinical Research, and Quality Improvement Research— Opportunities for Integration." *Pediatric Clinics of North America* 56 (4): 831–41.

Martimianakis, M. A., J. M. Maniate, and B. D. Hodges. 2009. "Sociological Interpretations of Professionalism." *Medical Education* 43 (9): 829–37.

Martin, S., P. Sutcliffe, F. Griffiths, J. Sturt, J. Powell, and A. Adams. 2011. "Effectiveness and Impact of Networked Communication Interventions in Young People with Mental Health Conditions: A Systematic Review." *Patient Education and Counseling* 85 (2): e108–19.

Martin-Sanchez, F., and I. Hermosilla-Gimeno. 2010. "Translational Bioinformatics." *Studies in Health Technology and Informatics* 151: 312–37.

Martinsons, M. G., and P. K. C. Chong. 1999. "The Influence of Human Factors and Specialist Involvement on Information Systems Success." *Human Relations* 52 (1): 123–52.

Mathieu, J. E., T. S. Heffner, G. F. Goodwin, E. Salas, and J. A. Cannon-Bowers. 2000. "The Influence of Shared Mental Models on Team Process and Performance." *Journal of Applied Psychology* 85 (2): 273–83.

Mayo Clinic. 2012. Center for Innovation. Accessed March 18. http://centerforinnovation.mayo.edu/transform/.

McAfee, A., and E. Brynjolfsson. 2008. "Investing in the IT That Makes a Competitive Difference." *Harvard Business Review* 86 (7/8): 99–107.

McDaniel, A. M., D. L. Schutte, and L. O. Keller. 2008. "Consumer Health Informatics: From Genomics to Population Health." *Nursing Outlook* 56 (5): 216–23.

McDermott, R. 1999. "Why Information Technology Inspired But Cannot Deliver Knowledge Management." *California Management Review* 41 (4): 103–17.

McFedries, P. 2006. "Technically Speaking: It's a Wiki, Wiki World." *Spectrum IEEE* 43 (12): 88.

McKay, H. G., E. G. Feil, R. E. Glasgow, and J. E. Brown. 1998. "Feasibility and Use of an Internet Support Service for Diabetes Self-Management." *Diabetes Education* 24 (2): 174–79.

McMahon, F. J., C. J. Thomas, R. J. Koskela, T. S. Breschel, T. C. Hightower, N. Rohrer, C. Savino, M. G. McInnis, S. G. Simpson, and J. R. DePaulo. 1998. "Integrating Clinical and Laboratory Data in Genetic Studies of Complex Phenotypes: A Network-based Data Management System." *American Journal of Medical Genetics* 81 (3): 248–56.

McNab, C. 2009. "What Social Media Offers to Health Professionals and Citizens." *Bulletin, World Health Organization* 87 (8): 566–67.

Mechanic, D. 2008. "Rethinking Medical Professionalism: The Role of Information Technology and Practice Innovations." *Milbank Quarterly* 86 (2): 327–58.

Medicomp Systems, Inc. 2004. "MEDCIN." *Medicomp Systems*. Cited September 29, 2008. www.medicomp.com.

Medina-Borja, A., and K. Pasupathy. 2007. "Uncovering Complex Relationships in System Dynamics Modeling: Exploring the Use of CHAID and CART." Proceedings of the System Dynamics Conference, Boston, August.

Melville, N., K. Kraemer, and V. Gurbaxani. 2004. "Information Technology and Organizational Performance: An Integrative Model of IT Business Value." *MIS Quarterly* 28 (2): 283–322.

Mercer, J. 2007. "Wikipedia and 'Open Source' Mental Health Information." *The Scientific Review of Mental Health Practice* 5 (1): 88–92.

Metzger, J., E. Welebob, D. W. Bates, S. Lipsitz, and D. C. Classen. 2010. "Mixed Results in the Safety Performance of Computerized Physician Order Entry." *Health Affairs* 29 (4): 655–63.

Middleton, B., and J. Janas, III. 2008. "Identifying and Understanding Business Processes in Clinical Practice." In *Electronic Health Records: A Guide for Clinicians and Administrators,* 2nd edition, by J. Carter, 143–67. Philadelphia: ACP Press.

Milardo, R. M. 2000. "Family and Social Network." *Journal of Marriage and the Family* 62 (3): 861–63.

Miles, R. 2011. "Lessons Learned, Ignored, Forgotten, and Reborn: Organizations and Management 1960 to Today." *Journal of Management Inquiry* 20 (1): 4–7.

Miles, R. E., and C. C. Snow. 1978. *Organizational Strategy, Structure and Process.* New York: McGraw Hill.

Miller, J., and J. Wechsler. 2011. "Private Market ACOs." *Managed Healthcare Executive* 21 (12): 22–29.

Mintzberg, H. 1979. *The Structuring of Organizations.* Englewood Cliffs, NJ: Prentice-Hall.

Mitchell, S. M., and S. M. Shortell. 2000. "The Governance and Management of Effective Community Health Partnerships: A Typology for Research, Policy and Practice." *Milbank Quarterly* 78 (2): 241–89.

Mooney, B. L., and A. M. Boyle. 2011. "10 Steps to Successful EHR Implementation." *Medical Economics* 88 (9): S4–S6, S8–S11.

Moore, J. H. 2007. "Bioinformatics." *Journal of Cellular Physiology* 213 (2): 365–69.

Moreno, M. A., M. R. Parks, F. J. Zimmerman, T. E. Brito, and D. A. Christakis. 2009. "Display of Health Risk Behaviors on MySpace by Adolescents: Prevalence and Associations." *Archives of Pediatrics and Adolescent Medicine* 163 (1): 27–34.

Morlion, B., C. Knoop, M. Paiva, and M. Estenne. 2002. "Internet-based Home Monitoring of Pulmonary Function After Lung Transplantation." *American Journal of Respiratory and Critical Care Medicine* 165 (5): 694–97.

Morris, A. H. 2002. "Decision Support and Safety of Clinical Environments." *Quality and Safety in Health Care* 11 (1): 69–75.

Murphy, J., E. Harper, E. Devine, L. Burke, and M. Hook. 2010. "Case Study: Lessons Learned When Embedding Evidence-Based Knowledge in a Nurse Care Planning and Documentation System." In *Evidence-based Practice in*

Nursing Informatics: Concepts and Applications, by A. Cashin and R. Cook, 174–90. Hershey, PA: IGI Global.

Murray, M., and D. M. Berwick. 2003. "Advanced Access, Reducing Waiting and Delays in Primary Care." *JAMA* 289 (8): 1035–40.

Muzio, D., S. Ackroyd, and J. F. Chanlat. 2008. *Redirections in the Study of Expert Labour.* New York: Palgrave MacMillan.

Muzio, D., and I. Kirkpatrick. 2011. "Professions and Organizations: A Conceptual Framework." *Current Sociology* 59 (4): 389–405.

Naditz, A. 2008. "Medicare's and Medicaid's New Reimbursement Policies for Telemedicine." *Telemedicine Journal and E-Health* 14 (1): 21–24.

Nakata, C., Z. Zhu, and M. L. Kraimer. 2009. "The Complex Contribution of Information Technology Capability to Business Performance." *Journal of Managerial Issues* 20 (4): 485–506.

National Alliance for Health Information Technology. 2008. "Defining Key Health Information Technology Terms." Accessed May 17, 2012. www.nahit.org/ images/pdfs/HITTermsFinalReport_051508.pdf.

National Cancer Institute. 2010. *Cancer Data Standards Registry and Repository (caDSR).* Accessed June 7, 2011. https://cabig.nci.nih.gov/concepts/ caDSR/.

National Center for Healthcare Leadership (NCHL). 2011. "Health Leadership Competency Model: Summary." Accessed May 20. http://nchl.org/static .asp?path=2852,3238.

National Center for Health Statistics (NCHS). 2011. *International Classification of Diseases, 10th Revision, Clinical Modification (ICD-10-CM).* Atlanta: Centers for Disease Control and Prevention.

National Information Standards Organization. 2005. *Guidelines for the Construction, Format, and Management of Monolingual Controlled Vocabularies.* Bethesda, MD: NISO Press.

National Library of Medicine. 2011. *PubMed.* Accessed June 7. www.ncbi.nlm.nih .gov/pubmed/.

———. 2010a. *Introduction to MeSH—2011.* Accessed June 6, 2011. www.nlm.nih .gov/mesh/introduction.html.

———. 2010b. MeSH Browser. Accessed June 7, 2011. www.nlm.nih.gov/ mesh/2011/mesh_browser/MBrowser.html.

———. 2009. *UMLS Reference Manual.* Bethesda, MD: National Library of Medicine.

Nelson, G. S. 2010. "The Healthcare Performance Dashboard: Linking Strategy to Metrics." SAS Global Forum, April 11–14, Seattle, Washington.

Nonaka, I., and H. Takeuchi. 1995. *The Knowledge Creating Company.* New York: Oxford University Press.

Noordegraaf, M. 2011. "Remaking Professionals? How Associations and Professional Education Connect Professionalism and Organizations." *Current Sociology* 59 (4): 465–88.

North, M. 2009. "The Hippocratic Oath." *National Library of Medicine, National Institutes of Health.* Accessed February 2. www.nlm.nih.gov/hmd/greek/greek_oath.html.

Noy, F. N., D. L. Rubin, and M. A. Musen. 2004. "Making Biomedical Ontologies and Ontology Repositories Work." *IEEE Intelligent Systems* 19 (6): 78–81.

O'Conaill, B., and S. Whittaker. 1997. "Characterizing, Predicting, and Measuring Video-Mediated Communication: A Conversational Approach." In *Video Mediated Communication,* edited by K. E. Finn, A. J. Sellen, and S. B. Wilbur, 107–31. Mahwah, NJ: Lawrence Erlbaum.

O'Connor, K. 2002. "What Every CIO Should Know About Technology Contracting." *Annual HIMSS Conference Proceedings: Educational Sessions,* Session 76.

Office of the National Coordinator for Health Information Technology (ONC). 2011. "Electronic Health Records and Meaningful Use." Accessed June 10. http://healthit.hhs.gov/portal/server.pt?open=512andobjID=2996andmode=2.

———. 2008. *Nationwide Privacy and Security Framework for Electronic Exchange of Individually Identifiable Health Information.* Washington, DC: Office of the National Coordinator for Health Information Technology.

Oliver, D. P., and G. Demiris. 2010. "Comparing Face-to-Face and Telehealth-Mediated Delivery of a Psychoeducational Intervention: A Case Comparison Study in Hospice." *Telemedicine and e-Health* 16 (6): 751–53.

O'Malley, A. S., J. M. Grossman, G. R. Cohen, N. M. Kemper, and H. H. Pham. 2009. "Are Electronic Medical Records Helpful for Care Coordination? Experiences of Physician Practices." *Journal of General Internal Medicine* 25 (3): 177–85.

O'Neil, E. H., and the Pew Health Professions Commission. 1998. *Recreating Health Professional Practice for a New Century: The Fourth Report of the Pew Health Professions Commission.* San Francisco: Pew Health Professions Commission.

Organisation for Economic Co-operation and Development (OECD). 1980. "Guidelines on the Protection of Privacy and Transborder Flows of Personal Data." September 23, 1980. *OECD.* Accessed March 1, 2012. www.oecd.org/document/20/0,3746,en_2649_34255_15589524_1_1_1_1,00.html.

Orsini, M. 2010. "Social Media: How Home Health Care Agencies Can Join the Chorus of Empowered Voices." *Home Health Care Management and Practice* 22 (3): 213–17.

Osheroff, J. A., D. E. Forsythe, B. G. Buchanan, R. A. Bankowitz, B. H. Blumenfeld, and R. A. Miller. 1991. "Physicians' Information Needs: Analysis of

Questions Posed During Clinical Teaching." *Annals of Internal Medicine* 114 (7): 576–81.

Ozdemir, Z., J. Barron, and S. Bandyopadhyay. 2011. "An Analysis of Adoption of Digital Health Records Under Switching Costs." *Information Systems Research* 22 (3): 491–503.

Paez, J. G., P. A. Janne, J. C. Lee, S. Tracy, H. Greulich, S. Gabriel, P. Herman, F. J. Kaye, N. Lindeman, T. J. Boggon, K. Naoki, H. Sasaki, Y. Fujii, M. J. Eck, W. R. Sellers, B. E. Johnson, and M. Meyerson. 2004. "EGFR Mutations in Lung Cancer: Correlation with Clinical Response to Gefitinib Therapy." *Science* 304: 1497–500.

Pamela, W., and B. Lorraine. 2007. "Private Payer Reimbursement for Telemedicine Services in the United States." *Telemedicine Journal and E-Health* 13 (1): 15–23.

Pare, G. 2002. "Implementing Clinical Information Systems: A Multiple-Case Study Within a US Hospital." *Health Services Management Research* 15 (2): 71–92.

Parente, S. T. 2009. "Health Information Technology and Financing's Next Frontier: The Potential of Medical Banking." *Business Economics* 44 (1): 41–51.

Parton, R., and R. Subbu. 2012. "ACO Rule Has Big Implications for IT." *Health Management Technology* 33 (4): 12–15.

Pasupathy, K. 2010. "Transforming Healthcare: Leveraging the Complementarities of Health Informatics and Systems Engineering." *International Journal of Healthcare Delivery Reform Initiatives* 2 (2): 34–54.

Patil, R. 1981. "Causal Representation of Patient Illness for Electrolyte and Acid-Base Diagnosis." Unpublished thesis, Massachusetts Institute of Technology.

Pavlou, P. A., and O. A. El Sawy. 2010. "The 'Third Hand': IT-Enabled Competitive Advantage in Turbulence Through Improvisational Capabilities." *Information Systems Research* 21 (3): 443–71.

Pearlson, K. E. 2001. *Managing and Using Information Systems: A Strategic Approach.* New York: Wiley.

Pince, H., R. Verberckmoes, and J. L. Willems. 1990. "Computer Aided Interpretation of Acid-base Disorders." *International Journal of Biomedical Computing* 25 (2–3): 177–92.

Pollak, A. 2012. "Growth and Convergence When Technology and Human Capital Are Complements." *Economic Enquiry.* Online version available at http://onlinelibrary.wiley.com/doi/10.1111/j.1465-7295.2012.00454.x/abstract.

Potash, D. L. 2011. "Accountable Clinical Management: An Integrated Approach." *Healthcare Financial Management* 65 (10): 94–98.

Powell, T. C., and A. Dent-Micallef. 1997. "Information Technology as Competitive Advantage: The Role of Human, Business, and Technology Resources." *Strategic Management Journal* 18 (2): 375–405.

Pratt, W., K. Unruh, A. Civan, and M. Skeels. 2006. "Personal Health Information Management." *Communications of the ACM* 49 (1): 51–55.

President's Council of Advisors on Science and Technology. 2010. *Report to the President Realizing the Full Potential of Health Information Technology to Improve Healthcare for Americans: The Path Forward.* Washington, DC: President's Council of Advisors on Science and Technology.

ProQuest Information and Learning. 2011. *AB/INFORM.* Ann Arbor, MI: ProQuest.

Pruitt, K. D., and D. R. Maglott. 2001. "RefSeq and LocusLink: NCBI Gene-Centered Resources." *Nucleic Acids Research* 29 (1): 137–40.

Quadagno, J. 2010. "Institutions, Interest Groups, and Ideology: An Agenda for the Sociology of Health Care Reform." *Journal of Health and Social Behavior* 51 (2): 125–36.

Raghuram, S., P. Tuertscher, and R. Garud. 2010. "Mapping the Field of Virtual Work: A Cocitation Analysis." *Information Systems Research* 21 (4): 983–99.

Rajnish, K. R. 2011. "Knowledge Management and Organizational Culture: A Theoretical Integrative Framework." *Journal of Knowledge Management* 15 (5): 779–801.

Ramnarayan, P., A. Tomlinson, G. Kulkarni, A. Rao, and J. Britto. 2004. "A Novel Diagnostic Aid (ISABEL): Development and Preliminary Evaluation of Clinical Performance." *Studies in Health Technology and Informatics* 107 (Pt 2): 1091–95.

RAND Compare. 2012. "Overview of Bundled Payment: Increase the Use of 'Bundled' Payment Approaches." Accessed March 21. www.randcompare.org/policy-options/bundled-payment.

Ray, G., J. B. Barney, and W. A. Muhanna. 2004. "Capabilities, Business Processes, and Competitive Advantage: Choosing the Dependent Variable in Empirical Tests of the Resource-based View." *Strategic Management Journal* 25 (1): 23–37.

Real, K. 2010. "Health-Related Organizational Communication: A General Platform for Interdisciplinary Research." *Management Communication Quarterly* 24 (3): 457–64.

Reich, J., F. Zhao, and J. Shin. 2002. "Information-Driven Dynamic Sensor Collaboration." *IEEE Signal Processing Magazine* 19 (2): 61–72.

Riva, A., R. Bellazzi, and M. Stefanelli. 1997. "A Web-based System for the Intelligent Management of Diabetic Patients." *M.D. Computing: Computers in Medical Practice* 14 (5): 360–64.

Robertson, M., and G. O. Hammersley. 2000. "Knowledge Management Practices within a Knowledge-Intensive Firm: The Significance of the People Management Dimension." *Journal of European Industrial Training* 24 (2/3/4): 241–54.

Robey, D., M. C. Boudreau, and G. M. Rose. 2000. "Information Technology and Organizational Learning: A Review and Assessment of Research." *Accounting Management and Information Technologies* 10 (2): 125–55.

Roehling, M. V., and P. M. Wright. 2006. "Organizationally Sensible Versus Legal-Centric Approaches to Employment Decisions." *Human Resource Management* 45 (4): 605–27.

Ross, J. W. 2003. "Creating a Strategic IT Architecture Competency: Learning in Stages." MIT Sloan School of Management, Working Paper No 4314-03. Cambridge, MA: Massachusetts Institute of Technology.

Ross, J. W., C. M. Beath, and D. L. Goodhue. 1996. "Develop Long-term Competitiveness Through IT Assets." *Sloan Management Review* 38 (1): 31–45.

Rothschild, S. K., S. Lapidos, A. Minnick, L. Fogg, and C. Catrambone. 2004. "Using Virtual Teams to Improve the Care of Chronically Ill Patients." *Journal of Clinical Outcomes Management* 11 (6): 346–50.

Rozental, T. D., T. M. George, and A. T. Chacko. 2010. "Social Networking Among Upper Extremity Patients." *The Journal of Hand Surgery* 35 (5): 819–23.

Rubin, R. J., K. A. Dietrich, and A. D. Hawk. 1998. "Clinical and Economic Impact of Implementing a Comprehensive Diabetes Management Program in Managed Care." *The Journal of Clinical Endocrinology and Metabolism* 83 (8): 2635–642.

Ruona, W. E. A., and S. K. Gibson. 2004. "The Making of Twenty-First-Century HR: An Analysis of the Convergence of HRM, HRD, and OD." *Human Resource Management* 43 (1): 49–66.

Russell, K. 2010. "SMI Supply Chain Leaders Focus on Transformation." *Healthcare Purchasing News* 34 (1): 48.

Sachs, M. A. 2005. "Transforming the Health System from the Inside Out." *Frontiers of Health Services Management* 22 (2): 3–12.

Sackett, D. L., W. Rosenberg, J. A. Frau, R. B. Haynes, and W. S. Richardson. 1996. "Evidence-based Medicine: What It Is and What It Isn't." *British Medical Journal* 312: 71–72.

Sarkar, I. N., A. J. Butte, Y. A. Lussier, P. Tarczy-Hornoch, and L. Ohno-Machado. 2011. "Translational Bioinformatics: Linking Knowledge Across Biological and Clinical Realms." *Journal of the American Medical Informatics Association* 18 (4): 354 –57.

Sauer, C., and L. P. Willcocks. 2002. "The Evolution of Organizational Architecture." *Sloan Management Review* 43 (3): 41–49.

Scanfeld, D., V. Scanfeld, and E. L. Larson. 2010. "Dissemination of Health Information Through Social Networks: Twitter and Antibiotics." *American Journal of Infection Control* 38 (3): 182–88.

Schaefer, A. J., M. D. Bailey, S. M. Shechter, and M. S. Roberts. 2004. "Medical Treatment Decisions Using Markov Decision Processes." In *Operations*

Research and Health Care: A Handbook of Methods and Applications, edited by M. L. Brandeau, F. Sainfort, and W. P. Pierskalla, 595–614. Boston: Kluwer Academic Publishers.

Schneider, B., and S. S. White. 2004. *Service Quality: Research Perspectives.* Thousand Oaks, CA: Sage Publications.

Schopp, L. H., J. W. Hales, J. L. Quetsch, M. J. Hauan, and G. D. Brown. 2004. "Design of a Peer-to-Peer Telerehabilitation Model." *Telemedicine Journal and E-Health* 10 (2): 243–51.

Scott, W. R., M. Ruef, P. J. Mendel, and C. A. Caronna. 2000. *Institutional Change and Healthcare Organizations: From Professional Dominance to Managed Care.* Chicago: The University of Chicago Press.

Sear, N. 2011. "Healthcare Reform: Aligning Clinicians and Supply Chain." *Healthcare Purchasing News* 34 (3): 70.

Segars, A. H., and V. Grover. 1998. "Strategic Information Systems Planning and Success: An Investigation of the Construct and Its Measurement." *MIS Quarterly* 22 (2): 139–63.

Selznick, P. 1992. *The Moral Commonwealth: Social Theory and the Promise of Community.* Berkeley, CA: University of California Press.

Senge, P. M. 1990. *The Fifth Discipline.* New York, NY: Currency Doubleday.

Sharp, J. W. 2011. *Desert Food Chain: The Insects, Part 12.* Accessed June 7. www.desertusa.com/mag06/jan/food12.html.

Shaw, J. 2005. "Managing All of Your Enterprise's Risks." *Risk Management* 52 (9): 22–29.

Shea, S., R. S. Weinstock, J. A. Teresi, W. Palmas, J. Starren, J. J. Cimino, A. M. Lai, L. Field, P. C. Morin, R. Goland, R. E. Izquierdo, S. Ebner, S. Silver, E. Petkova, J. Kong, and J. P. Eimicke. 2009. "A Randomized Trial Comparing Telemedicine Case Management with Usual Care in Older, Ethnically Diverse, Medically Underserved Patients with Diabetes Mellitus: 5 Year Results of the IDEATel Study." *Journal of the American Medical Informatics Association* 16 (4): 446–56.

Sherry, S. T., M. H. Ward, M. Kholodov, J. Baker, L. Phan, E. M. Smigielski, and K. Sirotkin. 2001. "dbSNP: The NCBI Database of Genetic Variation." *Nucleic Acids Research* 29 (1): 308–11.

Shimshak, D. G., D. Gropp Damico, and H. D. Burden. 1981. "A Priority Queuing Model of a Hospital Pharmacy Unit." *European Journal of Operational Research* 7 (4): 350–54.

Shortliffe, E. H. 2005. "Strategic Action in Health Information Technology: Why the Obvious Has Taken So Long." *Health Affairs* 24 (5): 1222–33.

———. 1976. *Computer-based Medical Consultations: MYCIN.* New York: Elsevier.

Shortliffe, E. H., and E. J. Sondik. 2006. "The Public Health Informatics Infrastructure: Anticipating Its Role in Cancer." *Cancer Causes and Control: CCC* 17 (7): 861–69.

Shu-Mei, T. 2010. "The Correlation Between Organizational Culture and Knowledge Conversion on Corporate Performance." *Journal of Knowledge Management* 14 (2): 269–84.

Silvert, W. 2001. "Modeling As a Discipline." *International Journal of General Systems* 30 (3): 261–82.

Sinnett, W. M. 2012. "In the Cloud and Beyond." *Financial Executive* 28 (1): 48–51.

Sittig, D. F., A. Wright, J. A. Osheroff, B. Middleton, J. M. Teich, J. S. Ash, and D. W. Bates. 2008. "Grand Challenges in Clinical Decision Support." *Journal of Biomedical Informatics* 41 (2): 387–92.

Skeels, M. M., K. T. Unruh, C. Powell, and W. Pratt. 2010. "Catalyzing Social Support for Breast Cancer Patients." Paper presented at the Proceedings of the 28th International Conference on Human Factors in Computing Systems, April 10–15.

Smith, H. L., W. I. Buller, Jr., and N. F. Piland. 2000. "Does Information Technology Make a Difference in Healthcare Organization Performance? A Multiyear Study." *Hospital Topics* 78 (2): 13–22.

Smith, B. K., H. Nachtmann, and E. A. Pohl. 2011. "Quality Measurement in the Healthcare Supply Chain." *Quality Management Journal* 18 (4): 50–60.

Smith, P., and R. Peck. 2010. "Beyond Genetics, Stratified and Personalized in Medicine Using Multiple Parameters." *Pharmaceuticals* 3 (5): 1637–51.

Smith, C. A., and P. J. Wicks. 2008. "PatientsLikeMe: Consumer Health Vocabulary as a Folksonomy." In *AMIA Annual Symposium Proceedings, Volume 2008*, 682–86. Bethesda, MD: AMIA.

Sonnad, S. S. 1998. "Organizational Tactics for the Successful Assimilation of Medical Practice Guidelines." *Health Care Management Review* 23 (3): 30–37.

Spetz, J., and D. Keane. 2009 "Information Technology Implementation in a Rural Hospital: A Cautionary Tale." *Journal of Healthcare Management* 54 (5): 337–47.

Staggers, N., C. A. Gassert, and D. J. Skiba. 2000. "Health Professionals Views of Informatics Education." *Journal of the American Medical Informatics Association* 76 (6): 550–58.

Starr, P. 1984. *The Social Transformation of American Medicine.* New York: Basic Books.

Stead, W. W. 2005. *Challenges in Informatics. Building a Better Delivery System: A New Engineering/Health Care Partnership*, 193–94. National Academy of Engineering and Institute of Medicine. Washington, DC: National Academies Press.

Stein, L. 2003. "Bioinformatics: Gone in 2012." The O'Reilly Bioinformatics Technology Conference, February 3–6.

Sterman, J. D. 2002. "All Models Are Wrong: Reflections on Becoming a Systems Scientist." *System Dynamics Review* 18: 501–31.

———. 2000. *Business Dynamics, System Thinking and Modeling for a Complex World*. New York: Irwin McGraw-Hill.

Stone, T. T., and G. D. Brown. 2005. "Information Strategy Related to Enterprise and Organizational Strategies." In *Strategic Management of Information Systems in Healthcare*, by G. D. Brown, T. T. Stone, and T. B. Patrick, 31–50. Chicago: Health Administration Press.

Strange, K. C., R. L. Ferrer, and W. L. Miller. 2009. "Making Sense of Health Care Transformation as Adaptive-Renewal Cycles." *Annals of Family Medicine* (7): 484–87.

Street, R. L. 1992. "Communicative Styles and Adaptations in Physician–Parent Consultations." *Social Science and Medicine* 34 (10): 1155–163.

Stronge, A. J., W. A. Rogers, and A. D. Fisk. 2007. "Human Factors Considerations in Implementing Telemedicine Systems to Accommodate Older Adults." *Journal of Telemedicine and Telecare* 13 (1): 1–3.

Suntharalingam, G., J. Cousins, D. Gattas, and M. Chapman. 2005. "Scanning the Horizon: Emerging Hospital-wide Technologies and Their Impact on Critical Care." *Critical Care* 9 (1): 12–15.

Swan, M. 2009. "Emerging Patient-driven Health Care Models: An Examination of Health Social Networks, Consumer Personalized Medicine and Quantified Self-Tracking." *International Journal of Environmental Research and Public Health* 6 (2): 492–525.

Swisher, J. R., S. H. Jacobson, J. B. Jun, and O. Balci. 2001. "Modeling and Analyzing a Physician Clinic Environment Using Discrete-Event (Visual) Simulation." *Computers and Operations Research* 28 (2): 105–25.

Tan, J., H. J. Wen, and N. Awad. 2005. "Health Care and Services Delivery Systems as Complex Adaptive Systems." *Communications of the ACM* 48 (5): 36–45.

Tataw, D. 2012. "Toward Human Resource Management in Inter-Professional Health Practice: Linking Organizational Culture, Group Identity and Individual Autonomy." *International Journal of Health Planning and Management*. Online version available at http://onlinelibrary.wiley.com/doi/10.1002/hpm.2098/abstract.

Taylor, K., and B. Dangerfield. 2005. "Modeling the Feedback Effects of Reconfiguring Health Services." *The Journal of the Operational Research Society* 56: 659–75.

Teece, D. J. 2007. "Explicating Dynamic Capabilities: The Nature and Microfoundations of (Sustainable) Enterprise Performance." *Strategic Management Journal* 28 (13): 1319–50.

Teece, D. J., G. Pisano, and A. Shuen. 1997. "Dynamic Capabilities and Strategic Management." *Strategic Management Journal* 18 (7): 509–33.

Terry, N. P. 2000. "Structural and Legal Implications of E-Health." *Journal of Health Law* 33 (4): 605–14.

Theodoridis, S., and K. Koutroumbas. 2009. *Pattern Recognition*. London: Academic Press.

Thomas, J. C., W. A. Kellogg, and T. Erickson. 2001. "The Knowledge Management Puzzle: Human and Social Factors in Knowledge Management." *IBM Systems Journal* 40 (4): 863–84.

Tierney, W. M., M. E. Miller, J. M. Overhage, and C. J. McDonald. 1993. "Physician Inpatient Order Writing on Microcomputer Workstations. Effects on Resource Utilization." *JAMA* 269 (3): 379–83.

Timmons, S. 2011. "Professionalization and its Discontents." *Health* 15 (4): 337–52.

Toffler, A. 1984. *The Third Wave*. New York: Bantam Books.

Tresolini, C. P., and the Pew-Fetzer Task Force. 1994. *Health Professions Education and Relationship-centered Care*. San Francisco: Pew Health Professions Commission.

Tricoci, P., J. M. Allen, J. M. Kramer, R. M. Califf, and S. C. Smith, Jr. 2009. "Scientific Evidence Underlying the ACC/AHA Clinical Practice Guidelines." *JAMA* 301 (8): 831–41.

Trivedi, M. H., E. J. Daly, J. K. Kern, B. D. Grannemann, P. Sunderajan, and C. A. Claassen. 2009. "Barriers to Implementation of a Computerized Decision Support System for Depression: An Observational Report on Lessons Learned in 'Real World' Clinical Settings." *BMC Medical Informatics and Decision Making* 9: 6.

Tsai, C. C., S. H. Tsai, Q. Zeng-Treitler, and B. A. Liang. 2007. "Patient-Centered Consumer Health Social Network Websites: A Pilot Study of Quality of User-Generated Health Information." In *AMIA Annual Symposium Proceedings, Volume 2007*, 1137. Accessed May 17, 2012. www.healthcare integrationadvisors.com/files/CMS%20Telemedicine%20Final%20Rule%20 %2800495611%29.PDF.

Tseng, S.-M. 2011. "The Effects of Hierarchical Culture on Knowledge Management Processes." *Management Research Review* 34 (5): 595–608.

Tufts Clinical and Translational Science Institute (CTSI). 2012. "What Is Translational Science?" Accessed April 7. www.tuftsctsi.org/About-Us/What-is-Translational-Science.aspx.

Tyson, P. 2001. "Hippocratic Oath Today." *NOVA*. Accessed March 16, 2012. www.pbs.org/wgbh/nova/body/hippocratic-oath-today.html.

US Congress. 2010. *Public Law 111-148, Patient Protection and Affordable Care Act (PPACA), 111th Congress, March 23, 2010*. Accessed March 6, 2012. www.gpo.gov/fdsys/pkg/PLAW-111publ148/pdf/PLAW-111publ148.pdf.

———. 2001. "Standards for Privacy of Individually Identifiable Health Information." 45 CFR Parts 160 and 164, April 14, 2001. Accessed March 1, 2012. http://aspe.hhs.gov/admnsimp/final/pvcguide1.htm.

———. 1974. "The Privacy Act of 1974." 5 U.S.C. 552a. Accessed March 1, 2012. www.justice.gov/opcl/privstat.htm.

US Department of Health and Human Services (HHS). 2012. *Notice of Proposed Rulemaking to Implement HITECH Act Modifications*. Accessed March 6. www.hhs.gov/ocr/privacy/hipaa/understanding/coveredentities/hitech-nprm.html.

———. 2010. "Health Information Technology: Initial Set of Standards, Implementation Specifications, and Certification Criteria for Electronic Health Record Technology; Final Rule." *Federal Register,* July 28.

———. 2009. *Information Technology for Economic and Clinical Health Act of 2009.* Accessed March 1. www.hhs.gov/ocr/privacy/hipaa/administrative/enforcementrule/hitechenforcementifr.html.

———. 2003. "Health Insurance Reform: Security Standards; Final Rule." 45 CFR Parts 160, 162, and 164 (SecRule 2003). *Federal Register* 68 (34).

———. 2000. *Final Privacy Rule Preamble.* Accessed March 27, 2011. http://aspe.hhs.gov/admnsimp/final/PvcPre01.htm.

US Department of Health and Human Services and Centers for Medicare and Medicaid Services (HHS and CMS). 2011. *CMS Telemedicine Final Rule.* Accessed May 17, 2012. www.healthcareintegrationadvisors.com/files/CMS%20Telemedicine%20Final%20Rule%20%2800495611%29.PDF.

US Department of Health, Education, and Welfare (HEW), Secretary's Advisory Committee on Automated Personal Data Systems (Code 1973). 1973. *Records, Computers, and the Rights of Citizens.* Accessed March 1, 2012. http://aspe.hhs.gov/DATACNCL/1973privacy/tocprefacemembers.htm.

US Department of Veterans Affairs. 2012. "My HealtheVet." Accessed May 17. www.myhealth.va.gov.

US Federal Trade Commission (FTC). 2007. "Fair Information Practice Principles." *Federal Trade Commission.* Accessed March 1, 2012. www.ftc.gov/reports/privacy3/fairinfo.shtm.

———. 1998. "Privacy Online: A Report to Congress." *Federal Trade Commission.* Accessed March 1, 2012. www.ftc.gov/reports/privacy3/toc.shtm.

US Supreme Court. 1928. *Olmstead v. U.S.* 277 U.S. 438. June 4, 1928. Dissenting opinion from Justice Louis Brandeis.

Vaccaro, A., F. Veloso, and S. Brusoni. 2009. "The Impact of Virtual Technologies on Knowledge-based Processes: An Empirical Study." *Research Policy* 38 (8): 1278–87.

Van de Ven, A., R. C. Leung, J. P. Bechara, and K. Sun. 2012. "Changing Organizational Designs and Performance Frontiers." *Organization Science* [forthcoming in 2012].

Venter J. C., et al. 2001. "The Sequence of the Human Genome." *Science* 291 (5507): 1304–51.

Verner, J., S. Overmyer, and K. McCain. 1999. "In the 25 Years Since the Mythical Man-Month What Have We Learned About Project Management?" *Information and Software Technology* 41: 1021–26.

Vest, J. R. 2009. "Health Information Exchange and Healthcare Utilization." *Journal of Medical Systems* 33 (3): 223–31.

Violino, B. 2009. "Analyze This." *Baseline Magazine.* Accessed May 20, 2012. www.baselinemag.com/c/a/Business-Intelligence/Analyze-This/.

Von Nortdenflycht, A. 2010. "What Is a Professional Service Firm? Toward a Theory and Taxonomy of Knowledge-Intensive Firms." *Academy of Management Review* 35 (1): 155–74.

Weiner, B. J., L. A. Savitz, S. Bernard, and L. G. Pucci. 2004. "How Do Integrated Delivery Systems Adopt and Implement Clinical Information Systems?" *Health Care Management Review* 29 (1): 51–66.

Weiss, J. B., and N. M. Lorenzi. 2007. "Challenges of Social Networking Technologies for Cancer Care and Social Support." In *AMIA Annual Symposium Proceedings, Volume 2007,* 1151. Bethesda, MD: AMIA.

Weiss, J. W., and A. Thorogood. 2011. "Information Technology (IT)/Business Alignment as a Strategic Weapon: A Diagnostic Tool." *Engineering Management Journal* 23 (2): 30–42.

Wells, J. D., and D. H. Gobeli. 2003. "The 3R Framework: Improving E-Strategy Across Reach, Richness and Range." *Business Horizons* 46 (2): 5–15.

White, J. A., and G. Wehlage. 1995. "Community Collaboration: If It Is Such a Good Idea, Why Is It So Hard To Do?" *Educational Evaluation and Policy Analysis* 17 (1): 23–38.

Wickramasinghe, N., R. K. Bali, B. Lehaney, J. L. Schaffer, and C. M. Gibbons. 2008. *Healthcare Knowledge Management Primer.* New York and London: Routledge, Taylor and Francis Group.

Wicks, P., M. Massagli, J. Frost, C. Brownstein, S. Okun, T. Vaughan, R. Bradley, and J. Heywood. 2010. "Sharing Health Data for Better Outcomes on PatientsLikeMe." *Journal of Medical Internet Research* 12 (2): e19.

Wilson, K., and J. Keelan. 2009. "Coping with Public Health 2.0." *Canadian Medical Association Journal* 180 (10): 1080.

Witten, I. H., and E. Frank. 2005. *Data Mining: Practical Machine Learning Tools and Techniques.* San Francisco: Morgan Kaufmann.

World Health Organization. 2012. *International Classification of Diseases.* Accessed March 6. www.who.int/classifications/icd/en.

———. 2007. *International Statistical Classification of Diseases and Related Health Problems, 10th Revision,* Version for 2007. Accessed June 13, 2011. http://apps.who.int/classifications/apps/icd/icd10online/.

Wright, A., and D. F. Sittig. 2008. "A Four-Phase Model of the Evolution of Clinical Decision Support Architectures." *International Journal of Medical Informatics* 77 (10): 641–49.

Wright, A., D. F. Sittig, J. S. Ash, J. Feblowitz, S. Meltzer, C. McMullen, and B. Middleton. 2011. "Development and Evaluation of a Comprehensive Clinical Decision Support Taxonomy: Comparison of Front-End Tools in Commercial and Internally Developed Electronic Health Record Systems." *Journal of the American Medical Informatics Association* 18 (3): 232–42.

Yahoo! 2011. "Smartphone Health Apps Are Changing Health Care." *Yahoo Voices.* Published March 16. www.associatedcontent.com/article/7821236/smartphone_health_apps_are_changing.html?cat=15.

Yang, H., W. Li, K. Liu, and J. Zhang. 2012. "Knowledge-based Clinical Pathway for Medical Quality Improvement." *Information Systems Frontiers* 14 (1): 105–17.

Yeager, T., and P. Sorensen. 2006. "Strategic Organization Development: Past to Present." *Organization Development Journal* 24 (4): 10–17.

Yeh, C. H., G. G. Lee, and J. C. Pai. 2012. "How Information System Capability Affects E-Business Information Technology Strategy Implementation: An Empirical Study in Taiwan." *Business Process Management Journal* 18 (2): 197–218.

Yokota, F., and K. M. Thompson. 2004. "Value of Information Literature Analysis: A Review of Applications in Health Risk Management." *Medical Decision Making* 24 (3): 287–98.

Youndt, M. A., and S. A. Snell. 2004. "Human Resource Configurations, Intellectual Capital, and Organizational Performance." *Journal of Managerial Issues* 16 (3): 337–60.

Young, S. D., and E. Rice. 2011. "Online Social Networking Technologies, HIV Knowledge, and Sexual Risk and Testing Behaviors Among Homeless Youth." *AIDS Behavior* 15 (2): 253–60.

Zammuto, R. F., T. L. Griffith, A. Majchrzak, D. J. Dougherty, and S. Faraj. 2007. "Information Technology and the Changing Fabric of Organization." *Organization Science* 18 (5): 749–62.

Zander, K. 1992. *Critical Pathways: Total Quality Management,* 305–15. Chicago: American Hospital Association Publishing.

Zarraga, C., and J. Bonache. 2005. "The Impact of Team Atmosphere on Knowledge Outcomes in Self-Managed Teams." *Organization Studies* 26 (5): 661–81.

Zhang, B., and K. Pasupathy. 2009. "Integration of Simulation Modeling Into Hospital Pharmacy Delivery Network Planning." INFORMS, Conference Proceedings, San Diego.

Zhang, J., and M. F. Walji. 2011. "TURF: A Unified Framework for Defining, Evaluating, Measuring, and Designing EHR Usability." *Journal of Biomedical Informatics* 44 (6): 1056–67.

Zhao, Y., A. S. Ash, J. Haughton, and B. McMillan. 2003. "Identifying Future High-Cost Cases Through Predictive Modeling." *Disease Management and Health Outcomes* 11 (6): 389–97.

Zoe, J., and A. Court. 2010. "Reconstructing Consumer Participation in Evidence-based Health Care: A Polemic." *International Journal of Consumer Studies* 34 (5): 558.

Zolkos, R. 2000. "Insurers Stymied in Managing Enterprise Risk." *Business Insurance* 34 (16): 1–2.

INDEX

ABOUT THE EDITORS

Gordon D. Brown, PhD, is professor emeritus and was (for 28 years) chair of the Department of Health Management and Informatics, School of Medicine at the University of Missouri. He served as scientist for the World Health Organization, Division of Epidemiology and Communications Science, developing integrative models for health systems, and has consulted on health system development and global health systems. In addition, he was the chair of the Accrediting Commission on Education for Health Services Administration (now the Commission on Accreditation for Health Management Education). Dr. Brown is a recipient of the Gary L. Filerman Prize for Educational Leadership from the Association of University Programs in Health Administration. He was a founding director and faculty member of the National Center for Managed Health Care Administration and is the author of numerous articles and books, including *Strategic Management of Information Systems in Healthcare*. He has held faculty appointments at the Pennsylvania State University and the Universidad del Valle in Cali, Colombia. He earned his MHA and PhD from the University of Iowa.

Timothy B. Patrick, PhD, is associate professor and chair of the Department of Health Informatics and Administration, College of Health Sciences at the University of Wisconsin-Milwaukee. He received an MS in computer science and a PhD in philosophy/logic and completed post-doctoral studies in medical informatics through a National Library of Medicine Post-Doctoral Fellowship at the School of Medicine of the University of Missouri-Columbia. His research includes metadata schema for representing questions and answers, measurements of the quality of translation of evidence into practice, readability of healthcare information for laypersons, and ontology mapping.

Kalyan S. Pasupathy, PhD, is an assistant professor in health management and informatics at the School of Medicine, University of Missouri. He earned a PhD in industrial and systems engineering, and his research involves modeling systems for performance measurement and process improvement, using optimization-based and nonparametric models to discover patterns in large data sets. He has published several articles and a book chapter in this area. His work has been commended, and he was awarded the Goodeve Medal by the Operations Research Society.

ABOUT THE CONTRIBUTORS

Dixie B. Baker, PhD, is a senior vice president and Technical Fellow at Science Applications International Corporation, where she serves as the chief technology officer for the health and life sciences business. She is an internationally recognized leader in information assurance, health information technology (HIT), and critical systems architecture. She speaks and writes on a number of technology and health-related areas, including information protection, high-assurance architecture, electronic medical records, and Internet safety. Dr. Baker is a member of the national HIT Standards Committee and chairs its Privacy and Security Workgroup. In addition, she serves on the Privacy and Security Policy Tiger Team of the HIT Policy Committee. She is a Fellow of the Healthcare Information Management and Systems Society (HIMSS) and the HIMSS Privacy and Security Committee. She holds a PhD in special education and an MS in computer science from the University of Southern California as well as MS and BS degrees from Florida State University and The Ohio State University, respectively.

Karen R. Cox, PhD, RN, is the manager of quality improvement and patient safety at University of Missouri Health Care and is an investigator in the Center for Health Care Quality at the University of Missouri Health Care in Columbia, Missouri. Her areas of practice and research include patient safety reporting and organizational learning, population-specific clinical outcomes studies, redesign for healthcare delivery process improvements, and health profession curriculum design and implementation (specific to quality improvement and safety).

George Demiris, PhD, is a professor of biomedical and health informatics at the University of Washington. He is the graduate program director of the Biomedical Informatics Graduate Program at the School of Medicine and the director of Clinical Informatics and Patient Centered Technologies at the School of Nursing. He is a Fellow of the American College of Medical Informatics. His research interests include the use of technology to support older adults and improve home and hospice care.

Yang Gong, MD, PhD, is assistant professor of clinical informatics in the Department of Health Management and Informatics, School of Medicine at the University of Missouri in Columbia. He received his PhD from the University of Texas Health Sciences Center and is a member of the MU Informatics Institute. Dr. Gong's research interests include human–computer interface and clinical decision support systems.

Lanis L. Hicks, PhD, is professor at the Department of Health Management and Informatics at the School of Medicine, University of Missouri. Dr. Hicks is a health economist. Her research has focused on the cost effectiveness of technologies in the delivery of healthcare, rural health, and workforce issues.

Mark A. Hoffman, PhD, is vice president of Life Sciences Solutions and is responsible for Cerner's Life Sciences development initiatives, including genomics, clinical trials, Galt, and the Cerner Discovere™ solutions. In his current role, he is charged with reducing the barriers between patient care and clinical research and with accelerating the pace at which new insights are available in clinical practice. Dr. Hoffman joined Cerner in 1997 and has served as a software engineer, team lead, manager, solution manager, and director. During his Cerner tenure, he led a team that incorporated genomic information into the electronic medical record, positioning Cerner as a leader in personalized medicine. He led the Cerner Flu Pandemic Initiative to connect more than 800 healthcare facilities for influenza surveillance. He earned a BS in molecular biology from William Jewell College and a PhD in bacteriology from the University of Wisconsin-Madison, and he completed a bioethics study at Oxford University.

Naresh Khatri, PhD, is a faculty member in the Department of Health Management and Informatics at the School of Medicine, University of Missouri-Columbia, where he teaches strategic human resource management and transformational leadership. Before joining the University of Missouri, he was faculty at the Nanyang Business School, Nanyang Technological University in Singapore for seven years. Dr. Khatri's research and teaching interests focus on unleashing the human potential in organizations.

William C. Kinney, MD, is a practicing third-generation otolaryngologist. He received an MD from Case Western Reserve University and completed surgical training at the Cleveland Clinic Foundation. He earned an MHA from the University of Missouri while practicing medicine full-time at the University of Missouri Health Care. Dr. Kinney is now in private practice and is the president of SurgeryFlow, Inc., a health information technology company that focuses on presurgical patient preparation.

Norma M. Lang, PhD, has authored numerous publications. Her pioneering work in identifying standards and measures to evaluate the quality of nursing care has served as a basis for nursing policy throughout the world. Her research expertise includes quality assurance, nursing standards and outcome measures, peer review, the Nursing Minimum Data Set, and the International Classification for Nursing Practice. She is a Fellow of the Institute of Medicine, the American Academy of Nursing, and the College of Physicians of Philadelphia; she is also an honorary Fellow of the Royal College of Nursing in London and an Honorary Member of the American Association of Colleges of Nursing. She was named to the governor's board of directors for the Wisconsin Relay of Electronic Data for Health (now called Wisconsin Statewide Health Information Network) and now serves on its policy committee. She is a member of the Office of the National Coordinator for Health Information Technology Quality Measurement Workgroup as well as a member of the Professional Leadership Group of the RWJF Aligning Forces for Quality Initiative in Wisconsin. Dr. Lang has served in several advisory capacities for the American Nurses Association and the American Medical Informatics Association work groups. She received the American Nurses Association's First President's Award, the Distinguished Membership Award, and the Jessie Scott Award. In addition, she was recognized by the North American Nursing Diagnosis Association with an Outstanding Leadership Award and by The Joint Commission with the prestigious Ernest A. Codman Individual Award. In 2010, her lifetime achievements were honored when she was inducted as a Living Legend in the American Academy of Nursing. Currently, she leads the knowledge-based nursing initiative at the University of Wisconsin-Milwaukee. Dr. Lang received a BSN from Alverno College and an MSN and a PhD from Marquette University. She also holds honorary doctorates from the State University of New York and Marquette University and an honorary master's from the University of Pennsylvania.

Ricky C. Leung, PhD, is assistant professor of health management in the Department of Health Management and Informatics, School of Medicine, University of Missouri. He obtained a PhD from the University of Wisconsin-Madison, and he held visiting appointments at Brown University and the City University of Hong Kong. Dr. Leung's research interests include organization and management theory, health economics, research methods, international health, and sociology of science and technology. He has published in high-impact journals, such as *Organization Science* and *Health Care Management Review*.

Win Phillips, PhD, is a clinical assistant professor in the Department of Health Management and Informatics at the University of Missouri. He is also affiliated with the MU Informatics Institute and Center for Health Ethics. He teaches courses in health informatics, health policy and politics, and health ethics. Outside of academia, Dr. Phillips has held information technology positions at Scott & White Hospital and Austin Heart at the Heart Hospital of Austin. He also has industry experience in systems development and project management.

Mihail Popescu, PhD, is an associate professor in the Department of Health Management and Informatics at the University of Missouri-Columbia. He received an MS in medical physics, an MS in electrical engineering, and a PhD in computer science from the University of Missouri-Columbia. He is a senior member of the Institute of Electrical and Electronics Engineers and a member of the MU Informatics Institute. His research interests include eldercare technologies, fuzzy logic, and ontological pattern recognition.

Blaine Reeder, PhD, is a Research Fellow at the School of Nursing, University of Washington in Seattle. He obtained his PhD in biomedical and health informatics at the School of Medicine, University of Washington. His research interests include public health interventions for chronic disease management and technology and aging.

Peter J. Tonellato, PhD, is a professor in the Zilber School of Public Health at the University of Wisconsin-Milwaukee, and a visiting professor in the Department of Pathology at Beth Israel Deaconess Medical Center. He is also the director of the Laboratory for Personalized Medicine at the Center for Biomedical Informatics at Harvard Medical School. Dr. Tonellato oversees the development of strategies, methods, bioinformatics tools, and analyses to study and test the accuracy and clinical efficacy of genetic discoveries and accelerate their translation to practical clinical use. In addition, he is a professor of computer science in the College of Engineering and Applied Science at the University of Wisconsin-Milwaukee and is the founder and codirector of the Biomedical and Health Informatics Research Institute.